Trends in
Nursing History

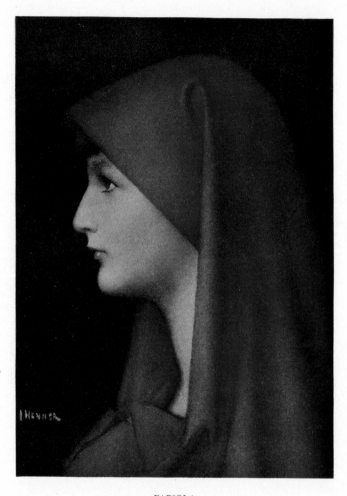

FABIOLA

An Early Christian Nurse

Trends in

Nursing History

Their Relationships to World Events

Fourth Edition, Illustrated

ELIZABETH M. JAMIESON, B.A., R.N.

*Late Director of Nursing, Fabiola Hospital, Oakland,
California, Assistant Director, Bureau of Registration
of Nurses, California, Instructor, Lakeside Hospital,
Cleveland, Ohio*

MARY F. SEWALL, B.S., R.N.

*Formerly Director of Nursing Education, Methodist
Hospital of Southern California, Los Angeles. Instructor,
Fabiola Hospital, Oakland, California. Educational
Director, San Joaquin General Hospital, School of
Nursing, Stockton, California*

W. B. SAUNDERS COMPANY
Philadelphia   London

Preface to the Fourth Edition

In this fourth edition of *Trends in Nursing History*, changes have been made chiefly in the last three chapters. Information relative to the United Nations, its principal organs and specialized agencies, has been revised as it pertains to nursing. A new chapter, "Modern Trends in Nursing," tells of research projects, completed and under way, as well as of changes in the structure of organized nursing. A new introduction and accounts of the Police Action of the United Nations in Korea and of the humanitarian work of Dr. Albert Schweitzer in French Equatorial Africa have been added to the chapter on "International Relationships."

For the purpose of portraying the times and nursing during each phase of the latter's development, emphasis has been placed on the general trend of events rather than on details in regard to them. The history of women has been emphasized since nursing has been identified with woman's life and work since the beginning of time, although men in great numbers entered the field through the religious orders of the Middle Ages and again today are being attracted into the profession.

Since the chief objective of a course in nursing history is the development of desirable attitudes toward the place occupied by nursing throughout the ages and in the total picture of world affairs today, it differs from other subjects in the curriculum. Considerable adjustment on the part of the student is often necessary in the beginning, but as the course progresses there comes an appreciation of its unique cultural value and of its ability to provide patterns for high standards of personal and professional living. A feeling of pride develops in the accomplishments of the profession under the guidance of its capable leaders as well as a sense of responsibility for helping to shape its future.

Due to the fact that considerable ground must be covered from the first glimpses of nursing in the relatively static periods, throughout the ages, to the dynamic present, it may be found expedient to reserve the last two or three chapters of the book for use as an introduction to the advanced course in Professional Adjustments. On the foundation provided eventually may be built a portrayal of the composite structure of nursing history as it assumes broader proportions and greater harmony with other structures arising from man's necessity.

With the broadening of man's viewpoint to include world health as a fundamental of the human race, the nurse assumes a new role as instrument of social progress. Boundless opportunities present themselves for utilizing her special knowledge and skills and for exerting the influence of her character in building a democratic world in which each of the earth's inhabitants will find opportunity for his own growth and development. As the student of today prepares to take her place in a more complicated, a more intimately acquainted, and a more interdependent world than did her sister of yesterday, knowledge of her relationship to the whole process of social growth becomes a necessity.

An acknowledgement of indebtedness is made to other books on nursing history, especially "A History of Nursing" by Dock and Nutting and "A Short History of Nursing" by Dock and Stewart, both of which represent authentic information without which it would be impossible to build other histories with varying emphases. Sincere appreciation is expressed to Leila I. Given, associate executive secretary of the American Nurses' Association, 1947-1952, for constructive criticism in relation to the chapter on "Modern Trends in Nursing." Gratitude is due also to Helen F. Hansen, executive secretary of the California Board of Nurse Examiners, 1933–1947, for valuable suggestions.

MARY FRANKLIN SEWALL

Pacific Grove, California

Contents

PART ONE   ANCIENT CIVILIZATIONS
                     Circa 5000 B.C. to 500 A.D.

I. LIFE AMONG PRIMITIVE PEOPLES   3

   Animism   4
   Primitive Medicine   6
   Summary 10
   Topics for Discussion 11
   References 11

II. BEGINNINGS OF CIVILIZATION 12

   The Near East 12
      Egypt 12
      The Fertile Crescent 21
      Persia (Iran) 34
   The Far East 35
      India 35
      China 41
   Summary 45
   Topics for Discussion 48
   References 50

III. BEGINNINGS OF CIVILIZATION (Continued) 52

   The Mediterranean World 52
      Greece 52
      Rome 66
   The Far West 73
      The Americas 73

Summary of Conditions at 1 A.D.   75
Topics for Discussion   76
References   78

IV. EARLY CHRISTIAN ERA, 1–500 A.D.   79

Christ, the Redeemer   80
Saul of Tarsus   83
Early Christian Orders of Women   86
    Deaconesses   86
    Widows and Virgins   88
Persecution of Christians   90
Influence of Constantine the Great   91
Roman Matrons   92
Diakonia and Xenodochia   95
Status of Medicine and Nursing   98
The Fall of Rome in 476 A.D.   102
Summary, 1 to 500 A.D.   104
Topics for Discussion   109
References   111

PART TWO   *THE MIDDLE AGES*

Circa 500 to 1500 A.D.

V. THE EARLY MIDDLE AGES: *Society in Small Cooperative
   Units*   115

Christian Monasticism   117
    Rise of Benedictine Monasteries   118
    Women of Monasticism   124
Feudalism and Chivalry   127
Guilds   132
Islam, A Rival of Christianity   134
Charlemagne Promotes Social Recovery Through
    Education   142
Medicine and Nursing   143
Summary of Early Middle Ages   146

Topics for Discussion............................ 148
References..................................... 149

VI. The Late Middle Ages: *Society Becoming Mobile; Detachment of Individuals*..................... 151

Pilgrimages to Palestine.......................... 152
William the Conqueror........................... 154
The Crusades, 1096–1271......................... 155
    Orders of Military Nurses.................... 158
    Medieval Social Problems.................... 163
    Rise of Mendicant Orders.................... 165
    Rise of Secular Orders...................... 170
    Gains and Losses of the Crusaders............ 174
    Social Changes Associated with the Crusades... 175
    Chivalry Influences the Position of Women..... 177
Great Plagues of the Fourteenth Century........... 179
Saint Catherine of Siena; Hospital Nurse and Visiting Nurse... 182
Medicine during the Late Middle Ages............. 185
    Growth of Hospitals....................... 190
    Nursing of the Late Middle Ages............. 194
Summary of Late Middle Ages.................... 199
Topics for Discussion............................ 201
References..................................... 204

PART THREE   *THE MODERN ERA: SCIENTIFIC, ECONOMIC, AND SOCIAL EVOLUTION*

Beginning Circa 1500 A.D.

VII. Renaissance, Reformation, and a Decline in Nursing, 1500–1860 A.D. 207

The Renaissance................................ 207
    The Classic Revival........................ 208
    Political Revolution........................ 211

Industrial Revolution........................ 213
The Reformation........................... 214
Transfer of European Culture to America..... 215
Medicine of the Renaissance................. 219
Medicine in America........................ 222
Public Health Movement: Era of Sanitation........ 227
Women of the Renaissance...................... 228
Education of Women........................ 231
Rise of Feminism........................... 233
Women of the Industrial Revolution........... 236
A Decline in Nursing............................ 238
Summary, 1500 to 1860......................... 244
Topics for Discussion........................... 246
References...................................... 247

VIII. EARLY HOSPITALS AND NURSING IN AMERICA........ 249

New Spain..................................... 249
New France.................................... 254
Canada.................................... 254
Louisiana.................................. 265
New England................................... 266
American Revolution (1775–1783)................. 273
Philadelphia Dispensary.................... 274
Nurse Society of Philadelphia.............. 275
Summary....................................... 277
Topics for Discussion........................... 281
References...................................... 282

IX. SPORADIC EFFORTS AT SOCIAL REFORM.............. 283

Catholic Social Reform......................... 283
Social Service Established.................... 283
Protestant Social Reform....................... 289
Prison Reform.............................. 291
Reform in Care of the Mentally Ill........... 295
Prevailing Nursing Methods Exposed.......... 297
Order of Modern Deaconesses Founded........ 299

Florence Nightingale: Reformer of Hospitals and
    Nursing.................................... 311
        Early Life............................... 311
        First Position........................... 316
        Crimean War Service...................... 317
        Post-War Activities........................ 326
    Summary..................................... 331
    Topics for Discussion.......................... 333
    References................................... 334

X. MODERN DEVELOPMENT OF SOCIAL AGENCIES, 1860–1893 336

    Nonsectarian Reform in Nursing................. 336
    Modern District Nursing....................... 341
    Workhouse Infirmary Reform................... 343
    Birth of the Red Cross in 1864.................. 345
    Nursing in the American Civil War, 1861–1865..... 349
        Work of the Sanitary Commission........... 349
        Volunteer Nursing........................ 352
        Organization of Army Nursing.............. 355
    Founding of American Red Cross Society, 1882.... 357
    Reform of Nursing in America.................. 358
        Pre-Nightingale Reform.................... 359
        Nightingale Reform....................... 360
        First Preliminary Courses.................. 372
        First Textbooks.......................... 374
        Prevailing Methods....................... 375
        Adoption of Uniforms..................... 376
    Other Evidences of Social Reform............... 378
        Salvation Army.......................... 378
        Settlement Houses........................ 379
        Y.M.C.A. and Y.W.C.A.................... 379
        Medical Missionaries...................... 380
    The New Nurse.............................. 381
    Medicine Enters a Revolutionary Period.......... 382
    Summary, 1860–1893......................... 386
    Topics for Discussion......................... 389
    References................................... 391

XI. GROUP CONSCIOUSNESS DEVELOPS WITH GROWTH OF
SCHOOLS, 1893–1920......................... 393

Growth of Nursing Associations.................. 394
Wars of Late Nineteenth Century................ 400
    Nursing in the Spanish-American War........ 401
    Nursing in the South African War........... 402
Army and Navy Nurse Corps Established......... 403
American Red Cross Nursing Service Established... 404
Advanced Education for Nurses.................. 405
Nursing During World War I, 1914–1918......... 411
    Royal College of Nursing................... 419
Postwar Reconstruction........................ 419
    League of Red Cross Societies.............. 419
    League of Nations......................... 420
General Trend in Nursing from 1893 to 1920...... 422
Broader Aims in Medicine...................... 423
Summary (1893–1920)......................... 427
Topics for Discussion......................... 430
References.................................... 432

XII. NATIONAL SURVEYS OF NURSING AND MEDICINE, 1920–
1939.. 433

The Rockefeller Survey, 1920–1923.............. 434
The Grading of Nursing Schools, 1926–1934....... 437
Registration and Licensing..................... 446
A Critical Survey of Medical Practice, 1927–1932.. 448
Social Security Act of 1935.................... 450
    Implementing the Act...................... 451
Summary, 1920–1939.......................... 452
Topics for Discussion......................... 454
References.................................... 455

XIII. WORLD WAR II, 1939–1945.................... 457

Medical Problems.............................. 458
    Procurement of Nurses..................... 460
Rehabilitation................................. 468

United Nations Relief and Rehabilitation Administration...................... 470
The Four Freedoms...................... 471
The Atlantic Charter...................... 472
The United Nations...................... 472
Post-war Developments...................... 479
American Red Cross Nursing Services............ 481
The Rise of Psychiatry...................... 482
Summary, 1939–1945...................... 485
Topics for Discussion...................... 488
References...................... 488

XIV. MODERN TRENDS IN NURSING...................... 490

Nursing Research...................... 490
Research and Statistics Unit of the A.N.A...... 491
Carnegie Study of Nursing Schools............ 494
Other Postwar Studies of Nursing............ 497
Nursing Technicians...................... 499
The School Data Survey of 1949.............. 500
National Accreditation of Nursing Schools..... 501
Changes in Structure of Organized Nursing........ 502
Revision of Nursing Practice Acts................ 508
A New Status for Women...................... 509
Summary...................... 510
Topics for Discussion...................... 513
References...................... 514

XV. INTERNATIONAL RELATIONSHIPS...................... 515

Relationship of I.C.N. to Other International Organizations...................... 515
Exchange of Nurses...................... 516
Regional Associations 518
France...................... 519
Germany...................... 525
Belgium...................... 530
Northern Europe...................... 531
Sweden...................... 533

Italy...................................... 534
The Balkans and the Middle East................ 535
    Greece.................................. 535
    Palestine................................ 536
Africa...................................... 536
The Orient.................................. 538
    China................................... 540
    Japan................................... 540
    Korea................................... 542
Mexico..................................... 544
South American Republics..................... 547
The International Council of Nurses.............. 550
The Florence Nightingale International Foundation. 556
Summary.................................... 558
Topics for Discussion......................... 558
References.................................. 560

INDEX.. 561

List of Illustrations

Fabiola..*Frontispiece*

1. Rough Stone Implements of Primitive Man............... 4
2. Prehistoric Skull Showing Trephine Openings Made during Life... 7
3. A Pharaoh... 15
4. Imhotep, Egyptian Deity, and First Physician of History. 16
5. In the Nile Valley................................... 18
6. Reconstruction of the Great Hypostyle Hall in the Temple of Karnak at Thebes, Egypt......................... 20
7. Fertile Crescent of the Pre-Christian Era.............. 22
8. Babylonian Medical Prescription in Cuneiform Writing.. 24
9. Moses.. 29
10. The Far East of Today.............................. 38
11. Caduceus... 53
12. Temple of Aesculapius at Athens.................... 56
13. The Theater of Epidauros........................... 58
14. Hippocrates.. 60
15. The Roman Empire at Its Greatest Extent............. 67
16. Saint Peter and Saint Paul......................... 85
17. Celsus.. 100
18. Barbarian Kingdoms in Western Europe after the Fall of Rome, 476 A.D.................................... 105
19. Medicine and Nursing of Ancient Civilizations........ 108
20. General Plan of a Monastery........................ 119
21. A Medieval Scribe at Work on His Manuscript........ 123
22. A Castle of Northern France Built in the Thirteenth Century... 129
23. Hall of the Clothmakers' Guild at Ypres, Belgium...... 133
24. Arabs in the Desert................................ 136
25. Crusaders... 157

26. A Knight Hospitaller of St. John of Jerusalem.......... 160
27. A Knight Hospitaller of St. John in Convent Dress...... 161
28. St. Francis of Assisi................................ 167
29. St. Elizabeth of Hungary............................ 171
30. St. Catherine of Siena.............................. 184
31. St. Hildegarde..................................... 186
32. A Ward in the Santo Spirito Hospital of Rome, Seven-
    teenth Century..................................... 190
33. "Knights Hospitallers Ministering to Patients in the Great
    Ward of the Sacred Infirmary at Valetta, Malta, in the
    Sixteenth Century"................................. 192
34. Nursing of the Middle Ages......................... 200
35. New England, New France, and New Spain............ 216
36. An Augustinian Nun................................ 243
37. A Sick-Room in the Hôtel Dieu, Paris............... 244
38. Hospital of Jesus of Nazareth, Mexico City........... 251
39. Santa Barbara Mission, Santa Barbara, California...... 252
40. Two Friars of the Franciscan Order of Santa Barbara
    Mission... 253
41. Early Canadian Settlements......................... 256
42. Hôtel Dieu of Quebec in 1825 Showing Stockades as Pro-
    tection Against Indian Attack...................... 259
43. Statue of Jeanne Mance Tending a Wounded Soldier.... 263
44. Old Charity Hospital, New Orleans.................. 265
45. St. Vincent de Paul................................ 285
46. Elizabeth Fry Reading to the Prisoners at Newgate Prison. 294
47. Modern Deaconess in the Nursery.................... 306
48. Places Associated with the Life of Florence Nightingale. 319
49. Florence Nightingale............................... 323
50. Statue of Florence Nightingale in Lincoln Park, Los
    Angeles... 325
51. Main Entrance to St. Thomas' Hospital.............. 337
52. Student Nurses of Today at the Liverpool Royal Infirmary 341
53. Henri Dunant...................................... 347
54. Clara Barton....................................... 355
55. Linda Richards..................................... 360
56. A Class in Bandaging at the Philadelphia General about
    1890.. 362

57. Isabel Hampton Robb............................. 365
58. Bellevue Head Nurses, 1891........................ 366
59. Mary Agnes Snively............................... 367
60. Miss Loveridge and an Early Group of Students, Good
     Samaritan Hospital, Portland, Oregon.............. 368
61. Nora Livingstone................................. 369
62. Anna Caroline Maxwell............................ 372
63. Mrs. Bedford Fenwick............................. 373
64. Mrs. Rebecca Strong, the Centenarian, (1843–1944)...... 374
65. Mrs. Estelle Massey Riddle, R.N.................... 399
66. Mary M. Roberts................................. 400
67. M. Adelaide Nutting.............................. 406
68. Lillian D. Wald.................................. 407
69. Isabel M. Stewart................................ 408
70. A Member of Princess Mary's Royal Air Force Nursing
     Service....................................... 412
71. Edith Cavell.................................... 414
72. A Member of the U. S. Army Nurse Corps during World
     War I.. 415
73. Three Pioneers of the Red Cross.................... 417
74. Jean Isabel Gunn, O.B.E., LL.D.................... 445
75. Dame Katherine H. Jones, D.B.E., R.R.C., S.R.N....... 458
76. Colonel Elizabeth L. Smellie, C.B.E., R.R.C........... 459
77. A Volunteer Nurse's Aide Assists the Nurse........... 461
78. Trio of Army Nurses............................. 463
79. A Member of the United States Cadet Nurse Corps during
     World War II................................. 464
80. Two Navy Nurses on a Hospital Ship in the North Atlantic 465
81. A Hospital Train................................ 467
82. An Evacuation Hospital near a Battlefront............ 467
83. A British Hospital after Raiders Passed............... 469
84. A WHO Field Mission in China Supervises Relief and
     Medical Care Provided for Children at the Nanking
     General Hospital.............................. 476
85. Nursing of the Modern Era, 1500–   484
86. Fewer Schools of Nursing but More Students.......... 494
87. A Team Leader and Her Nursing Team Clarify Their As-
     signments Before Starting the Day's Work........... 496

88. Elizabeth K. Porter, Ruth Sleeper.................... 504
89. Student Nurses Attending the Biennial Convention of 1952
    at a Party Given by the New Jersey State Student
    Organization...................................... 507
90. At a Meeting of the WHO Expert Committee on Nursing. 517
91. Nursing is Dedicated.............................. 518
92. Dr. Anna Hamilton................................ 521
93. Mademoiselle Chaptal............................. 522
94. The American Nurses' Memorial, Bordeaux, France, as
    It Looked Before World War II.................... 523
95. Sister Agnes Karll................................ 527
96. German Red Cross Nurse in Working Uniform........ 528
97. A German Red Cross Nurse Ready for Service......... 529
98. Mrs. Frances Payne Bolton with Representatives of Nor-
    way and India, Congress of I.C.N., 1947............ 532
99. Student Nurses at Sophiahemmet, Stockholm, Sweden... 533
100. A West Africa Nurse Instructor Checks the Work of Some
     African Student Nurses........................... 537
101. Two Trained Nurses of the Gold Coast, Africa, Acting as
     Welfare Workers................................. 539
102. St. Luke's International Medical Center and College of
     Nursing, Tokyo.................................. 541
103. Colonel Mary G. Phillips, Chief of the U. S. Army Nurse
     Corps, Arrives at Seoul, Korea.................... 543
104. Entrance to the Hospital De Jesus Nazarens, Built by
     Cortez in 1524.................................. 546
105. Daisy C. Bridges of England........................ 549
106. Gerda Hojer, Former President of the I.C.N............ 556
107. Lillian Wu of China and Anna Rypackova of Czecho-
     slovakia with Katharine Densford at the I.C.N. Congress
     in Atlantic City, New Jersey...................... 557

PART ONE

Ancient Civilizations

Circa 5000 B.C. to 500 A.D.

Life Among Primitive Peoples

Available historical records of man's life upon the earth show early division into small, well-defined tribes built up around the nucleus of family relationship. The solidarity of these scattered groups was marked, for mutual protection was a basic reason for development. Although stronger or more intelligent members took natural precedence over those who were not their equals, each individual expected to serve, to his utmost capacity, the common welfare. As an individual, he received little consideration, and failure to be useful was sometimes cause for his elimination. Expediency excused, on occasion, extermination of the infant, the aged, or the sick. The primitive group was organized for convenience in management of human affairs, and for strength in holding its own in a difficult world. It survives in some far distant parts of the earth, in Australia, and in Africa, and remnants of it may be seen in the Scottish clan or in the Indian groups of America.

Customs or *mores* peculiar to each tribe constituted one of the chief means of perpetuating it. They were, in reality, habits of action that had proved expedient, and had come to be looked upon as the only right way of doing things. Children brought up in the mores of one group accepted them. If, now and then, an individual rebelled against what experience made desirable for the good of all, he was destroyed or sent out to meet hostile nature alone. This strong tendency to adhere to customs that proved themselves satisfactory gave, eventually, to some of them, the fixity of law.

Man's world in these first days of his existence on the earth did not permit him a self-contained life within any group. He had not learned to subdue nature and make her provide for his needs. Cattle, horses, birds, and other sources of animal food were not

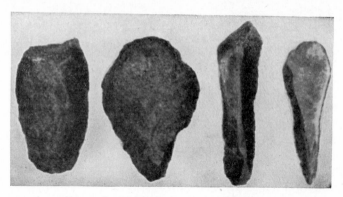

Rough Stone Implements of Primitive Man
(Courtesy of the Metropoiltan Museum of Art.)

domesticated. Plants were still growing wild and where they listed. If he was to survive, man must find the answer to his varied needs by searching for it among nature's offerings, and experimenting with them. As he consumed what might lie near him, he must go farther afield for more. No settled home could be his. Necessity made him a nomad. He lived in caves in order to escape wind and storm.

Gradually, man acquired knowledge which enabled him to distinguish the harmful from the useful. Empirically, through tasting, he learned food and medicinal values in plants. Animals he must kill. Fish he must catch. The stone became his implement. At first he simply picked up one of these detached pieces of rock and threw it, just as it was. In time, he adapted its shape to many purposes and used the stone with such skill that this earliest period of human habitation of the earth is known as the *Old Stone Age*. The first manufactured implement of man has been given the name "fist hatchet." It has been found in caves as a rough stone of a size convenient for holding, and with sharpened point for piercing that which was dangerous to life or was desirable as food.

ANIMISM

In the roving existence which was man's, constantly changing experiences were met. All about him—besides rocks, fish and animals, rivers, trees, mountains and birds—were myriad forms of life with which natural science has made us familiar but toward knowledge of which he had no science to guide him. It was to be expected that he should ascribe to all such forms of nature, qualities of which he became conscious in himself. We cannot be surprised to find him endowing them with human faculties. His rivers, trees, and sky, his rocks, plants, animals, birds, and fishes moved with life, and must also feel and make similar responses to his own. The sounds produced in nature resembled those of the language that he invented eventually to make known his wants. In his possession of physical senses, he saw reason for corresponding senses in all natural life. These things could deliberately help or hurt him. This *animism*, as we call it, has been delightfully expressed in "Hiawatha," Longfellow's conception of primitive living and thinking:

> And the West-Wind came at evening,
> Walking lightly o'er the prairies,
> Whispering to the leaves and blossoms,
> Bending low the flowers and grasses.
> . . . .
> That is but the owl and owlet,
> Talking in their native language,
> Talking, scolding at each other.
> . . . .
> Then the little Hiawatha
> Learned of every bird its language,
> Learned their names and all their secrets.
> . . . .
> Of all beasts he learned the language,
> Learned their names and all their secrets.
> . . . .
> Talked with them when'er he met them.
> Called them "Hiawatha's Brothers."

Animism thus opened up to man a still greater world—that of his imagination. In the end he found himself surrounded with a veil of superstition that he has not yet been able to destroy completely. While it brought much of added beauty into life, it brought, also, fear and unnecessary ugliness. Spirits were good or evil as he grew familiar with them, and to their influence he came to assign the catastrophes, as well as the benefits of every-day life. While certain acts or happenings brought happiness, added strength, or new life to the little bands of human wanderers, others meant sadness, weakness, or death. Disasters like storm, earthquake, drought, flood, lightning, fire, or illness, were explained by the presence of evil spirits.

PRIMITIVE MEDICINE

From some natural phenomena man might escape by changing his location; from the ravages of disease he had to learn to protect himself and to find means of cure. The comforting effects of applying water externally had been experienced early in river bathing. It is possible that the first idea of using water in medical treatment was obtained from animals, for these cleanse their wounds by licking, and they have also been known to keep them submerged in water until inflammation subsides. His own wonderful invention of fire-making by means of friction acquainted primitive man with the comforting value of heat. Both water and heat he diverted to his use when incapacitated by any illness. In his use of stones, warmed by contact with fire, lies the origin of later methods of searing and counter-irritation by hot stones or by iron bars.

In the vegetable world, experiences of emesis or catharsis following attempts to use certain plants for food doubtless underlay his discrimination in choice. It is possible that some of his knowledge was gained also from observation of creatures in the animal kingdom. These, it is believed, existed on the earth before human beings, and methods of treatment of disease may have been developed by them before man's advent. Primitive man, moreover, was much closer to animals in nature and act than he is today. He moved among them as another animal, one with themselves, and fear of them was a matter of gradual breeding. In any case, examples of animal instinct in selection of plant remedies with which to meet the misfortune of accident or disease are not unknown.

Stumbling as he was toward an understanding of maladies which made him uncomfortable and sometimes even thinned his numbers alarmingly, primitive man did not find, among the beasts or birds of creation, treatment that cured all of the ailments that befell him. In his dilemma he turned for explanation to the spirits which he believed he had discovered. His next step was to imagine the migration of evil ones among these into his body. The symptoms apparent —excessive pain, convulsions, mental aberration—were to him explicable only as their work. In time he found it possible to refer

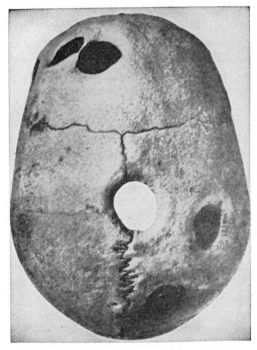

Prehistoric Skull Showing Trephine Openings Made During Life

"The rounded edges of the openings show that the bone has grown after the wound was made. Thus we know they were made while the owner was living. Excavated in Peru." (Clendening, Logan: Behind the Doctor. Alfred A. Knopf, New York.)

certain types of symptoms to the work of particular spirits, and was led to devise means of driving these away. The following of a very natural impulse gave to him his earliest method. He sought to destroy by mechanical force. With his fist he struck the offending body in the part in which the spirit seemed to be lodged. Repeated blows in the area thus inhabited led to a pummeling which has been tempered in our time to the movements of massage.

Knowledge of plants which had unpleasant effects was turned to account. Concoctions, nauseating or otherwise disagreeable to spirits, were made. Their expulsion through the intestinal tract was accomplished by the administration of herbs which caused purging;

expulsion by way of the mouth followed a choice of herbs which acted as emetics. When the evil one had lodged in the head, which nature encased in a covering of bony plates, trephining was resorted to—and not uncommonly. Evidence of this extreme measure is to be found among the skeletons of many primitive peoples.

Human ingenuity thus early was developing to meet the requirements of existence. Immediate needs of the family in health had been met by a natural division in occupation, determined by sex. To woman was allotted the home tasks and the care of children; to man, the hunting necessary to provide food. With increasing numbers and new desires came a never-ending stream of new duties for both. The incidence of illness was an added burden which mankind is still trying to shake off. Life was to become, in time, the complicated existence that we know today, and treatment and prevention of illness were to consume the energies of many people. In the beginning, however, it meant that care of those who were incapacitated became, logically, an additional task to be assumed by those who remained in camp with them. Women became nurses.

The Medicine Man   Healthy men traveled far afield and brought back new remedies. Some of them became very expert in divining symptoms and making application of special remedies to them. As the world went on and further division of labor became possible, such experts were charged with the responsibility of interpreting available knowledge of disease and its cure. It became necessary for each of these men who became wise in medical lore, to assume an ever-increasing intimacy with the spirits which men had learned to blame or exhort when they failed to solve the mystery surrounding cause and effect in disease. In degrees of importance varying with his success in freeing men from evil spirits, the *Medicine Man* became an outstanding figure in his tribe.

On the initiative and resourcefulness of the Medicine Man devolved the business of restoring men to usefulness. Imagination of necessity exceeded wisdom in his equipment, for the limits of human knowledge were very narrow. Invention of methods more and more strange, and the creation of startling impressions became characteristic of his work. With his use of the senses of touch and taste above alluded to, he included in his instruments those of sound, smell, and sight. He mumbled words, the power of which was magic because their meaning was to be divined by spirits alone. He contrived to make noises louder and more disagreeable than those which usually aroused fear in people that he knew. He produced the stifling effect of smoke and the unpleasantness of some odors in strength sufficient to hasten the departure of a spirit made too uncomfortable to linger.

The Medicine Man discovered, by adopting strange disguises, that the sight of his own body might be expected to inspire fear in the supernatural. His choice of materials for such disguise being limited to objects more or less familiar to all about him, he made unusual combinations of skins or hoofs of animals, horns, feathers, grasses, snakes, or toads. Attired thus, he was able to strike awe into the hearts of those who beheld him. He satisfied himself, his audience, and his patient of his ability to frighten off an evil spirit. To enhance his effect, he danced and indulged in antics tending to extremes limited only by the originality of his invention.

Two further requirements devolved on him who would be set apart as a specialist for the cure of disease or dispelling of misfortune. He must demonstrate his ability to invoke the help of good spirits to drive off evil ones, and he must prove his power to bring disaster or disease on enemies. Development of these two separate functions gave rise to a distinction in the kind of magic adopted. *White magic* was designed for kindly, helpful purposes. *Black magic* was hostile and destructive in its aims. Humanity's confidence in the presence of light, with its corresponding fear in darkness, may account for the origin of the names. As system gradually invaded all these experiments in penetration of the unknown, the cure of sickness took on the quality of ritualistic religious ceremony, and the Medicine Man was set apart from ordinary men as a functionary of corresponding holiness.

The Priest-physician   Ceremonial rites gave to men an added support in presence of sickness. In both patient and onlookers there was induced a firmness of faith that had great influence on the outcome. The Medicine Man elaborated the rites. As time went on he mingled imagination with experience, and finally passed over to the *Priest-physician,* who succeeded him, a strange mixture of superstition and fact.

SUMMARY

The history of man is a record of successive changes to which it has been necessary for him to find means of adjustment. In early times these changes came about with exceeding slowness, for they were largely dependent on ideas, and new ideas were rare. That period of time which precedes the five or six thousand years of written history dates back indefinitely. Relics of stone implements, cave markings, or skeletons constitute our source of information about these earliest times.

The primitive group was developed on a basis of family relationship. It originated in a need for greater safety, and the all-importance of group welfare submerged the cause of the individual. Mutual aid within the group was, for a long time, the limit of helpfulness.

Survival in primitive times was dependent on available vegetation, and on hunting. Tribes, therefore, were nomadic. They followed the supply of food. In time they developed implements to further the efficiency of hunting. Wood clubs were used; but, as the greater number of implements were of stone, this age of man came to be known as the *Old Stone Age*, as well as the Age of Hunters. It lasted for thousands of years.

Primitive man endowed natural objects with those qualities that he found in himself. All of them were to him animate, and the beliefs which grew up about this basic belief constitute what we all *animism*. Through animism he explained natural phenomena, including those causing disaster or disease. On this basis, also, he built up a mass of superstition and a system of empiric medicine, both of which still influence men of today.

The incidence of disease affected the history of man profoundly. To offset its ravages he made haste to appease spirits that he thought might be angry, and to invoke the aid of those who were friendly. He turned to account what he knew of the effects of physical force, water, heat, or vegetable products. A man who attained prestige through his use of these various agents rose to the position of *Medicine Man*. By him were developed systems of *black* and *white magic*. As treatment of disease became associated with religion, these systems were organized into ritualistic ceremonies and the Medicine Man was succeeded by the *Priest-physician*.

The first division of labor was a natural one. To women fell the lot of caring for children. Men hunted for food. Their work was hazardous, and accidents were probably frequent. Disease invaded tribes. People became old. Another duty was assumed by women; they did the nursing. This was confined to their own families, in the beginning. Long after, as the conception of hospitality was broadened, their help was extended to outsiders.

TOPICS FOR DISCUSSION

1. Name some difficulties that you would have been likely to encounter if you had been a member of a primitive tribe.
2. Do you think that primitive mores were a help or a hindrance toward a satisfactory way of life?
3. What two terms are used to describe this prehistoric period, and why?
4. Discuss animism as it is expressed in Longfellow's "Hiawatha."
5. Give examples of animism as you have discovered them in literature or elsewhere.
6. How did primitive man explain the presence of disease?
7. At what was treatment directed, and what were some of the earliest methods?
8. Give illustrations of the influence of superstition today on (*a*) everyday life, (*b*) cure of disease.
9. Differentiate between the Medicine Man and the Priest-physician, and between the black and white magic practiced by both of them.
10. Show how responsibility for care of the sick came to be assumed by women rather than by men.
11. From what sources is knowledge of the prehistoric period obtained?

REFERENCES

Benedict, Ruth: Patterns of Culture. New York, Houghton Mifflin Co., 1934.
Breasted, J. H.: Ancient Times. Boston, Ginn & Co., 1916.
Frazer, Sir James George: The Golden Bough—A Study in Magic and Religion. New York, The Macmillan Co., 1940.
Masters, Edgar Lee: The New World. New York, D. Appleton-Century Co., 1937.
Reinach, Salomon: Orpheus: A History of Religions. New York, Liveright, Inc., 1930.
Sumner, W. G.: Folkways. New York, Ginn & Co., 1907.

Beginnings of Civilization

The nomadic manner of life followed by primitive man brought about constant changes in location of tribes. People naturally followed directions indicated by the presence of food. They tended to move toward the south where moisture, warmth of temperature, and luxuriance of vegetable growth made it possible for men to live with less effort and a greater degree of comfort than was possible in northerly sections. This movement, it is now generally believed, radiated from the interior of Europe and Asia toward the warm shores of the Mediterranean Sea, India, and China. A lesser migration led in the direction of western Europe and the British Isles. Travel and settlement usually followed the shores of great rivers.

As regions bordering on the Mediterranean Sea came to form the greater part of the known world, this body of water was believed to occupy the center of the earth, as its name implies. All areas to the east of it were known as *eastern*, those to the west, as *western*.

THE NEAR EAST

EGYPT

A very long, narrow valley lying on either side of the Nile River constituted what came to be known as Egypt. The people who settled on this fertile strip were destined to go through the same stages of development as other regions, but at an earlier period. Long after the Egyptians had reached the triumph of their pyramids and temples, the bulk of mankind was still barbarian and living in primitive huts and tents. By the year 5000 B.C., man had added to his early invention of stone implements other inventions which helped to bring radical changes into his manner of living. The grindstone enabled him to give his tools a sharpness and smoothness that facilitated the work for which they were intended. To the now greatly improved fist-hatchet some ingenious person added a handle, and the axe had been invented.

The effect of this simple change proved to be revolutionary. The axe gave mastery over the forest, and opened up the opportunity to make a new type of home to replace the ancient cave dwelling. It also led to ships, with all their possibilities in the way of carriage and human communication. From observation of the germination and growth of seeds dropped inadvertently near camps, man had learned that he might control his supply of edible plants and grains. He now tamed animals, the dog probably first. He taught dogs, donkeys, and oxen to carry his burdens. Cattle, sheep, and goats were then domesticated. The uses of tillage were learned. Man had arrived at the Age of Farmers or the *New Stone Age.*

No longer compelled to wander constantly and to spend the greater part of his energies in search for means of subsistence, man was enabled to turn energies into new channels. From this time, his inventions increased in number. The wheel and cart were among the earliest. These enabled him to transfer the load from the backs of men and animals, and transportation of goods and products was facilitated. By 4000 B.C., the observation and calculation of Egyptians had produced a calendar consisting of twelve months of thirty days each. Finding themselves with five extra days, they made these holidays, and used them to celebrate the birthdays of gods.

By 3000 B.C., writing had been introduced, at first in the form of pictures, later as signs or "hieroglyphics." The earliest of these were cut in stone. Hieroglyphics are found also in ink, on papyrus. This invention of writing was one of tremendous importance in the life of Egypt. By effecting a ready transfer of ideas, it became immediately an influence on public opinion. It enabled rulers to organize governments. Laws could now be set down and kept constantly in the minds of the people. It gave impetus to trade by making possible the transmission of other than verbal messages. It made possible both contracts and records.

This stimulation of the inventive spirit which characterized a settled mode of living was accompanied by an increasing prosperity. The rich, black soil of the valley chosen for settlement by the Egyptians was unusually fertile. They increased its productiveness by a system of irrigation. They built roads and boats. Assured now of a steady supply of food they found it possible to dispose of an excess of crops elsewhere. Trade flourished. The rewards of trade enabled these pioneers of civilization to express themselves in many ways. Buildings assumed the dignity of architecture, among a people for whom building must have had a special interest. Palaces, temples, and tombs arose over the land.

Growth of Religion   Into the growth of this new world went another force that was of great significance in all matters pertaining to health. Men had arrived at a stage in their beliefs where faith in the power of a human being to control spirits no longer satisfied them. They were building up a world outside their own—a world inhabited by gods whose wisdom and strength far exceeded theirs. Mythology was displacing animism as man became farther removed from contact with nature.

Among the people of Egypt a trinity of gods ultimately came into control of bodily and spiritual welfare. *Isis*, Mother Earth, gave her help to the sick. This she did, most frequently, through the medium of dreams. Her son, *Horus*, from whom the Pharaohs believed themselves descended, was taught the lore of medicine by his mother. *Osiris*, husband of Isis and father of Horus, was god of light or "sun-god." To Osiris and Isis, Egyptians referred the origin of agriculture which became sacred as the source of all the wealth that had come to them since they had begun to till fields along the Nile. Osiris, they empowered to sit in judgment on the souls of those who died; for man, induced by his experience of conversing in dreams with departed friends, had by now arrived at belief in immortality. He conceived a soul which inhabited the body, and which remained in it as long as the body was free of decay. In order to preserve the soul, he invented the technic of embalming.

Gods still inhabited animals, birds, and other living creatures, it is true. Inanimate nature continued also to provide abiding places for spirits, but men began to make objects to represent their gods. Figures of wood or stone were carved and set up in places accessible to all. These answered a need for close contact with beings hitherto afar off, and hidden behind an impenetrable veil of mystery. Idols became precious to men, and they gave to them the protection from natural elements that they had found necessary for themselves.

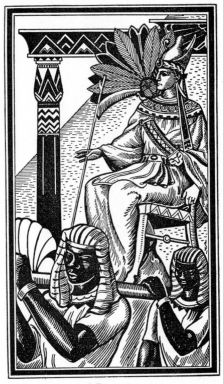

A PHARAOH

(From Reinach, Salomon: Orpheus—A History of Religions. New York, Liveright, Inc.)

Sheltering roofs were built over them. As their purposes became less simple, these first temples increased in size and beauty. Today their ruins bespeak to us the grandeur which they finally attained. Priests presided over them, appointed to the special task of maintaining a favorable relationship with the gods. Through the efforts of these human agents, the will of deities was interpreted, and appropriate ceremonies for their invocation or propitiation were devised. Among those who sought their help were many who came on account of sickness. The temple thus assumed the dual aspect of church and hospital, and the priest became a *Priest-physician.*

Priest-physician of Egypt   The office of the Priest-physician of

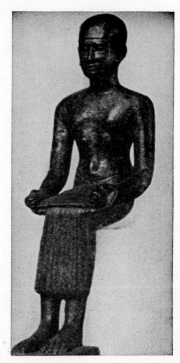

IMHOTEP, EGYPTIAN DEITY, AND FIRST PHYSICIAN OF HISTORY
(Pacific Coast Journal of Nursing, May, 1942.)

Egypt was a strengthening of the bond which already existed between medicine and religion. The man who held it became a representative of great power, and the temple a center of riches. It was necessary for him to live apart and to uphold an example of the utmost purity of life. This purity, he enhanced by cleanliness of body, and he is said to have bathed twice daily and twice during the night. In the absence of bacteriological science, he sometimes tested water for its acceptability by use of sacred birds who drank of it and bathed in it before he did. His office might be handed down by family inheritance and divine right. He was the envy of the Pharaohs, some of whom attempted, by study of medicine and intrusion on his power, to achieve his position.

In his methods of banishing sickness, this Priest-physician did not greatly differ from his predecessor, the Medicine Man, but the manners of his time did not permit the same grotesque behavior. In response to prayers, the public still received at his hands the benefit of empiric treatment and magic. From all Priest-physicians of Egypt, history singles out a man by the name of *Imhotep* as the greatest. So successful was he in healing the sick, and so strikingly generous and kindly in personality, that, after his death, the people elevated him to the rank of god. Among Egyptians, belief in Imhotep was so great that they erected statues and temples in his honor so that worshippers might address prayers to their wise and beloved physician.

The wisdom acquired by man through ages of experience was now ascribed to his gods. Deviation from their teachings became a crime. History would seem to indicate that priests of Egypt collected gradually, and arranged in systematic form, religious and other precepts and such mores as time had fixed into law.

Medicine in Early Egypt   Included in the forty-two "Sacred Books" eventually completed were six which represented the current knowledge of medical care. In them was gathered together much of that empiric medical lore tested out by primitive women, Medicine Men, and Priest-physicians. It has come down to us on rolls of papyrus. Of these first medical books, the one bought by Dr. Ebers of Germany in 1874, and known as the "Ebers' papyrus," is considered the best. It contains a classification and description of diseases. The complexity of its prescriptions, one of which contains thirty-five drugs, argues the need of specialists in compounding them. That such specialists did exist in the time of Moses, who lived about 1500 B.C., is shown by the following quotations from the thirtieth Chapter of Exodus:

"And thou shalt make it an oil of holy ointment, an ointment compounded after the art of the apothecary: it shall be an holy anointing oil."

"And the Lord said unto Moses, Take unto thee . . . these sweet spices with pure frankincense: of each shall there be a like weight. And thou shalt make it a perfume, a confection, after the art of the apothecary, tempered together, pure and holy."

The organization of human affairs thus begun must be acknowledged as a progressive step, but the finality of placing all decisions in the hands of the gods took away from man his initiative. His life was ordered for him. In medicine, all experimentation was dis-

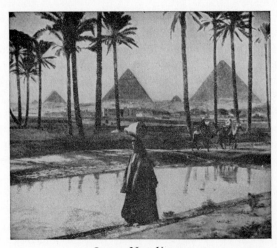

IN THE NILE VALLEY

(From "World History," by Hayes, Moon and Wayland, by permission of The Macmillan Co.)

couraged. Dissection was not permitted. If patients died following treatment which varied from that prescribed in the Sacred Books, the Priest-physician paid with his life. Further advance in medicine was checked.

Belief in Immortality   If the Egyptian has thus given us proof of his capacity for organizing affairs of the earthly life, he also has left behind him, in mummies and tombs, expression of an equal capacity and interest in arranging for a life after death. His belief in immortality led him to devise effective methods of preserving both body and soul. In order to provide a permanent home for the latter, an elaborate process was developed, the technics of which were so effective that his mummified bodies may be seen today. His art of embalming remains a mystery, but to the medical world has been given a knowledge of diseases existing at that time, and of some treatments then in use. There are splendid examples of the art of fine bandaging. As many as a thousand yards of linen, in various widths and bandage patterns, might be used on one mummy. Bandages were moistened with some gluey substance which hardened to form an impervious case for an aseptically cleansed body from which the internal organs had been removed.

Assured of the preservation of body and soul for all time, the next step was to provide a safe repository for them. Coffins were made, as well as sarcophagi. Tombs of stone were erected. As prosperity grew, expenditure for these increased. As much as possible of the property necessary for comfort in life was buried with the dead. The extent of men's interest in the future of the soul may be gauged by the determination of their Pharaohs or rulers to spare no expense in assuring for themselves an everlasting life. The pyramid type of tomb was their choice and some of the pyramids erected for the mummies of themselves and their families still stand in the vicinity of the old capital city, Memphis. The Cheops Pyramid covers thirteen acres at its base, and is nearly 500 feet high. It is estimated to have taken twenty years in building, and to have consumed the labor of 120,000 men. It was built for the Pharaoh, Cheops, and stands as a memorial also to a civilization then at the height of its greatness. Before 1 A.D., the people of Egypt were to lose wealth, power, and even freedom, in humiliating defeat at the hands of their neighbors.

In 330 B.C. came the invasion under Alexander the Great. As a fortunate aftermath of this disaster, a new and great city flourished on the Nile delta. Alexandria was, in time, to be celebrated as the home of Cleopatra, Queen of Egypt; but the real fame of the new city rested on things more substantial than luxury or beauty. In Alexandria was accumulated a great library of ancient manuscripts which attracted the scholars of the world. Thousands of men employed as copyists made possible dissemination of the knowledge contained in these first books. A *museum* which was, in reality, a university, drew teachers of eminence and became renowned among students. Distinguished physicians from many countries were among them and scientific medicine was studied, for the culture introduced by Alexander was Greek, and the methods of Hippocrates were in use in the school which he founded. The Museum achieved honor throughout the world for its work in medicine, mathematics, geography, and astronomy.

The glory of the Alexandrian Empire was not to last. A greater empire was already on the horizon of world affairs and in 30 B.C. the Romans came to Egypt, led by Octavius, successor to Julius Caesar. Cleopatra, its queen, found herself at the head of a country

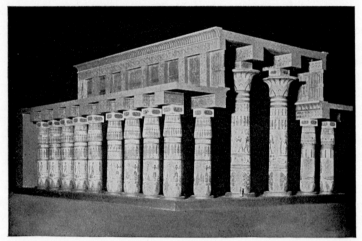

RECONSTRUCTION OF THE GREAT HYPOSTYLE HALL IN THE TEMPLE OF KARNAK
AT THEBES, EGYPT
(Courtesy of the Metropolitan Museum of Art, New York City.)

too weak to withstand him. In order to avoid shame at the hands
of a conqueror, she committed suicide. Roman organization and
Roman tyranny succeeded the culture of Greece along the banks of
the Nile where man's luxurious living had, so far, only followed
Nature's prodigality in his behalf.

Temples   The significance of the temple as a moulding influence in all early civilizations cannot be overestimated. Beginning as
a meager shelter of crudest form built to protect a god from the
eroding effect of weather, the temple became a center of community
and national life. It arose to a magnitude and attained a magnificence
that forced it into towering contrast to the early simplicity of human
existence. On the *Temple of Karnak* at Thebes, the largest in Egypt,
were spent nearly two thousand years of effort. The walls of its
front gate are forty-nine feet thick. A court inside is said to be
eight thousand square feet greater than the entire area of St. Paul's
Cathedral in London.

In the temples frequented by those in search of health, Priest-
physicians shared their tasks with a group of *temple-women*. These
women were often of high social position, and they held the rank
of *priestess*. That they may have performed some nursing duties for

those who sought priestly intercession with the gods is possible, but history fails to make this point clear. It is probable that nursing care was chiefly the responsibility of the mother or daughters in the home. The mother in ancient Egypt occupied a position of authority, and the level of woman's place in Egyptian society was relatively high.

All ethical standards, by this time, were determined by a select group of priests. Sympathetic treatment of the unfortunate was enforced by law. Food, water and clothing must also be provided for the needy. Justice, truth, and humanity were extolled as virtues. Humane expression, however, was limited to friends. Consideration was not expected where enemies were concerned.

THE FERTILE CRESCENT

The three ancient countries of *Babylonia*, *Assyria*, and *Palestine* formed a crescent-shaped strip of land extending from the Persian Gulf in the east to the Mediterranean Sea in the west. Babylonia occupied the eastern end of the crescent, just north of the Persian Gulf, Assyria was in the center, and in the west was Palestine, on the southeast coast of the Mediterranean. Because of the presence of three great rivers, the Tigris, the Euphrates and the River Jordan, together with good soil, this whole region was extremely fertile and became known as the "Fertile Crescent." Its fertility was the more marked because to the north of it lay a great mountainous region that was more or less uninhabitable, and to the south was the vast area of Arabian Desert. For centuries nomads of the desert, moving from one region to another in search of pasturage for their flocks and herds, drifted into these fertile valleys. In time they became agriculturists, and in time, also, wealth and economic changes led them to the building of cities. Their success was to arouse the envy of numerous other peoples, while it kept alive long-continued struggles between them and their nomad brethren, as well as with the mountaineers from the north.

Babylonia   The region between the Tigris and Euphrates valleys was originally known as Mesopotamia, or "the land between the rivers." Here the beginnings of civilization appeared as early as 4000 to 3000 B.C., with so rich a development of morals, learning, and the arts that it has been called by some, "The Cradle of All Culture."

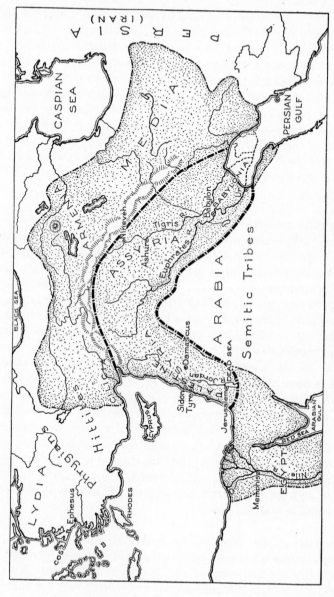

FERTILE CRESCENT OF THE PRE-CHRISTIAN ERA

About 2100 B.C., Babylonians had reached a status of such importance that their lands were known as the "Babylonian Empire." Their king, *Hammurabi*, followed the long-continued policies of warfare with a constructive program that was distinctive in its originality, and would carry his name through the ages of history. A very religious man, he built temples for his people. He also developed systems of irrigation. His fame, however, rests chiefly on his collection of all the older laws and customs of business, legal, and social life, and his systematic arrangement of these into a comprehensive Code of Law. This he caused to be engraved on a great shaft of black stone which was placed in one of the temples of Babylon. Today, it is the oldest preserved code of ancient law. The sense of justice for that time displayed in it is surprising, as well as the consideration shown for the poor and defenseless classes.

The code afforded protection to business by making a contract before witnesses an essential in all buying and selling. In many ways, it offered protection also to agriculturists in both the landowning and the renting classes. Death was the penalty for stealing children or slaves. The child whose father was killed in the service of his country was heir to the father's property. Men who hired mercenaries to fight in their places received the death penalty if they failed to pay their substitutes. Death also was dealt to a robber; if he escaped, the community was called upon to compensate the man whom he had robbed.

Medicine in Babylonia. Hammurabi's code also provided for the regulation of the arts of medicine and surgery, and differentiated between fees for operation on a "gentleman" and those chargeable to a freedman or a slave. Severe penalties fell upon the surgeon whose work was not successful. In case of failure to cure a gentleman, the operator's hands were to be cut off; in the case of an uncured servant, he must pay the owner the current price of a slave. Both these and the punishments inflicted upon criminals and those guilty of minor delinquencies seem harsh, but account must be taken of the fact that religion at that time did little to soften men's hearts, and that the value placed on life several thousand years ago was inestimably less than the value placed on it today. That the Code of Hammurabi advanced the common good of Babylonia is substanti-

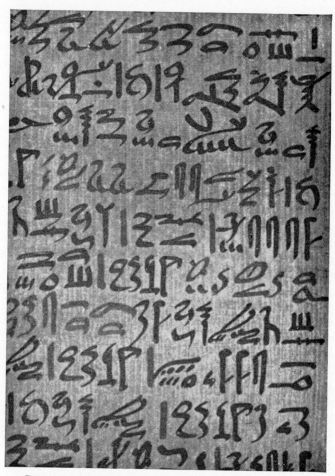

BABYLONIAN MEDICAL PRESCRIPTION IN CUNEIFORM WRITING
(Museum of the University of Leipzig.)

ated by the fact that for nearly three centuries after his reign his country knew increasing prosperity.

The practice of medicine was considered of utmost importance at this early date of Babylonian history. Surgery was in advance of internal medicine which concerned itself mainly with magical formulas to banish demons, the general belief being that gods of evil spirits avenge themselves upon erring human beings by visiting disease upon them. Babylonians had an unusual sense of sin, and were fair-minded enough to acknowledge that their first duty lay, therefore, in conducting themselves as their gods and good spirits, dwelling in earth, sky, or sea, would desire. This, for them, was preventive medicine. It also protected them in a future life when well-served gods would rescue them from the dreary life in Hades which followed death otherwise.

Their surgeons understood nasal tamponing for bleeding, cataract couching, blood letting, and the use of facial applications in cases of erysipelas. Bodies of sacrificed animals supplied the only opportunity for anatomical research. Babylonian priests were astrologists and diviners. They ascribed the source of epidemics to inauspicious astral influence. They diagnosed human ailments by examining the livers of dead animals. Indeed, their system of medicine placed noteworthy reliance on *divination*, that weak, human attempt to unveil obscured knowledge through supernatural methods. "Divining" or ascertaining was attempted by many means. Communion with the dead, crystal-gazing, palmistry, card-reading, omens, portents, falling of meteors—even the instinctive acts of birds or animals—all were used as its medium. In Babylonian life and religion it played an important part, and especially in that country did it take the form of astrological interpretation.

Progress. Among people of Babylonia were those who had knowledge of the elements of science. Some men were learned astronomers. The science of mathematics was understood and applied practically. The division of the year, the week, the day, the hour and the minute as we use it today is traced to its origin in this country. Babylonia cultivated the arts of music, pottery-making, glass-blowing, weaving, and carried on an important trade, especially with Egypt. The world learned to recognize her as an efficient military power. These descendants of nomad tent dwellers even became skilled architects. Babylonians handed down the story of man's creation, and from them was derived the tradition of that Deluge which scientific men of our day have established as an actual fact. They may have built the Ark which survived it.

Women were never held in high regard in Babylonia. Polygamy was practiced. Women's opportunity was strictly domestic. The upper classes of women enjoyed less freedom of action than was accorded those of the middle and lower groups of society.

Assyria   The little kingdom of Assur or Assyria arose in the middle portion of the Fertile Crescent. Its climate was more invigorating than that of the hot Babylonian plain, and its position with mountain ranges on three sides, and a river on the fourth, was better adapted to defense of its frontiers against mountaineer or nomad. As Assyrians acquired culture, they passed it on to other peoples, and Nineveh, their capital city, became the center of art and commerce in the East. Its great walls stretched for two and one-half miles along the Tigris. Here lived their king in dazzling splendor, surrounded by a throng of officials who assisted him in his administrative work.

The Assyrians were a hardened, warlike race of practical bent who built up the greatest empire that the world had yet known. Their one supreme god was a "god of battles." Their armies were first to use weapons of bronze. A library of clay tablets recently unearthed reveals them as a superstitious people believing in the influence of lunar changes and using charms and amulets. So sacred to them was the number seven that the seventh day was reserved for rest.

Sickness represented punishment for sin, and was curable by repentance, while medical practice otherwise confined itself to magic and empiricism. So much time was occupied with war that little was left for education in anything but military tactics. Education of the higher kind was restricted to the priesthood. Needless to say, Assyrian womanhood did not achieve a high position.

Palestine   At the same time that members of Semitic tribes were drifting into Babylonia and Assyria from the arid regions of the Arabian Desert, other members of the same tribes were making their way into the region of Palestine at the western end of the Fertile Crescent. The natives whom they overran gave to these people the name "Hebrews," which, in translation, means "the people from beyond."[1] By the time Hammurabi became king of Babylonia, the Hebrews

[1] Reinach, Salomon: Orpheus: A History of Religions. New York, Liveright, Inc., 1930, p. 182.

were well established in their walled towns, and were going forth from them to practice agricultural pursuits. Then migrating to Egypt, they were taken into captivity, and remained as slaves in that country for more than four hundred years, when they were permitted to leave under the leadership of Moses in the fifteenth century B.C. After forty years of wandering, they reentered Palestine, and the country was divided up among their twelve tribes.

The mountainous character of this part of the Fertile Crescent, and its comparative lack of richness in minerals, made it less desirable than Babylonia or Assyria. Its location between Egypt and these countries was a dangerous one. In case of war, it was the pathway between them. Not for many years were the Hebrews permitted to grow into a strong nation, but about 1100 B.C., when Egypt had become weakened, we find a kingdom in Palestine with *Saul* as its first ruler. In many ways, its people remained true to their desert origin, and Saul was no exception, but he went further than most in his refusal to live in a fixed home. The chosen abode of Palestine's ruler was a tent which could be moved readily within the bounds set by his kingship.

The Hebrew people were well fitted to undertake the stupendous task of reclaiming a land of some desert characteristics, for Palestine, besides being mountainous with narrow, gorge-like valleys, lacked adequate rainfall and water supply. It was a task that strengthened patience and accentuated persistence—qualities which have been theirs to a notable degree throughout the ages since they settled there. They learned to build towns high above the plain, to collect water in cisterns, to cultivate the olive and the grape, both of which find a way to be productive in hot, dry climates. The olive, in particular, because of its extreme slowness in growth and its need of care while young, requires the utmost industry, patience, and foresight. This tree, which has made itself the symbol of peace and civic virtues, exacted all of them in the fifteen to twenty years that it took to reach full development. The Hebrew people waited, and nurtured orchards which eventually became known throughout the world. Olive trees, once grown, have tremendous longevity, and produce oil sufficiently precious to be used in anointing kings. The grapes went into desirable wines, and wool for clothing was contributed by the sheep that found pasture on dry hillsides.

Under *David*, Saul's successor, the country flourished and the city of Jerusalem became the center of its political and religious activities. *Solomon*, who inherited the throne in order of succession, is remembered chiefly for his love of oriental luxury and showy display, the cost of which burdened the people with taxes. In his own day, however, Solomon won an international reputation for wisdom and justice in administration, which was sufficiently influential to bring about the famous visit of the *Queen of Sheba*.[2] A woman of initiative and determination, this lady organized a royal caravan and set out on the long journey from southern Arabia to Palestine with the avowed purpose of proving with hard questions this man of whom she had heard so much. Solomon extended to her every kingly courtesy, and answered all her inquiries. At the conclusion of her stay she made a speech of thanks which, in its graciousness of expression, equals that of the successful woman speaker of the modern world who has enjoyed the distinction of being publicly entertained. The queen summed up her personal conclusions regarding her host's claims to fame as follows:

"It was a true report which I heard in mine own land of thine acts, and of thy wisdom: Howbeit, I believed not their words until I came, and mine eyes have seen it: And, behold, the one half of the greatness of thy wisdom was not told me."[3]

Religion was to constitute the chief contribution of the Hebrews to the betterment of a world that had come to have sore need of it. During centuries of confusing uncertainty, they had held with considerable loyalty to the one Father, God, who had emerged supreme from an early polytheism. In his organization of a code of laws which must yet be in harmony with the needs of his times, Moses developed the Mosaic Law around the worship of this one ethical Father God who demanded obedience from his children. The debt of mankind to the Hebrews came not through the adoption of any new ritual, but through the acceptance of this idea of one God, Jehovah, Maker of all things, who sat in judgment of human actions, a beneficent Being from whom all good could be expected to come, and with whom men might use their intelligence in individual communion through the spirit of prayer. By 1 A.D., this religion had been

[2] I Kings, X.
[3] II Chronicles, IX: 5–6.

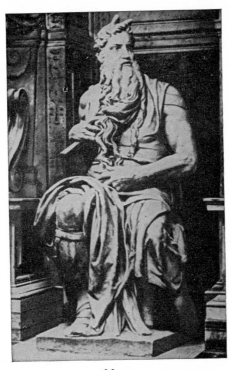

MOSES

(By Michelangelo from "Famous Statues and Their Stories," by Edwin Rayner, Grosset and Dunlap, 1936.)

set down in what we know as the Old Testament. It was written by many authors and, mainly, in the Hebrew language.

In an age in which people had inherited so many gods that religious worship was fast becoming a mechanical and meaningless official routine, and which knew not at all the significance of a life of the spirit, the Hebrew religion pointed out to them a way to begin all over again in the search for the eternal. Its emphasis on the *brotherhood of man* made all men equally eligible to the favor of a strict but kindly Father. All who carried out His wishes could hope for good to come; all were given an incentive to live which other religions had not offered. Its teaching of charity toward others, and the dignity with which it clothed human life, softened human attitudes and broadened human outlook. Individually and collectively, the followers of one God of goodness felt the power to progress to better things. It proved to be a power that changed the whole course of civilization. Indeed, the Old Testament of the Hebrews, combined with the New Testament, written in the early Christian era, "contain the germ of the great ideas of modern civilization, and checking it by history, we see how deeply modern civilization is indebted to it."[4]

Rising empires seized Palestine, each in its turn, and by 1 A.D. the country was under the rule of Rome. In that day, her religion shared, in common with other religions of the time, a nullifying burden of routine ceremonial, while its low invasion by idolatry had become very apparent. Prophets had long since foretold the coming of a Christ or Messiah. During captivity and wandering they had seen the good as well as the evil in human beings, and had learned to conceive a sphere, the bounds of which were not set by any one nation. This was the kingdom of God.

Medicine in Palestine. From a medical standpoint, the Hebrews have a wonderful record of achievement in the practice of hygiene and sanitation, and of systematic, organized control of prevention of disease. Doubtless, much of their medical treatment was learned during captivity in Egypt. The laws ascribed to Moses, who undertook the responsibility of their leadership on the post-exilic journey from Egypt to Palestine, were designed to cover the camp life of more than half a million people who had to have an abode sufficiently settled in character to permit them to find subsistence along the way. They took into account almost every detail of personal and public hygiene. Inspection of food, regulation of diet, slaughtering of animals for food, diagnosis and reporting of communicable disease, isolation and quarantine—all were provided for. Circumcision as a religious practice was ensured as a sanitary measure. The Priest-physicians took on the function of health inspectors. The reporting of disease was compulsory. Orders for treatment and isolation, if warranted, were received from the priest, who also saw to the disinfection of body, clothing, and habitation. Persons excluded from the

[4] Reinach, Salomon: Orpheus: A History of Religions. Liveright, Inc., New York, 1930, p. 186.

camp because of disease were compelled to secure permission from the priest before reentering it.

Under Hebrew law, religion and medicine combined to control the public health, and responsibility for it centered on the Priest-physician. The wisdom and common-sense thinking which developed health laws in an age which lacked the help of either bacteriology or refrigeration will be apparent. To the Hebrews we owe the introduction of prophylaxis. It was prompted by the need of national protection, not only in the face of nearly a half century of camping, but also by the need of national fighting strength, and the hope of national prestige—the two most prominent ideals of the time.

Women of Palestine. Biblical stories in which women appear portray impartially all types common to feminine human nature. *Ruth* exemplifies loyal friendship, *Jezebel* has been called the prototype of Lady Macbeth, *Huldah* was a prophetess, *Deborah* a judge and a Joan of Arc, *Delilah* utterly treacherous, and *Vashti* defied a royal husband's command, thereby raising alarm among his courtiers lest all women might follow her example and become difficult to manage. Her action, indeed, led to an ordinance declaring men to be rulers in their homes. The sweetness of all romance, however, enters into the story of *Rebekah*, a heroine of decision and action. In the twenty-fourth chapter of Genesis, we see her setting out by camel train with her nurse, another Deborah, to meet Isaac, who was to become her husband. Although Deborah was a child's nurse and a companion, no doubt at times she was called upon to perform some nursing duties, and, therefore, represents the first nurse to have her name come down to us in history.

Hebrew women, like all others, held a relatively better position in the early days of tribal clans than in later times. Divorce and polygamy brought various restrictions upon them. At times they were sold into captivity. However, the home atmosphere, as interpreted in general, was an exemplary one. The family bond was strong. Children were taught to honor both parents, as shown in one of the ten commandments of Moses which reads, "Honor thy father and thy mother; that thy days may be long upon the land which the Lord thy God giveth thee." Parents shared responsibility for children's education. Morality, health, habits which affect physical or mental welfare, and manners were taught with the assistance of biblical tradition and precept. Fathers must teach trades to sons, mothers must make daughters good housekeepers and homemakers. The virtues of that mother whose "children will rise up and call her blessed" show her to be wise, kindly, capable, and business-like. The mother of a king taught her son to expect such a woman to organize her life as follows:

"She seeketh wool, and flax, and worketh willingly with her hands.
She is like the merchants' ships; she bringeth her food from afar.
She riseth also while it is yet night, and giveth meat to her household, and a portion to her maidens.
She considereth a field, and buyeth it: with the fruit of her hands, she planteth a vineyard.
She girdeth her loins with strength, and strengtheneth her arms.
She perceiveth that her merchandise is good: her candle goeth not out by night.
She layeth her hands to the spindle, and her hands hold the distaff.
She stretcheth out her hand to the poor: yea, she reacheth forth her hands to the needy.
She is not afraid of the snow for her household: for all her household are clothed with scarlet.
She maketh herself coverings of tapestry; her clothing is silk and purple.
Her husband is known in the gates when he sitteth among the elders of the land.
She maketh fine linen, and selleth it: and delivereth girdles unto the merchant.
Strength and honour are her clothing: and she shall rejoice in the time to come.
She openeth her mouth with wisdom; and in her tongue is the law of kindness.
She looketh well to the ways of her household; and eateth not the bread of idleness.
Her children arise up, and call her blessed; her husband also, and he praiseth her.
Favour is deceitful, and beauty is vain; but a woman that feareth the Lord, she shall be praised.
Give her of the fruit of her hands; and let her own works praise her in the gates."[5]

With wealth and luxury, some of the ideals of home life and some of their pride in housekeeping were lost by Hebrew women. Isaiah understood the shortcomings of the fashionable among them, and frankly addressed them as follows:

"Because the daughters of Zion are haughty, and walk with stretched forth necks and wanton eyes, walking and mincing as they go, and making a tinkling with their feet: therefore the Lord will smite—the daughters of Zion. . . . In that

[5] Proverbs XXXI: 13–31.

day the Lord will take away the bravery of their tinkling ornaments about their feet. . . . The chains, and the bracelets, and the mufflers, the bonnets, and the ornaments of the legs, and the headbands, and the tablets, and the earrings, the rings, nose jewels, the changeable suits of apparel, and the mantles, and the wimples, and the crisping pins, the glasses, and the fine linen, and the hoods, and the veils. And it shall come to pass, that instead of sweet smell there shall be a stink; and instead of a girdle, a rent; and instead of well-set hair, baldness; and instead of a stomacher, a girding of sackcloth; and burning instead of beauty."[6]

The equality which their religion gave to the Hebrews as children sharing in common the gifts of a merciful Father, was, in itself, a stimulus to charity in their dealings with one another. Continual reminders are given by their leaders of their past condition of servitude in Egypt, and of the many experiences of lack of kindness among people of that country. The stranger, the fatherless, the widow, and the poor are not allowed to be forgotten. The borrower who is unable to redeem his pawned clothing before night must have it returned that he may use it as a sleeping garment (Deuteronomy XXIV: 12–13). Usury is chargeable to strangers, but no usury may be charged to a Hebrew "brother" (Deuteronomy XXIII: 20). The hired servant is not to be oppressed whether he be Hebrew or of alien birth. He is also to receive his pay promptly, "for he is poor and setteth his heart upon it."[7] Owners of vineyards must leave some fruit on the vines, those who have olive orchards must refrain from beating down the olives more than once, corners of grain fields must be left unreaped, and forgotten sheaves or gleanings are not to be gathered from the open fields. The way is thus opened to the poor who followed harvesters (Deuteronomy XXIV: 19–22). Consideration is urged even for an enemy, "if thou meet thine enemy's ox or his ass going astray, thou shalt surely bring it back to him."[8]

In addition to these privileges, a system of tithing gave into the hands of the church, for clerical support and distribution to the poor, one-tenth of each property owner's profit after the second year and one-tenth of his harvest annually. "When thou hast made an end of tithing all the tithes of thine increase the third year, which is the year of tithing, and hast given it to the Levite, the stranger, the fatherless, and the widow, that they may eat within thy gates, and be filled; then shalt thou say before the Lord thy God, I have

[6] Isaiah III: 16–24.

[7] Deuteronomy XXIV: 15.

[8] Exodus XXIII: 4.

brought away the hallowed things out of mine house, and also have given them unto the Levite and unto the stranger, to the fatherless, and to the widow, which thou hast commanded me: I have not transgressed thy commandments, neither have I forgotten them."[9] On this tithing system depended for support the *xenodochia* or lodging houses provided for strangers. These institutions later developed, as an accessory to their service, the care of the sick, and in this way became predecessors of the modern hospital.

PERSIA (IRAN)

To the east of the Fertile Crescent, and running between the Persian Gulf and the Caspian Sea, lay the Plateau of Iran occupied in ancient times by peoples known respectively as Medes and Persians. By the fifth century B.C., the Persians had not only conquered their neighbors, the Medes, and carried the boundary of Persia eastward to the Indus River in India, but had extended her rule westward in the greatest empire yet known to mankind. Persia had already won a reputation for tyranny, and the energies of her aristocracy were wholly devoted to war and the acquisition of wealth through plunder and the levy of tribute. Fortunately for Europe, Greece was able to turn the tide of farther advance, and the imperial greatness of a people whose aims were purely selfish, and whose influence was almost wholly destructive, lasted only about two hundred years.

Into religion the Persians brought belief in a god of goodness, and another of evil. The Zendavesta or sacred books of Persia owe their authorship, in the main, to one *Zoroaster* who lived about 600 B.C. The world, according to the Zendavesta, is ruled by two Creators, one making light and good, the other darkness and evil. Good and evil are at constant war for mastery, and good is always triumphant. Fire, earth, and water are sacred elements, and, of these, fire is purest. Earth and water must be kept free from pollution by man's observance of religious law. Immortality is a mental, rather than a physical, state, its happiness or unhappiness dependent on the righteousness or evil of the lives of men on earth. The principal virtues are those of veracity, virility and hard work. Celibacy and

9 Deuteronomy XXVI: 12–14.

fasting are decried as weakening influences. Asceticism made no appeal to the Persian.

It has been said that Persians and Hebrews contributed more than any other ancient peoples to the elevation of standards of human morality. The resemblance between their religious ideals will be seen readily. Both make *good* their guiding star. Both reward good living in an afterlife. Both essayed to control physical health by religious law and practice. To medicine, Persia contributed little in comparison with Palestine. Like the religion of the Hebrews, Zoroastrianism sank into ritualistic routine, but the dignity with which it endowed labor in an age of slavery is important. The god of good was as busy as he expected those to be who worshipped him. His work was to shape the universe and his industry sanctified all work. His followers, like him, worked and fought.

THE FAR EAST

While great civilizations of ancient times were developing in the Near East, a vast continent lay so far beyond them as to be almost unknown. Asia, as it came to be called, comprised the region covered in our day by India, China, and Japan. Modern geographers and historians, on the basis of distance and location, distinguish the combined areas of these countries by the inclusive name of *Far East* or *Orient*. Little information is available of the progress of men as they lived here in primitive days, but they are believed to have had stages of development similar to those passed through by other men; that is, an Age of Hunters, a Pastoral Age, and an Age of Farmers.

INDIA

India, in the form of a triangular peninsula, lies in the southern part of the Far Eastern continent. Two chains of mountains along its upper border cut it off almost completely from the rest of Asia. Nature has effected a further isolation by providing access to it on its two remaining sides by way of the ocean only.

People who migrated from central Asia in ancient times filtered through the mountain passes on the north. They found in India a race darker in color than themselves, enjoying a warmer climate and a richer vegetation than they had known. In time, these northern

Aryans took the country away from its Negroid and Mongoloid inhabitants by conquest. In her social development, India shows the influence of this early mixture of races which merged old and new without assimilation. Her caste system with its characteristic acceptance of inequality in birth and uneven division of wealth originated in these early days.

What is known of primitive India has come down to us in the form of folklore, a type of history popular among Aryan tribes. Handed down among the people, most frequently through the mother who sings or tells it to her children, folklore is a mixture of truth and fiction. It serves the double purpose of instruction and entertainment, and usually it exalts the glory of the past. The folklore of India is considered particularly fascinating, and was told in a style which so appealed to Arab fancy that it was borrowed for the "Arabian Nights." Animism and nature worship permeate what is the work of many story tellers. The mysticism which entered it later, and which has been so characteristic of India, may have been due in part to an enervating climate which reduced physical activity to a minimum. The people of India are dreamers. At the same time, what has come down to us from their shadowy past indicates a considerable degree of civilization.

Brahmanism   Preeminent in influence on the outlook of India has been that part of its folklore which its priests gathered together eventually and preserved for the use of succeeding generations. Upon these men, to whom was accorded a position in the highest caste, rested the obligation of memorizing ancient hymns and prayers which were a part of India's worship. When the art of writing came into use, they transcribed this learning into sacred books known as "Vedas." The Vedas represent an accumulation of man's most valued knowledge as developed in his Asiatic environment during the earliest period of which we have record. They became the Bible of India. Their content was law.

To animism, nature worship, and magic, the Veda owes its source. It is imbued with belief in sacrifice to kind spirits and to gods, as man's protection from the ills of life and his hope of a satisfactory reincarnation. It gives some evidence of the spirit of *asceticism* which was to become, in the course of time, a dominant influence throughout the world. For students of medicine and nursing, there is especial significance in the fact that, in the Vedas, man is pictured as free from sin and disease at birth. One in particular, known as the *Ayur Veda*, or the Veda of Longevity, is medical in viewpoint and content, and stresses hygiene and prevention of sickness. It teaches man to preserve a perfect body by his own determination to practice precepts that have been culled from general experience. Inoculation against smallpox is mentioned. Curative practice in medicine, surgery, and pediatrics is discussed. Materia medica is included.

As time goes on we find the mass of the people of India becoming dissatisfied with the religion of the Vedas as interpreted to them by their priests. More and more effort and sacrifice was demanded of the worshipper if he was to satisfy his gods. The thought of transmigration of his soul after death was kept before him continually, while the finality of caste closed the door to all hope of opportunity in the present world. At best, life could be but burdensome and work a hardship in this marshy, tropical country, the dampness and heat of which were unalleviated by any modern methods of sanitation, ventilation, or refrigeration. Men began to look for a compensatory change in belief and mode of living.

Asceticism In the development of civilization there had long been those who chose the life of the recluse in an effort to escape the sordidness of life, and attain a closer relation with the spiritual. People of India turned, therefore, to asceticism in the hope of attaining that peace of soul which is a human need. As ascetics they practiced extreme self-denial. Withdrawal from family and friends, torture of the body, and a system of diet that approached starvation expressed their renunciation of physical pleasures, and thereby brought them nearer to infinite spiritual good. Asceticism brought into the life of man a narrow severity in ideals of piety which persists to this day, and which people of today are endeavoring to transmute into ideals that will ensure fullness of life in the present, while they harmonize with a variety of beliefs concerning the future. Successively, asceticism was to find renewed expression among early Christians, in the monasticism of the Middle Ages, in the harshness of life under the influence of beginning Protestantism, and in the puritanical ideals of early America.

Rise of Buddhism About 500 B.C., there was born in India a child who was to become its outstanding exponent of asceticism up

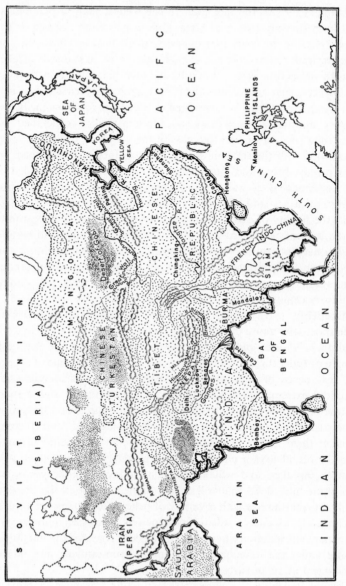

THE FAR EAST OF TODAY

to that time. *Gautama*, who came to be known as *Buddha* or the "enlightened one," belonged to the caste of princes. While yet a young man he abandoned his wife, his child, and a life of ease amid beautiful surroundings, to become one of a group of hermit ascetics. Unsatisfied by the Brahmin religion, which accentuated caste differences and induced fear of a lowered caste after death, Buddha set out alone as a mendicant monk, inspired to bring content to all men. The religion which he offered had no gods and required no sacrifices.

By disregarding caste, Buddhism made possible for everyone the practice of a system of self-education which would destroy all material desire. Release from worldly evils would thus be achieved while on earth, and the perfect Buddhist need have no fear of life after death. He would enter here into a state of "Nirvana" or perfect peace in which he would avoid the misery which is a major part of living. Complete renunciation of self with charity toward all men was further expression of a kindly though pessimistic religion to which India turned eagerly. Images of Buddha gave his spirit, eventually, the concrete form familiar in our time. The figure was not intended to represent a god, but, rather, that perfection of character which is attainable, through work, by the individual Buddhist.

The Reign of King Asoka   About 250 B.C., in the very beginning of a long reign which was to make him one of the foremost rulers in history, *King Asoka* of India became a convert to Buddhism. Reared in the tradition of war, he had entered upon a campaign of invasion with the aim of acquiring territory, but his remorse for the human suffering that he caused was so real that he refused to fight again. Instead, he introduced methods of arbitration that brought him fame among potential enemies. War, he told men, should be a spiritual conquest. "It is in the conquests of religion that the gods take pleasure."[10] As a Buddhist, peaceful penetration became his aim in the future, and the influence of his gentle spirit was felt far beyond his realm.

In proclamations inscribed upon rock, King Asoka urged his people to study the new religion. He exhorted them to show kindness to slaves, and to give alms to the poor. In a world which set little value upon life, he succeeded in organizing what amounted to

[10] Steel, F. A.: India Through the Ages. New York, E. P. Dutton & Co.

a national society for the prevention of cruelty to animals. By his own example, as well as by precept, he persuaded the people of India that all living things are worthy of respect.

The wise rule of "Good King Asoka" brought prosperity. Improved buildings were provided for the use of travelers in India. These compare with the hotel and garage of today, for they gave shelter to animals as well as to their owners. Hospitals were founded. Monasteries of great magnificence were built for the men and women who wished to retire from the work-a-day world to pass lives of purity in study and contemplation. Buddha had founded similar religious communities during his life-time, and some of them had attained public regard as well as lands and wealth. They were now a source of help to King Asoka, whose chief desire was to give to all the world the doctrines of peace and love inherent in Buddhism.

Medicine in Early India   India set high moral standards for those who would choose the care of the sick as a life work. Her exaction of a king's permission for right to practice medicine was akin to our license system. Prevention of disease was traditionally a matter of first importance, and care of the body a religious duty. Compulsory hygienic measures were adopted. Bathing twice a day was a regulation that must have been readily enforced in a climate of distressing heat. The crude massage of early times had refined itself into a form of treatment that was in high favor. Trustworthiness and skill were demanded of midwives who, in common with doctors, were admonished to have short fingernails. Clean lying-in rooms with cross ventilation were requisite for deliveries. Operations were preceded by religious ceremony and prayer. By 1 A.D., the methods prescribed by magic already had been altered to conform with more up-to-date practice, although the Priest-physician still controlled the field of medicine, and retarded it considerably by his refusal to come into contact with blood or pathological tissues. As in Egypt, dissection of the human body was forbidden.

Position of Women   Socially, the women of India in the period preceding 1 A.D. held a relatively high position. Monogamy was the general rule, although polygamy was practiced. King Asoka had shown interest in their education, and the higher castes enjoyed some privileges that approach those accorded to Western women today. Their status, in fact, presents a sharp contrast to that to which they were to be reduced in later times. In any consideration of woman's position, however, the fact must be faced that the place held by them among Western peoples has never been reached in Asiatic countries. Woman's activities were, in the main, those connected with management of her home. Doubtless she performed the duties of a nurse when sickness befell a member of her family. In institutions, these duties were entrusted to old women and to men.

CHINA

Ancient China lay across the great range of the Himalaya Mountains, far to the northeast of India. Like India, it was cut off from the Mediterranean world, and lacked the stimulation of ideas which accompanies a freer intercourse among peoples. The Chinese are thought to have come from central Asia about 3000 B.C. Their earliest settlement was made along the banks of the Yellow River where lies an area of very finely pulverized and fertile soil or loess, which reaches, in some places, a depth of several feet. No record has been found of their Stone Age, but they developed another of the great civilizations that record man's progress beyond the primitive. What knowledge has come down to us in regard to this civilization is, in the main, legendary. Little credence is given to available history of China until the twelfth century B.C., when the Chou dynasty began a rule which lasted nine hundred years. During this period, civilizations spread south from the Yellow River to the Yangtse River.

Just as we found in the Near East, and again in India, there developed among the people of Eastern Asia a mythology. Sacred books also were written which compare with the ancient Papyri of Egypt and the Vedas of India.

Confucianism   About 500 B.C., and toward the end of the Chou dynasty, there came into the world of the Far East an influence which affects its life and customs to the present time. While the teachings of Buddha were changing the outlook of men in India, *Confucius* entered the life of China. As a child, he studied her sacred books and learned to revere their teachings. As a man, he turned to them for inspiration that was to make him one of the greatest reformers and teachers the world has known.

Born into a period of political disturbance and unhappiness that had been induced by corruption in its governing group, Confucius sought means of relieving oppression in his country by going back to ancient customs for the basis of a governmental ideal. He hoped to solve the problem of clean politics by demanding fair and kind dealing on the part of a ruler in exchange for the respect and veneration of his people. The empire would be an ideal family in which the emperor took the place of both father and mother, and guided the destiny of subjects bound together by ties of brotherly love.

The patriarchal rule, which China had developed in common with other peoples, appealed to Confucius as a fundamental factor in the attainment of a good life for all. The sacred books held record of this system, still in force but greatly weakened. With their help he revived it. The family became the unit of society. The father assumed responsibility for the welfare of all persons comprising the family. Owner of all property, and endowed with supreme authority, he was expected to rule with wisdom and kindliness. On the foundation of such family units, each organized under authority of the person most likely to govern it happily, and all subject to the rule of an emperor, also wise and kind, Confucius, the reformer, hoped to build up a contented, peaceful empire. The emphasis which Confucius placed on ancestor worship as a part of the patriarchal system proved a lasting influence, for ill as well as good, on the development of China.

Ancestor Worship   Ancestor worship has been a phase of religious growth among all human beings. It rests upon a genealogy traced back to the founder of the family line who may be a man, a woman, a god, a hero, or even a bird or an animal. In China, the descent was traceable through fathers of families only. No worship was accorded to female ancestors, for the mother's share in the honors of descent was ignored. Through the efforts of Confucius, ancestor worship attained great strength, a strength which was to resist the passage of time in this distant stronghold much longer than it had elsewhere. Ultimately, it became the backbone of political organization in China. The home of the Confucianist still treasures its Hall of Ancestors, and, if sufficiently wealthy, supports its temple for their worship.

The philosophy passed down to us by disciples of Confucius is composed of precepts and rules of etiquette. Great emphasis was placed on the value of knowledge in solving life's problems. Right conduct could be expected to follow naturally a careful study of acts performed by men of wisdom. Faithfulness and sincerity were chief among virtues. Energy, perseverance, family affection and reverence for age were others. Confucius urged men to think good thoughts, and to treat each other as brothers, doing nothing unto others that they would not have others do unto them. The Confucian formulary made its strongest appeal to men of his own aristocratic and more enlightened class.

On the whole, and especially through its glorification of the past, the influence of Confucian teaching on Chinese development was arresting. It failed to stimulate ambition for better things. Nevertheless, it was China that invented the mariner's compass, and discovered how to make gunpowder. She made use of bronze money as early as 1100 B.C., and European missionaries of a later era were surprised to find that she had not only collected great libraries, but was able to demonstrate, in addition to paper making, the art of printing on paper with wood blocks, from which was developed the indispensable art of modern paper printing.

The descendants of Confucius, who had one son and one grandson, have been likened to the Jews who trace their lineage to Abraham. Both leaders are now represented by groups aggregating many thousands of people. Traditionary influence has constituted the binding tie in each group. Their customs and ideals have been the outcome of a patriarchal system which Abraham perfected, and on which Confucius set his hope.

By 200 B.C., or after about three centuries of Confucianism, another ideal of life was brought into the Far East from India. Buddhism became the religion of the populace. With its advent monasteries in charge of monks or nuns arose in China.

Position of Women   Although records have been found which would indicate a different status for women in China as early as 2000 B.C., their position, as ultimately defined by custom, and quite definitely by Confucius, was inferior to that of men. A woman was expected to become a fruitful and submissive wife. The education of her daughters, it is true, was in her hands. The daughters, however, were severed from connection with the family of father and mother when they married. Marriage automatically transferred them to membership of subordinate character in the families of husbands.

To this inevitable alteration in her allegiance are traceable at least two ideas which influenced the position of the Chinese woman for centuries later. The cost of rearing a female child came to stand out as useless expense because, in the end, no benefit would accrue to the family from which she was descended. Education beyond that required for home management was not necessary. Woman's work gradually confined itself to home keeping and family building. Highly valued for her fertility, her value became greatest when she produced sons. The reception awaiting her daughters was settled by the Chinese in the following terse expression of their sentiment: "Eighteen goddess-like daughters are not equal to one son with a limp."

Medicine in Early China   China's medical knowledge dates far back in her history. Before 2000 B.C., dissection was permitted. The Chinese made studies of the circulation, and placed great stress on the behavior of the pulse. Systematic methods of physical diagnosis were used, and four words in their teaching indicate the principles on which examination was based. The following guideposts were set for the physician, "Look, Listen, Ask, Feel." In common with other peoples, the Chinese had their system of massage, and they are said to have been willing to assign this form of treatment to operators who were blind. For reduction of fever, the bath was used, and as a means of helping an evil spirit to escape from the prison of the body, blood letting was resorted to.

Its religious beliefs were the means of making China preeminently a static country. The whole vast area was brought under the rule of custom by *Confucianism*, which regulated the conduct of everyday life, venerated the past, and evaded the future. *Buddhism* and *Taoism*, a form of stoicism, only helped to give strength to the bonds of tradition. None of the three religious influences offered incentive for purposeful advancement. Everything was settled. "What is gray with age becomes religion" in China, and her medical precedents remained, until recently, wholly under the spell of that ancient tradition which controlled her social and political life.

A study of variations in China from better known ideas and

standards makes two things stand out because of their reasonableness. China venerated both knowledge and age. She looked for knowledge as the reward of experience as well as of study. In knowledge, she hid the key to wealth and power. The basis of the honors that she accorded men were ability and merit, and her aristocracy was one of learning. For her old men, China demanded reverence for wisdom learned by living; to her old women she gave love and a position of high esteem in the families which her young married women entered as slaves. To have reached the age of sixty in China was not to have become useless, but to receive recognition for a greater usefulness than could be offered by youth. One earned honor and was expected to be a valuable counsellor if one had lived wisely and well.

SUMMARY

Egypt, the Fertile Crescent, and Persia, all regions of the Near East, are believed to have attained a considerable degree of progress toward civilization before any of their barbarian neighbors, and Egypt appears to have been ahead of the other two. In Egypt, about 5000 B.C., man invented the axe with which he could build stationary homes, and learned to plant crops that would supply him with food. His nomadic manner of existence could then be abandoned. The "New Stone Age" or the "Age of Farmers" had arrived.

About 4000 B.C., the Egyptians produced a calendar of twelve months of thirty days each, and five holidays to celebrate the birthdays of the gods. By 3000 B.C., another invention causing revolutionary advances in living and thinking was a method of putting ideas into writing, first in the form of pictures and later as hieroglyphics. A spirit world was developed which was inhabited by many gods, chief among whom were the trinity, Isis, Osiris, and their son Horus. Images were made to give concrete evidence of their presence, and then shelters to protect them. From these crude beginnings magnificent temples emerged, and to them came many seeking divine assistance in all manner of afflictions. The sick among them were received by Priest-physicians and temple women, the latter of whom are believed to have performed some nursing duties.

Of the three regions of the Fertile Crescent, Babylonia, Assyria, and Palestine, the only noteworthy progress of a humanitarian nature came through Babylonia and Palestine. In *Babylonia*, about 2100 B.C., reigned King Hammurabi, a religious and just man who is known for his uplifting social influence. His Code of Law, engraved on a pillar of stone in a large temple, is today the oldest known code of its kind in existence. It represented a revision of the laws in force when Hammurabi came into power and aimed at ensuring justice and protection for all classes of people. Among other things, the practice of medicine and surgery was regulated so as to discourage experimentation by unscrupulous persons.

Palestine, home of the Hebrews, made contributions toward world betterment through the channels of religion and charity. The Old Testament of the Christian Bible, with its emphasis on one God, an omnipotent and omnipresent Father of all men, proved to be a power great enough to change the whole course of civilization. The dignity with which it clothed human life softened human attitudes and broadened human outlook.

After wandering into Egypt and falling into captivity, where they remained as slaves for four hundred years, it was Moses, the lawgiver, who led the Hebrews back to Palestine. On the homeward journey, he regulated camp life by enforcement of principles of personal hygiene and public sanitation, while through the Ten Commandments direction was given to human conduct.

The hardships endured in Egypt and on the homeward journey created a compassionate people. A system of tithing was developed to provide money for charitable purposes, and xenodochia erected to shelter the traveler, the orphan, the aged, and the poor. In time, these institutions cared for the sick as well, and, therefore, are regarded as the forerunners of hospitals.

In *Persia*, to the east of the Fertile Crescent, the ethical principles of truthfulness and industry were emphasized in their sacred books, the Zendavesta. Written largely by Zoroaster, they gave promise of reward after death for a life of goodness and struggle upon this earth.

In the Far East, about the time of Zoroaster, there lived two other men who brought hope and happiness to their people. Confucius of *China* and Buddha of *India* both emphasized the need of brotherly love in man's troubled existence. While both men belonged to the aristocratic and more enlightened stratum of society, the one brought into being a philosophy of life that appealed to this group, and the other, who included all classes as human beings, attracted the masses who knew the cruel influence of caste.

No public worship characterized Confucianism while Buddhism encouraged the growth of temples and monasteries. The ancestor worship stressed by Confucius was ignored by Buddha. Confucius, indeed, strove only to show men how to reduce life in the present to a well-regulated, satisfactory scheme, and he advocated a middle road, or avoidance of extremes in all phases of living. Buddha taught that "Nirvana" or spiritual serenity can be achieved only by giving up all material desire and dwelling on spiritual things. His teachings of kindliness and brotherly love closely resemble those of the Christian religion.

Each man inhibited development in his own way. Both were interested in learning, but Confucius, by adherence to custom and by strict regulation of the earthly life, produced an ultra-conservatism. Buddha provided an escape from reality which destroyed ambition, and with it, progress. China, by her adoption of both religions, brought herself completely under the influence of a static policy.

The teachings of brotherly love and peace inherent in Buddhism were greatly promoted by "Good King Asoka" who ruled in India about 250 B.C. Medicine received special attention from him, and high standards were set for its practice. So well remembered and so beloved is King Asoka by the people of India that it has been said of him,

"If a man's fame can be measured by the number of hearts who revere his memory, by the number of lips who have mentioned and still mention him with honour, Asoka is more famous than Charlemagne or Caesar."[11]

History so far gives little mention of nursing as a separate occupation. From the earliest time, the midwife was accepted in her role of specialist to women during childbirth, and the child's nurse appears to have had some distinction in early Palestine. Priestesses are believed to have performed many functions now recognized as those of the nurse, for, in the temple, man's first center of community thought and activity, is disclosed the nucleus of his religious education, medicine, and nursing.

[11] Quoted in the Encyclopedia Britannica.

TOPICS FOR DISCUSSION
EGYPT

1. How does the period of development of Egypt compare with that of other ancient civilizations?
2. Compare the Old Stone Age of primitive man with the New Stone Age of the Egyptians.
3. Give the names and attributes of the trinity of gods that ultimately came into control of bodily and spiritual welfare of Egyptians.
4. (*a*) Tell something of the Priest-physician of ancient Egypt. (*b*) What name stands out as that of the greatest of these men?
5. (*a*) Into what books did the priests collect their religious precepts? (*b*) In which one of these is the medical world especially interested?
6. Name two circumstances which prevented progress in medical knowledge.
7. What do you know of the ancient city of Alexandria?
8. What is known of the position of women in Egypt during this early period?
9. Tell what you know of the medicine and nursing of ancient Egypt.
10. (*a*) Of what significance were the early temples? (*b*) What were the duties of temple women?
11. Make a chart showing outstanding events that occurred about every thousand years, beginning around 5000 B.C.
12. Procure from a college book store, or other source, an outline map of Europe, and fill in names of mountains, bodies of water, and cities as they are studied.

FERTILE CRESCENT

1. Give the geographical location of the Fertile Crescent, naming its rivers and the three ancient civilizations that developed within its boundaries.
2. Justify the statement that Hammurabi exerted a great social influence in the Babylonian Empire.
3. Name several drawbacks to the practice of medicine and surgery of that period.

4. What was the general position of Babylonian women?
5. Name several characteristics of the ancient Assyrians.
6. What were Assyrian attitudes toward sickness and medical practice?
7. What do you know of the position of Assyrian women?
8. Give a general description of the characteristics of the Hebrew people.
9. Name two great contributions of the Hebrews to religion.
10. (*a*) Give definite reasons for the fact that the Hebrews are credited with making great advances in the practice of hygiene and sanitation. (*b*) Why is Moses known as a "great sanitarian" and also as "the law-giver"?
11. What laws did Moses provide for the Hebrew people, and in what book of the Bible are they found?
12. Show how the virtues stressed by the Hebrew religion led to provision for institutional care of the sick?

PERSIA

1. Give the location of ancient Persia, and state the name by which it is known today.
2. What was the sacred book of the Persians, and who was its author?
3. How were the problems of the universe accounted for in the Zendavesta?
4. What is your estimate of the virtues that were highly esteemed by the Persians?
5. Why has it been stated that the Persians and the Hebrews made greater contributions than any other ancient peoples to the elevation of standards of morality?

THE FAR EAST

1. (*a*) Name two mountain ranges which separate India from the remainder of Asia. (*b*) How else is it isolated?
2. (*a*) Into what two bodies of water do the Indus and Ganges rivers empty? (*b*) Which of these rivers is considered sacred and capable of curing of disease those who bathe in it?
3. Compare the teachings of the Vedas of India with those of the ancient papyri of Egypt.

4. In India, what procedure similar to licensing was demanded of a physician before he would be permitted to practice?

5. In the interests of prevention of disease, what practices were required of doctors and midwives?

6. If you were a young person growing up in India, how do you think the caste system would affect your outlook on life?

7. What great man arose in India to point the way toward development of a more desirable mental attitude?

8. Give reasons for the fact that Buddhism is regarded as having characteristics in common with Christianity.

9. Through what channels did Good King Asoka exert an uplifting social influence?

10. Through reference reading, show how the following customs illustrate the unhappy and subordinate position of women in more modern India: Child-marriage. Infanticide. Suttee.

11. Describe and locate the Taj Mahal. Show how it represents an exception to the general regard in which women were held at the time it was built.

12. Give the geographical location of ancient China, with a description of the rivers and the soil that attracted early settlers.

13. Compare the causes for unhappiness of the people of ancient India and China.

14. (a) Compare the life and teachings of Confucius of China with those of Buddha of India. (b) Show how each affected general progress.

15. What is your opinion of the virtues emphasized by Confucius?

16. What was the status of Chinese medicine of this period?

17. Did China's attitude in regard to dissection compare favorably or unfavorably with that of other ancient countries?

18. (a) Describe the life of the average young girl of ancient China. (b) Under what circumstances might the women of China be called upon to do some nursing?

19. Make a chart showing the virtues held necessary for a good life in each of the regions studied.

REFERENCES

Ayscough, Florence: Chinese Women Yesterday and Today. Boston, Houghton Mifflin Co., 1937.

Breasted, James Henry: The Conquest of Civilization. New York, Harper & Brothers, 1938.

Brown, Lewis: The World's Great Scriptures. New York, The Macmillan Co., 1946.

Dock and Nutting: A History of Nursing. New York, G. P. Putnam's Sons, 1907, Vol. I, Chap. 5.

Durant, Will: Our Oriental Heritage. New York, Simon & Schuster, Inc., 1935.

Durant, Will: Caesar and Christ. New York, Simon & Schuster, Inc., 1944.

Hauswirth, Frieda: Purdah: The Status of India Women. New York, The Vanguard Press, 1932.

Hurd-Mead, Kate Campbell: A History of Women in Medicine. Haddam, Conn. The Haddam Press, 1938.

Marble, Annie Russell: Women of the Bible. New York and London, Century Co., 1923.

Old Testament:
>   Book of Ruth (love story of Ruth).
>   I Kings XVIII; XIX; XX (Jezebel).
>   II Kings IX (Jezebel).
>   II Kings XXII: 14–20 (Huldah).
>   Judges IV and V (Deborah).
>   Judges XVI (Delilah).
>   Esther I (Vashti).
>   Genesis XXIV (Rebekah).

Shorter, Alan W.: Everyday Life in Ancient Egypt. London, Sampson Low, Marston and Co., Ltd., 1932.

Steel, F. A.: India Through the Ages. New York, E. P. Dutton & Co., pp. 1–10 (Vedas), pp. 46–49 (King Asoka).

Storrow, Rev. E.: Our Sisters in India. New York, Fleming H. Revell Co. (Indian women in history, child marriage, infanticide, suttee.)

Wells, H. G.: Outline of History. New York, The Macmillan Co., pp. 354–371 (Buddha and King Asoka).

Williams, Edward Thomas: China Yesterday and Today. New York, Thomas Y. Crowell Co., 1932, Chap. 2 (Beginnings of China).

Yutang, Lin: My Country and My People. New York, The John Day Company, 1939.

Beginnings of Civilization

(Continued)

THE MEDITERRANEAN WORLD

GREECE

Jutting out into the Mediterranean Sea from the southeastern part of Europe is a peninsula which, at its outmost end, turns back upon itself. This is the country that we know as Greece, but we shall find that our tiny republic of the twentieth century is but a remnant of an ancient Greece. Its much indented coast line offers a few good harbors, and in early times lent itself readily to a trade which was carried on in small boats. The interior is mountainous, and of singular beauty, while the climate is warm and sunny. Sea breezes moderate the heat of southern summers. Winters are mild.

For their history, the mixture of peoples who later came to be known as Greek learned to rely upon the writings of *Homer* who recorded the deeds of ancient heroes in his poems, "The Iliad" and "The Odyssey." Written about 1100 B.C., these became the sacred books of Greece. Through mythology, they traced their origin to *Chiron*, strongest of a race of Centaurs, or men whose bodies were half human and half horse. Their gods became many, and besides war, natural forces, and animals, they represented abstract qualities such as strength, beauty, youth, and others which would inspire the imagination and veneration of men who, in time, proved that they were of notably artistic temperament.

Apollo, god of the sun, did more than provide food or supply ancestry for rulers who would have divine authority for their acts.

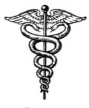

CADUCEUS

To the Greeks, Apollo was god of health—and of medicine, the supporter of health. His sister, Artemis, was acquainted with medical lore and assisted him in the instruction of Chiron the Centaur. Chiron, in turn, was made responsible for the education of Apollo's son *Asklepios*, "The Blameless Physician." Representation of Asklepios showed him holding the staff of the traveler, entwined with the serpents of wisdom—emblems still used by the medical profession in the caduceus. Asklepios' wife shared his work, for she was revered as "The Soothing One." Their children assisted them. One son was the possessor of hands which were an asset to him in surgical work. Another gave his attention to matters associated with internal medicine. Of their daughters, *Hygeia* served as goddess of health, while *Panacea* presided over the administration of medicine and was known as the healer of all ills.

The loveliness of their surroundings made a deep impression on the responsive Greek people. They enjoyed the opportunity given them for outdoor life. In meeting the exigencies of war, poverty, and disease they exhibited a practical bent. They planned systematically for the development of skill and strength for fighting, and they achieved a wise simplicity of life that accorded with their resources. Hospitality was to them a virtue and a religious duty, the demands of which they met by providing organized charity and care for those who were poor or sick. To be sure, they denied this care to incurable cases and to women in confinement, but it must be remembered that they were not alone in considering both death and birth sources of pollution. Their apparent indifference to suffering was closely allied to an intuitive sense of disease prevention on the part of primitive people. Technical knowledge of such prevention by methods that we now accept as nursing procedures was exceedingly meager. The prime reason, however, lay in the fact that the interest of the Greek people was not held by sickness and misery in which lies neither beauty nor perfection. They looked and worked for the positive states of health and happiness.

Institutional Care of the Sick   Care for the sick was provided by the *xenodochion* which was similar in function to the xenodochium of the Hebrews. After Christianity had awakened men to the extent of human misery and their responsibility for doing something about it, this type of institution was to be copied wherever the religion of brotherhood was preached. It became the hospice of the early church. Originally, the xenodochion was built for the purpose of providing lodging and refreshment for the strangers whose number increased with travel and commerce. Sickness among these wayfarers was inevitable and, in all likelihood, the functions of medical and nursing care were added before long. The work of the xenodochion, done as it eventually was under municipal management, might be considered a forerunner of that of the modern city and county hospital.

The *iatrion* was another civic undertaking of the Greeks. The work done in it would correspond most closely with that of the dispensary, or its outgrowth of the present day—the out-patient department or clinic of a hospital. Medical advice could be obtained at the iatrion by the ambulatory sick, operations were performed if necessary, and prescriptions were compounded and issued. No provision was made for hospitalization at the iatrion of those who needed care in bed.

Temples   The appreciative people of Greece found, in the topography of that country, opportunity for selection of lofty sites of unusual beauty for their temples. The artistic genius of architects and sculptors was not restrained. Neither money nor toil was spared in bringing to successful completion such conceptions as those of the Parthenon in Athens, which, twenty-five hundred years later, is "admittedly the most perfect building ever conceived by the mind or built by the hand of man."[1] Her *Temple of Epidauros*, in its beautiful mountain setting near Athens, bears especial interest for us because of the part that it has played in medical history. Its hospital aspect

[1] Magoffian and Davis: The Romance of Archaeology. New York, Henry Holt & Co., 1929, p. 118.

will be discussed later. It is quite easy to conjure up a picture of Epidauros after reading the following artist's conception of Delphi where stood another Greek temple. Epidauros, too, was the goal of many pilgrims. It was, in all probability, quite as effective in its beauty as the others.

"The pilgrims to Delphi saw the mountain at the base of which the shrines were situated long before arriving at the gates of the sacred enclosures. Stark cliffs of limestone, with deep and shadowy clefts penetrating their walls made a gray background for the spreading sacred groves of olive and cypress, silver gray and deep green, in the midst of which statues gleamed. From all parts of Greece, came all classes of men: Spartans, roughly attired; shepherds with goat skin capoted capes; Ionians, clad in spotless white, their tunics bordered with embroidered frets; here and there soldiers, or hoplites, with leathern cuirasses and shields and spears, and the priests and the priestesses of Apollo. They wandered towards the temple erected upon the highest eminence, its white colonnades casting deep shadows on its walls, its eaves and details sparkling in color and gold; and among marble and bronze statues of the famous athletes, and memorials, recording great deeds of the time. The white robes shone bright in the groves, processions passed with song and dancing, marble seats invited repose and contemplation of the numberless works of art, and outside the enclosure or temenos, great hostelries were bustling with guests arriving and departing, and the nude bodies of the athletes reflected the sunlight as they ran and wrestled and flung the javelin either in practice or in the games. The small clean-cut horses in the races were criticized and compared, and constantly the ceremonies of awarding the crowns to victors attracted an ever increasing crowd. There came also solemn embassies from far cities to consult the oracle, men of eminence dealing with pretentious subjects; these passed within the temple and listened for the decision of the gods."[2]

But the temple was more than a building, crude or beautiful as it might be. It was the pulse of national life. Its records are national history. Rulers made use of it for broadcasting information or laws. Its priests comforted, healed, exhorted, or swayed the public in this common gathering place. In the absence of microphones or radios, nature frequently supplied echoes, or exaggerated sound waves traveling through caverns, to help the human voice. Many functions besides that of worship occupied men in or near the temple. They made it a bank, a market, a social welfare society, a community recreation center, sometimes a school, always an object of lavish adoration and best creative effort. It is not to be wondered at, therefore, that high on mountain tops, on plains, or deserts, in cities, even buried under ruins of former civilizations, we find these memorials of their achievement and beliefs which men intended to last

[2] Committee on Education of the American Institute of Architects: The Significance of the Fine Arts. Marshall Jones and Company, Boston, 1923, pp. 30–31.

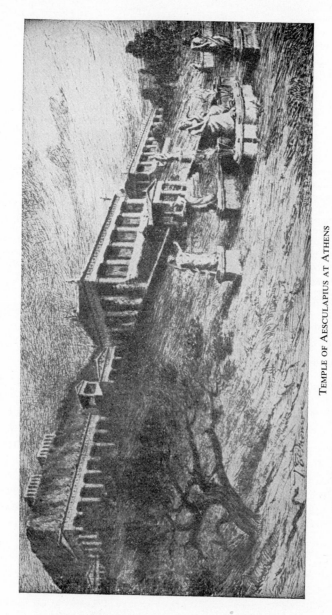

TEMPLE OF AESCULAPIUS AT ATHENS

(Dana, Charles L.: The Peaks of Medical History. Paul B. Hoeber, Inc., New York.)

forever. They were the centers from which radiated religion, education, medicine, and nursing.

Temples of Asklepios   The temples devoted to the worship of Asklepios (Æsculapius, as he was called later by the Latin people of Rome) were the main centers of medical work in Greece. *They illustrate the best development of that constant association between religion, medicine, and nursing that existed in early times.* Through them is represented a national effort to bring about physical and moral health among the people. Greek reverence for physical perfection retarded medical advancement when it prohibited marring the body by dissection. At the same time, it went far beyond the choice of a god to whom worship might be addressed in the hope of health as a reward for sacrifice. It brought about the development of a group of specialists who were preparing the way for a man destined to change medicine from primitive magic to science. These specialists were priests who attained skill in the care of the sick who came with the well to join in prayers to Asklepios. Asklepios may even have been, like Imhotep of Egypt, a human physician so beloved of those to whom he once gave his service in life that time brought about his deification after death. The traditions of medical care inherited by his representatives may have had an unusual basis of knowledge and common sense. In any case, the success of these priests of the Asklepian temples caused them to be set apart in a group known as the *Asklepiades*. They shared their wisdom with selected students, and, as early as the eighth century B.C. had originated a form of medical school in Greece. By 500 B.C., they were practicing in the xenodochion, the iatrion, and in certain temples of Asklepios which had been given over to them.

EPIDAUROS, A TEMPLE OF ASKLEPIOS. Some temples of Asklepiades assumed the character of health centers in which the core of activities was the Greek ideal of health as a balanced state of well-being in mind, body, and soul. The most celebrated of these was at Epidauros, a few miles from Athens. On a scenic site amid groves of trees, Epidauros offered to those who resorted thither places of worship, hotels, libraries, gymnasia, a stadium with a capacity of twelve thousand spectators, a theater, and a hospital. Sixteen thousand people could be accommodated in the theater, which has been proved by recent excavation to have been one of the most beautiful of the outdoor

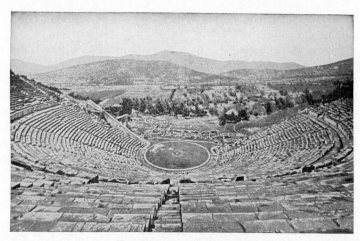

THE THEATER OF EPIDAUROS
One of the most beautiful in Greece. (Courtesy of The Amalgamated Press of
London, England. Photo by Messbildanstal.)

theaters of the Greeks. Like all the other buildings of Epidauros, it
was of white marble.

To the hospital men thronged in response to reports of miraculous
cures performed by Priest-physicians who interpreted treatment prescribed by Asklepios. We are told that, upon entrance, the patient
met the same assiduity of effort to induce confidence that charac-
terizes the reception of patients in our hospitals today. Until the
time of Hippocrates, it was not customary to make any physical examination, but priests endeavored to inspire hope by assurance of
the super-human skill of Asklepios. They arranged for the sacrifice
which would encourage his favor. Then the patient was bathed and
clad in white garments. Clean, relaxed, and probably quite tired out
after a journey, in all likelihood made on foot and followed by the
excitement of admitting routine in the haven for which he had
longed, he was assigned to a bed in a building or on a porch provided for the sick. Evening worship was conducted, and after that
he went to sleep. A message purporting to come from Asklepios was
delivered to him during the night. It has been suggested that the
Priest-physician made rounds when all was quiet, and talked to patients drowsy with sleep or drugs. No record verifies this. Treatments

defined by the dream oracle took the form of warm baths, massage, inunctions, catharsis, or blood-letting, with diet regulation and other hygienic measures. The aid of the sacred serpent might also be invoked. Snakes of nonpoisonous variety moved at will among the patients, and through licking wounds gave cleansing treatment which often enabled them to heal.

The opportunities offered to the sick at Epidauros bear considerable resemblance to those obtainable today at the many great sanitoria or "cures." The temple shared the soothing beauty of its site with others of its kind. It was the result of careful selection, and it had its own effect. The same care in choosing sites made indispensable a good water supply. Mineral springs were made use of whenever possible. The routine of care was largely hygienic and took full advantage of sunlight and fresh air available in rural surroundings. Ample provision was made for instruction, exercise, bathing, and entertainment. The worship of the god Asklepios, revered for his character as well as for his wisdom in matters pertaining to sickness, lifted patients above themselves, and increased their faith. The aura of magic which surrounded all the work of the Asklepiades may have been a concession to the times, but it met with popular approval, and was continued long after those who used it had acquired knowledge tending more and more toward the scientific. Only slowly did it disappear before the advent of rationalism about the fifth century B.C., and the wisdom of Hippocrates in whom medicine was to find its expression of the "Birth of Reason."

The "Birth of Reason"

Greek civilization continued to progress and many changes took place. Slavery increased as did poverty. Nevertheless, through the intellectual and artistic prestige of Athens, inspiration was to be given to the Greek people, and the privilege of kindling that flame of the spirit which lighted the path to fields that still beckon in art, literature, and science. To *Aristotle*, whose insatiable desire for knowledge of the meaning of life led him to dissect animals, men would owe the foundation of biology as well as the study of comparative anatomy. *Hippocrates* would lay the foundation of scientific medicine, *Socrates* and *Plato* those of philosophy and government. By the work of these and many other men of genius

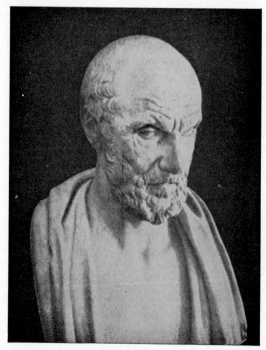

HIPPOCRATES

or scholarship Greece would be able to broadcast culture through-out a waiting world. Greek influence would mean not only a change from empiric to scientific methods; it would make apparent, forever after, a distinction between the sound and the unsound. Indubitably, it must affect the work of the nurse as well as that of the physician, although woman's assumption of duties considered by Hippocrates as part of medical care was a process through which succeeding ages must bring into being a second profession. Before this could be pos-sible, a complete change in her status had to be effected through social, economic, and educational processes.

Hippocrates   *Hippocrates* was the son of a Priest-physician and one of the Asklepiades. He was born on the island of Cos in 460 B.C. Here was a school of medicine already well known, and we may suppose that the youth grew up in the traditions surrounding the sacred cult of his father. Destiny pointed to him as the man who would dispel the mists of magic and expose to the light of knowledge all those superstitions which served to obscure the whole question of how to keep health in the human body. Hippocrates forced the transition from magic to science toward which the specialized skill of temple priests had been tending. He is said to have spent much time in observing symptoms, and in this way to have gleaned considerable knowledge regarding the ills of those who sought treatment. He found groups of symptoms shared in common by groups of people. If such were the case, he reasoned, there must be a common cause. He produced the disturbing theory that failure of health follows disobedience to certain laws of nature, and that prevention of disease depends on obedience to these laws. On man, not on spirits, must rest the burden of health maintenance. Present-day medicine dates its beginning from the work of Hippocrates which made it possible for scientific medicine to supersede the empiric. He is still known as the "Father of Medicine."

The new viewpoint which Hippocrates offered to physicians made necessary a searching inquiry into history and symptoms. Keen observation he decreed to be an inseparable companion of thoughtful reasoning before conclusions as to treatment were possible. Treatment must be individual, and dependent upon the diagnosis reached. Prevailing custom, up to his time, had not made such discrimination. No technics of physical examination and no systematic methods of recording history of symptoms existed. It was for him, and those who worked with him during a long life, to originate both, and to define principles on which they might be based. While no writings ascribed to the man who decided the fate of medicine were made public for fifty years after his death, the course to be taken in medical investigation and treatment for ages to come after him were, in their scientific trend, the work of this great scholar. The professional footing of medicine found a solid foundation in his ideals of ethical conduct and practice. Portions of the oath required of his students are still used in an oath taken by students graduating from medical schools today. It is the basis of the Nightingale Pledge so often mistakenly ascribed to the authorship of Miss Florence Nightingale, and now assumed by students graduating from some schools of nursing.

Strangely enough, the enviable place in history gained by this country of scholarly wisdom was reached in spite of, and actually through, political subjugation. In 338 B.C., Philip of Macedonia conquered Greece. The education of his son, Alexander, he placed in the hands of one of her scholars, and when this young man succeeded his father, he possessed an appreciation of Greek civilization so sincere that he included in his ambition to conquer the world a determination to endow it with the culture of Greece. His success was acknowledged when he became known as "Alexander the Great." Cities that he took from Greece became greater; cities that he built were Greek in character. The city of Alexandria in Egypt, which was named after him, became the gathering place of scholars from all over the world. In Alexandria, medical science received the encouragement of permissible dissection which it failed to receive in Greece. Greeks carried all that their country stood for in the way of scholarship or art to this and other foreign centers. At home, Greek culture expanded with the stimulus of appreciation and opportunity elsewhere. It was, indeed, a historic period of cultural flowering. It made the thinker a leader.

Some discontent was doubtless due to the insecurity of her political position. Alexander, who had elevated her so suddenly to a position of world fame, did not live long enough to stabilize her government. Without Alexander's leadership, it fell quickly to pieces, for a new power was rising in the West. After a series of disheartening attempts to maintain her prestige, Greece fell into the hands of her grasping neighbor, Rome, by 146 B.C. The civilization that had risen on the Tiber would eventually build a new empire to replace the old.

Long after the downfall of political prestige, the country of mountainous beauty was to hold the regard of man through her gift to them of a mental horizon. With advancing civilization, life was becoming everywhere more and more complicated. There was smaller demand for physical strength, and more leisure. The old mores in the Far East as well as in the West failed to function satisfactorily. Men found that they had to think more than was necessary in the days of greater simplicity and few ambitions. They were forced to turn inward for a new system of living that would serve as a foundation on which to build a life that was different from the old one, but that would prove to be a good life for all. This is a crossroads that has been reached a number of times in history since. In all such crises, there have been those who wished to follow the old road, and others who wished to take a new one.

The period about 500 B.C. marked more than a Golden Age for Greece. The Birth of Reason which brought her fame was bringing about changes in far-off India and China. Her philosophies had counterparts in other lands. In India, Buddhism was offering its hope of peace to discontented and suffering men. In China, Confucius was making his appeal to the intellectual class in the hope of working out a scheme of living which might systematize and render more agreeable the life of all men. When he failed to reach all men, Buddhism became the solace of the poor. Everywhere there was evident a striving to understand the meaning of life and death. Blind worship of old gods did not fill man's need. Worry, ambition, poverty, cruelty, and pain seemed to be taking an ever greater place in life. There must be some way of producing happiness. The doctrine of brotherly love had come out of India; asceticism and monasticism were well on the way. Nobody was satisfied, and many were thinking. The world was preparing for 1 A.D.

Greek Women   To this Birth of Reason which so stimulated thought and education, some have traced a decline in the status of women. She was not included by the Greeks in its benefits. We seem to lack evidence that more than a very few Greek women sought these benefits. The mores of the time kept woman strictly confined to home duties. When her men turned to mental interests, study and public life altered their attitude toward the home. Work became more and more specialized, ambitions changed, children became necessary only as they were needed to serve the state. Mere fertility was not as important as it had been in a simpler, agricultural society. There was born a desire to rise above the demands of a purely physical existence, to have freedom for contemplation, to use creatively the mental power of which men were now conscious.

Aristotle expressed the generally accepted feeling of his time when he wrote: "The slave has no deliberative faculty at all; the woman has, but it is without authority, and the child has it, but it is immature."[3] Plato anticipated the twentieth century when he said:

[3] Putnam, Emily: The Lady. New York and London, G. P. Putnam's Sons, 1921, p. 34.

"None of the occupations which comprehend the ordering of a state belong to woman as woman, nor yet to man as man, but natural gifts are to be found here and there in both sexes alike; and, so far as her nature is concerned, the woman is admissible to all pursuits as well as the man."[4]

The girl baby did not meet with a hearty welcome in Greece. When she came to marry, she was not free to choose her husband. She had a dower value. The higher her social position, the less free was she to mingle with other people. Her only alternative to the protection of marriage was slavery or prostitution. The law gave her no recognition, for during her whole life she was, legally, a minor. She was not even permitted to act as hostess to her husband's friends, but withdrew to a separate part of the house after she had seen that preparations for their entertainment were complete. The duties which fell to her lot confined her strictly to the family circle, and, probably, nursing was often an arduous task for the housewife who was responsible for the care of her men, so often called upon to be soldiers, for her children, and for varying numbers of slaves.

The customs which society exacts of its upper class women are always reflected on the life of other groups of women. The status that was theirs in ancient Greece was retained, in large measure, for centuries later. Traces of the restrictive mores which surrounded her may be seen in our own customs, and much more than traces of them are to be met in some countries today. The following quotation gives an admirable interpretation of this status as it has been handed down to us by a famous author:

"Ischomachos was a priggish young Athenian of good social position whom Xenophon has immortalized for us. When he married he made up his mind to educate his wife. She was a girl of fifteen, as brides often were in Athens, and, as he told Socrates, the greatest pains had been taken with her by her parents so that she might see as little as possible, hear as little as possible, and ask the fewest possible questions. Ischomachos had a well-ordered mind. When the wife had been broken in and had grown used to her husband's hand (the phrases are his own), he laid down for her the proposition that they had pooled their goods and formed a partnership for two purposes: to produce children and to keep house. The question of the rearing of children he postponed until they should have some, but in regard to the house he defined very clearly their mutual relations. God and custom, he said, concurred in delimiting these.

" 'Men are strong; therefore, they must go out to contend with the elements and, if need be, with other men to get a living for their families. Women are phys-

4 *Ibid.*, p. 36.

ically weak; therefore, God meant them to live in the house. They are timid, while men are bold; they must therefore be stewards while men are acquirers. Women are naturally fonder of babies than men are; by this discrimination God beckons women to the nursery.' Having apparently won his child-wife's consent to this familiar substitution of effect for cause, he explained her duties in detail. She was to organize the slaves, selecting some for out-door work, some for the house. She was to receive and store the supplies as they came in from the farm. Another department of her work was clothing the family. Every step from the reception of the raw wool to the turning out of the finished garment was to be taken under her eye. And this was to be one duty which the husband feared would be very diasgreeable,—the care of any slave that might fall ill. But to this the little newly tamed wife made a charming answer, an answer that casts forward many centuries to Elizabeth of Hungary and the frame of mind that we think of as 'Christian.' 'That will be the pleasantest task of all,' she said, 'if it will make them fonder of me.' . . . Ischomachos then describes in detail how he spent a whole day helping his wife to get her house in order, and teaching her the beauty of system, and methods by which she might attain it in household management.

" 'When all these arrangements were made,' Ischomachos continued, 'I told my wife that good laws will not keep a state in order unless they are enforced, and that she, as the chief executive officer under our constitution must contrive by rewards and punishments that law should prevail in our house. By way of apology for laying upon her so many troublesome duties, I bade her observe that we cannot reasonably expect servants spontaneously to be careful of the master's goods, since they have no interest in being so; the owner is the one who must take trouble to preserve his property. To this my wife replied that it was as natural to a woman to look after her belongings as to look after her children, and that I should have given her a more difficult task if I had bidden her give no heed to these matters.'

"Socrates liked this. 'By Hera,' he cried, 'your wife reasons like a man.' Ischomachos was emboldened to further confidences. 'One day I saw her with a lot of powder on her face to make her look whiter and a lot of rouge to make her look redder and high-heeled shoes to make her look taller. I pointed out to her in the first place that she was doing as dishonourable a thing in trying to deceive me about her looks as I should have done if I had tried to deceive her about my property. And then I remarked that though her arts might impose upon others, they could not upon me who saw her at all times. I was sure to catch her early in the morning before they had been applied, or tears would betray them, or perspiration, or the bath.'

"The little lady seems to have taken this also in good part, for she asked her husband how she should gain a genuine bloom if she must give up the semblance of it, and he gave her the following advice: 'I told her not to be forever sitting about like a slave girl but to stand at the loom, teaching what she knew and learning what she did not. I advised her to look on at the bread-making and stand by while the housekeeper dealt out supplies and go about inspecting everything. Thus she could practice her profession and take a walk at the same time. I added that excellent exercise could be had by making beds and kneading dough.' "[5]

The activities of woman were by this time well defined in the minds of men, and did not carry her beyond the confines of home unless

[5] Putnam, Emily: The Lady. New York and London, G. P. Putnam's Sons, 1921, pp. 5–10.

she were a priestess, a slave, or a harlot. She had quite lost the equality with man in the adventure of living with which she started out. The knowledge of the herb gatherer was still hers by hearsay, although it had, in the main, passed over to the use of priests, and, in the role of assistant to the priests of the Asklepian temples, woman probably retained what was to prove a loophole of escape to one of her earliest public occupations, nursing.

ROME

While Greece was developing into a world renowned home of art and thinking, there lived on a long peninsula beside her an agricultural people whom we know as Latins. These people were preparing to wield tremendous influence of a different nature over the future of mankind. The peninsula was Italy, separated from Greece by only a narrow sea, and divided down its middle by a chain of mountains. Level plains on the western side had been chosen by the Latins for their home.

In due time, a civilization grew up with a capital located near the mouth of the Tiber. Legend places the birth date of this city of Rome at 753 B.C., and enwraps the event with the uncertainty of a variety of mythological interpretations. Its site on seven hills appears to have been the choice of twin brothers, Romulus and Remus, themselves indebted for life to the nourishment and care given them by a kindly wolf who found them on a mountain top, abandoned by a goddess mother.

By 500 B.C., when Greece was entering upon her Golden Age, and the influence of Buddha and Confucius was dawning upon an unhappy India and an intellectual minority in China, the city of Rome had struggled into the status of a *republic* with a ruler chosen by election. Its citizens were still, in the main, farmers, and theirs was an honored occupation. The civilization of the world beyond had not touched the Latin state deeply. Even the temple, so characteristic a feature of other infant cultures, was not essential to the religion of the early Roman. Gods were borrowed, and temples built for worship later, but his deities were few, and their functions highly practical. Small images of them were used for worship, which could be carried on at home. *Jupiter* was charged with the welfare of the city, *Juno* was woman's patroness, *Mars* was god of war, and *Janus*

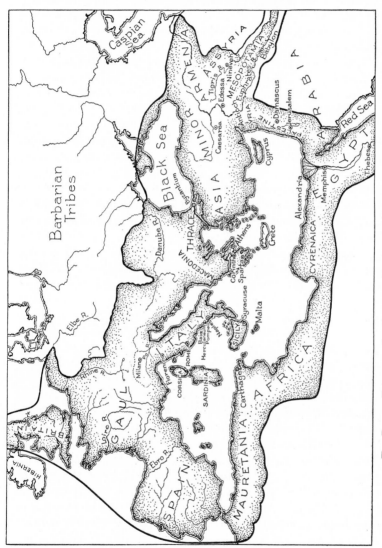

THE ROMAN EMPIRE AT ITS GREATEST EXTENT (Under Trajan, A.D. 98–117.)

was the god of openings or beginnings. He guarded the archway gate through which the soldiers marched to war. This arch, later replaced by the temple of Janus, remained open for the duration of war. Its closing announced peace.

Contacts with Greece gave Roman citizens some appreciation of its famous culture, and by 146 B.C., this country was under her control. Greek scholars were made Roman slaves and became teachers of men, women, and children in what was to be the Imperial City of the World. Greek physicians of the Hippocratic school, who were also slaves, introduced their ideas on the practice of medicine, and were impatient with the ignorant Latin who preferred, on the whole, to cling to superstitition and tradition. The policy of Rome, however, did not limit itself to bringing the best of Greek and Oriental civilizations as she found them, within reach of her people in Italy. As her empire grew, these civilizations were spread throughout the whole uncivilized Near West. For Rome not only proceeded to take the place of Alexander the Great in the eastern world, but she was on the way to subjugating a large part of Europe as well. Time would thoroughly Romanize Italy, Spain, and France. Her territory would spread from Britain to the Black Sea, and would encircle what was then the middle of the earth, the Mediterranean. Meanwhile, the gates of Janus seldom closed. Fighting satisfied Roman taste, as imaginative creation, scholarship, and art satisfied the Greek. Rome turned the eyes of the world her way. By the time Julius Caesar ruled her state in the first century B.C., men acknowledged her triumph by admitting that "All roads lead to Rome."

History has accepted *Julius Caesar* (100–44 B.C.) as a brilliant example of the Roman warrior statesman. Bent on conquest, swiftly decisive in thought and action, constructive in his attitude toward the conquered, ever alert to his own advancement as well as to his country's glory, Caesar has handed himself down to us in the Commentaries on his wars. During a lifetime, this "Father of his Country,"[6] as Romans came to know him, subjugated and introduced to civilization western Europe and Britain, while he rose to the position of Dictator in what was now the Roman Empire. His person was declared sacred. His office was considered divine. This did not prevent his assassination by close associates, who explained it as

[6] Hammerton and Barnes: The Illustrated World History, p. 264.

a "sacrifice" for the good of a state just emerging from its experiment in republican government and giving itself over reluctantly to one-man rule. Following immediately upon long years of conquest, the reign of Julius Caesar was necessarily one of imperial organization. It brought a semblance of peace and some security for commercial enterprise. Economic conditions were somewhat improved. Political privileges were extended more widely among the people.

Julius Caesar was not allowed to finish other social reforms that he planned, but he had proved himself well fitted for the difficult task of being the pioneer of Roman monarchy, and his succession in 29 B.C. by a grand-nephew to be known as *Augustus Caesar* brought a peace within the City of Seven Hills which was to last for two centuries.

Before the dawn of the Christian era, Rome was excessively rich. Her trade had become enormous. She was attaining a degree of culture. *Virgil* wrote the history of her ancestors in the Aeneid, *Horace* gave her a name in poetry, *Livy* and *Cicero* wrote her prose, while the latter also exemplified her best achievement in oratory. As she brought home slaves from conquered countries, those of her people who were in a position to become wealthy became also idle. The custom of bringing home art as well as treasure from dispossessed peoples put beauty into their hands. Their transition from the rugged life of the pioneer to a life of ease had been abnormally rapid. Old domestic virtues were being undermined. Divorce was common.

Unprepared as they were for the assimilation of the best in other cultures, Roman taste and opportunity were those of the new-rich of our own day. Work was given over to slaves, homes became more and more luxurious, fashions in dress were elaborate, and social functions extravagant. Both men and women assumed what was frequently a superficial interest in learning. Scholarly slaves read philosophy to them in the moments left after performance of multiple social duties. Some of them wrote. They patronized the arts. They vied with each other in library collection. Great public buildings began to be erected, and places of amusement. Elaborate public baths were introduced for all classes of society. In all of these, Rome demonstrated her ideal of size and solidarity with ornateness of decoration. Meanwhile, the chasm that civilization created everywhere between rich and poor was getting wider, and the land was passing into the hands of a few. These wasted its resources through faulty farming, while cities became the refuge of displaced farmers. The city of Rome was turning into a cosmopolitan center, not unlike New York, London, Shanghai, or Buenos Aires, where people of all races gathered, where all religions were tolerated, and where all human vices found a foothold.

Roman Medicine   In medical advancement, Rome fell far short of Greece. She appreciated hygiene as a foundation for the fighting strength that she could not do without. Her health work in the way of sanitation was marvelous. Sewer and drains, and pavement on their streets, made cities clean. Great aqueducts brought pure drinking water into them and supplied the citizens of Rome with bathing facilities. Baths with heated water appeared in her homes. Indeed, under the Empire, the bath, previously taken for the sake of cleanliness assumed the importance of a cult among the Romans who in their eagerness to enjoy long life, and their earnestness about bathing, came to believe that one day would lengthen into two, if two baths were taken. Some enthusiasts took as many as twelve in twenty-four hours, and disastrous results are said to have followed the custom of entering the water immediately after a substantial meal. A complete and luxurious technic involving the use of hot and cold water, inunctions, and massage, was developed. Both private and public bath houses took on the character of clubs or centers of social intercourse for men and women. They might contain gymnasia, libraries, and dining rooms.

Notwithstanding what would seem to have been a high degree of civic and individual cleanliness, the city was the prey of frequent epidemics of disease. Much of this was brought in with conquests, some of it was undoubtedly due to rapidity of growth, for Rome introduced the tenement which rose to the height of four stories and necessitated laws to prevent its becoming a skyscraper, or killing too many of the people in its collapse. The usual alley street separated these buildings, and the usual habits of crowding and discarding rubbish by throwing it into the street robbed the poor of fresh air and reduced their resistance to disease. Moreover, the marshes surrounding the city persisted in spite of drainage, and fostered the malaria to which history has ascribed Rome's ultimate downfall.

For help when sickness came, the Romans clung to their gods, to herbs, or to superstition which might even include the keeping of snakes in their houses. Although Greek physicians were allowed to do most of their work after 200 B.C., Hippocratic medicine failed to make much headway. Its earlier representatives were frequently mediocre or grasping and Romans met them with suspicion. No great physicians arose among Roman scholars themselves before the first century. Army hospitals were conducted well and Roman soldiers received good care wherever they might be. The dispensaries provided for the care of the public were badly managed. Weakness won contempt rather than pity. Sanitary ideals, also, did not prevent Romans from leaving their dead paupers and abandoned slaves unburied, for excavations have revealed the existence, within city limits, of huge puticuli or open pits into which these were thrown. Obviously, a condition was created here that must have nullified much engineering effort.

Roman Women   Turning to the women of Rome, we find them of a caliber that matched that of their men. Indeed, Romans are said to have conquered all people save their own women. Coarser in grain, stronger in personality, the Roman woman quite lacked the retiring submissiveness that characterized the typical Greek woman, and was never able to acquire her negative virtues. Both were minors in the eyes of the law, but that was a resemblance which custom failed to uphold. The Roman woman got around the law. She succeeded in making hers a better position, and actually acquired the right to hold property in her own name and to appear in court to give testimony. She has been compared in her early days to the American pioneer women of New England, or of the days of the covered wagon in America—companion worker with a busy husband, of enduring strength, physical and moral, a capable, resourceful housekeeper, and a good mother. Stoically, she sacrificed her sons to her country's growth.

When wars ceased, Roman women proceeded to enjoy with the men the fruits of conquest. They appeared in public, went to theaters, sports, and banquets. Their independence developed to such strength during the frequent absence of their husbands that it was a problem to subdue them in time of peace. On several occasions the women of Rome protested publicly against what they considered injustice. Once they refused to pay taxes to be levied on private incomes for support of civil war, although they insisted on their loyalty in support of a country endangered by enemy attack. They did work that would continue to be traditionally woman's work for centuries to come, but before the first century they were equipped beyond their predecessors in civilization with an independence of spirit that would enable them to emerge into other spheres at the first opportunity.

In her own home the Roman woman held acknowledged sway. Subordinate to her husband outside of it, she was addressed by him as "domina" in its privacy. She could come and go as she pleased under the protection of her "stola matronalis," a garment worn over her tunic on the street, and donned when she married. She entertained guests, and sat with them at table. She could nurse her household or turn that work over to Greek slaves if she had them. She could dally with philosophy if she chose to do so. When riches came, she might go in for "society," which frivolous institution she is credited with originating. But, as in all ages, those who indulge in extremes of conduct are remembered while those who adhere with faithfulness to the more substantial mores are forgotten, so there must have been great numbers of Roman women who did traditional work and represented traditional virtues in their "constantly changing world."

It is interesting to see how these conservative citizens lived. The typical home among the Latins opened through a vestibule into a common living room known as the "atrium." The name is believed to have been derived from the blackness of walls and ceiling continually smoked by a fire on an open chimneyless hearth at the back of the room. The importance of the atrium, however, lies in the fact that it was the pivot on which the household turned. Opposite its door stood the bridal bed, made useful by day as a couch. Rooms opened off the atrium at the sides, and in one of these, or over the hearth, or in an alcove, was a repository for the household gods and busts or wax masks of their ancestors. In order to conduct formal worship of these and the domestic gods, the father gathered his family together daily.

In the atrium the mother educated her children and told them stories of their ancestors. Here the spinning and weaving were done and the daughters of the household were instructed in these and other domestic arts. Here the entire family group, including slaves and children, might gather at meals cooked on the hearth. In the middle of the atrium stood a fountain or cistern comparable to our well or pump, but supplied with pipes under the floor to carry off water. Bedrooms might be upstairs, but the plan remained the same for all, and our inheritance is not difficult to discern. The atrium of the Roman, the great hall of the feudal knight, the kitchen of New England, or the living room of the western ranch of America—do they not all owe their origin to one human inspiration and a common need?

THE FAR WEST

THE AMERICAS

Empires of the Near East, the Far East and the Mediterranean World had risen and disappeared before their builders became aware that, far to the west, across what seemed an endless expanse of sea, lay riches far greater than any of those which they had spent centuries in wresting one from the other. In the light of the setting sun, there was being developed another civilization that might outshine any civilization thus far achieved. The earliest inhabitants of the unknown continent that was to be America are believed to have come from Central Asia, and to have crossed the relatively narrow and island-strewn strait of Bering into the territory that we know as Alaska. It must be recalled to mind that all such early great migratory movements of humanity usually began in a search for food, and continued to be movements, sometimes for centuries. This one is believed to have lasted until comparatively recent times.

These Indians, as *Columbus* named their descendants, filtered over the land, principally in easterly and southerly directions. Waterways were the natural lead, and traces of very early Indian occupation are said to have been found as far east as the Atlantic coast. Eventually they abandoned hunting and, as time went on, drifted into agriculture and established a settled mode of life, mainly in what is now called Mexico, Central America, and Peru, where the climate differed most from the homeland. Scientists differ in setting a period for the habitation of this area. Some place it as far back as ten, or even twenty thousand years ago, and some dare to say that men reached civilization in America earlier than they did in Egypt. In any case, it is thought that American Indians, as we now speak of them, progressed culturally very much as man has done elsewhere, from the Stone Age onward, slowly, and under the influence of varied climatic conditions.

Among these groups of pioneers from another continent, several attained a high degree of civilization. Some were still in the Stone Age in 1492 A.D. The *Toltecs*, the *Aztecs*, the *Mayas*, and the *Incas*, occupying the land from Mexico to Peru, not only acquired wealth, but left behind them monuments of man's achievement in the building of temples and palaces which challenge the art of the Egyptian. The Incas also built great highways, and are said to have been gifted beyond the others. Agriculture in the new land came to include cultivation of a grain known as "corn." Sweet and white potatoes, tobacco, tomatoes, pumpkins, strawberries, pineapples, and peanuts were also developed. Chocolate, capsicum, and vanilla were in use. Writing was known, and the Maya group invented a calendar which is thought to have reckoned time from August 6, 613 B.C. Some of the finest temples produced by early America originated between 1000 B.C. and 1 A.D.

As we have found customary among primitive people, the offices of religion, medicine, nursing, and pharmacy were combined in one individual who was set apart from other men. Medicine Man, and later, Priest, essayed to conquer Indian ills of body or mind. Little has been carried down to us except as folklore, but it is believed that sacred books were destroyed by Spanish invaders. With the stimulus of modern interest in archaeological study of these people, it is probable that we shall learn to value our inheritance from them proportionately to our knowledge. We owe to them the origin of various processes of commercial value. Their baskets still defy our skill and patience. They learned to utilize wood ashes as a cleaning powder, to tan leather with oak bark, and to develop glue from fish. They were the next people to be reached in the enlarging circle of acquaintanceship around the globe.

Among Indians in the tribal state, the position of the Indian woman was, in some respects, unusually good. Descent was sometimes traced through the female line, in which case this position rose correspondingly. While she obeyed certain restrictions set by tribal practice as masculine rights, she retained complete authority over her home. The children were in her charge until admitted to tribal membership, and, in at least one group, a woman's council took part in discussion of all affairs affecting the welfare of the tribe. The appointment of civil chief was dependent on their wishes, and, when war was agreed upon, women declared it.

SUMMARY OF CONDITIONS AT 1 A. D.

At the time of the birth of Christ, the major part of the world was under the rule of Rome. Her empire stretched from the Atlantic Ocean to the Black Sea. It penetrated Europe to boundaries set by the Rhine and the Danube rivers. It circled the Mediterranean Sea, center of the world, as the name implies. It included Britain, Asia Minor and the Fertile Crescent. The little city state on the Tiber had, in less than eight hundred years, made slaves of the greater part of humanity. Its harsh militarism had been somewhat tempered by the influence of Greek scholars who lived as slaves in Roman households. The city itself had become cosmopolitan in character, and Roman imperial policy under Caesar Augustus, seen in the perspective of the twentieth century, was unifying peoples and bringing about a greater understanding of human differences.

During the centuries leading up to culmination of this great empire of the west, other empires had come and gone. Civilizations had been developed in various parts of the world. As the light of history is shed on the obscurities of its past, we begin to understand that this world has never stood still. It is a world of life, a dynamic world. From its beginnings, man has been adjusting himself to constant changes. Now, in adjustment to a life of increased hardship, with cruelties such as slavery, constant demands for military service, and exorbitant tax levies, he was beginning to see that something must be done if he were to live happily. It was a time when reform had become necessary, and reformers arose. The men who came forward at that critical period of man's history were of a mental magnitude that enabled them to arrive at truths which not only aided the adjustment of human beings of their own time, but have influenced the life of men through all succeeding ages.

The Greek philosophers, principal of whom were Socrates, Plato and Aristotle, taught people to think and, through reasoning and well-ordered planning, to attain "The Good Life." Hippocrates, in the realm of sickness, threw his energies into dispelling men's ancient beliefs in magic, and endeavored to supplant them by honest effort to acquire knowledge of facts regarding symptoms. He built up, on principles of scientific observation, a system of medicine which still prevails in spite of the passage of many centuries. The ethical ideals which permeated it have served to strengthen a true safeguard for human health.

While progress toward civilization was being made in regions of the Near East, Far East, and the Mediterranean World, certain tribes of Central Asia are believed to have wandered through Bering Strait and Alaska, down into North, Central, and South America. A relatively high degree of culture was acquired by the Toltecs, Aztecs, Mayas, and Incas. In these tribes, the arts of medicine, nursing, and pharmacy were combined in the Medicine Man, and later in the Priest-physician. The position of their women was exceptional, in some instances, since they are said to have held complete authority over the home, to have taken part in a woman's council, and even to have declared war when occasion arose. Lineage was known to be traced through female ancestors.

As to who cared for the sick during this early period, very little has come down to us in history. Hippocrates, doubtless, was assisted in his work by many women, but he makes no mention of a definite assignment of duties. As far as woman in general was concerned, her position in society had remained rather low. Generally speaking, she had lost her primitive equality with man and become a "household drudge." The Roman woman had succeeded in wresting to herself some independence. Already, for nearly two centuries it had been possible for her to be independent financially. In her ranks were those who knew both riches and power as well as educational advantages. Strong in action, cooperative, brave in enterprise, she stood out among the women of her time. Dauntless, like her men, in the conquering of obstacles in her way, she was preparing herself for advancement to a new world which was about to beckon her outside the home.

TOPICS FOR DISCUSSION
GREECE

1. (a) Give a description of the location and climate of Greece. (b) Where is the island of Crete? (c) Of Cos?

2. Give the author, names, and date of writing of the sacred books of Greece.
3. Make an outline of Greek gods that influenced the practice of medicine, naming an outstanding characteristic of each.
4. Describe in detail the people of Greece, and their attitude toward illness, and toward birth and death.
5. Compare the functions of the xenodochion and the iatrion.
6. Show how the temples of Asklepios illustrate the close association between religion, medicine, and nursing.
7. Account for the statement that scientific medicine and ethical principles of the present day had their beginnings in ancient Greece.
8. Make a chart of the great men of all ancient civilizations who lived about 500 B.C., during the period known as the "Birth of Reason."
9. Show the effects of building of the Alexandrian Empire on the spread of Greek culture.
10. Tell what you know of Greek women before 1 A.D.
11. What do you think of the implications of the Greek ideal of "moderation in all things"?

ROME

1. Compare Greece and Rome in regard to geographical location, climate and people.
2. (a) How does the time of the founding of Rome compare with that of other ancient civilizations? (b) What is the legend in regard to it?
3. What gods were revered in ancient Rome?
4. What authors wrote the history, poetry, and prose of ancient Rome?
5. (a) Name several sanitary practices of the ancient Romans. (b) In what ways were these counterbalanced?
6. The development of Roman hospitals and medicine was directed toward what purpose?
7. How did Roman women compare with those of Greece?
8. Who was Emperor of Rome at the time of the birth of Jesus, the Christ?
9. After reference to a map in a general history, outline in red on

your map the border of the Roman Empire as it existed at its greatest extent.

FAR WEST

1. (*a*) The earliest inhabitants of America are believed to have come from what region? (*b*) What caused them to migrate? (*c*) What route did they take?

2. (*a*) What Indian tribes attained the highest degree of civilization? (*b*) Where were they located? (*c*) Name some of their achievements.

3. What evidence is there that the position of women in some tribes was exceptionally good?

4. (*a*) Outline a summary of the great personages who lived about 500 B.C. during the age of "The Birth of Reason." (*b*) What Hebrew prophets can be added to the list?

5. (*a*) What was the general condition of the known world at the beginning of the Christian era? (*b*) Give reasons for the fact that the average man and woman were not in a position where contentment was possible.

6. Of the women of the various regions studied, which group demonstrated a noticeable spirit of independence?

7. What is known of the nursing of this early period?

REFERENCES

Beard and Beard: A Basic History of the United States. New York, New Home Library, 1944.

Bury, J. B.: A History of Greece. New York, Modern Library.

Carcopino, Jerome: Daily Life in Ancient Rome. New Haven, Yale University Press, 1940.

Durant, Will: Life of Greece. New York, Simon and Schuster, 1935.

Gaer, Joseph: How the Great Religions Began. New York, Dodd Mead and Co., 1935.

Gibbons, Edward: The Decline and Fall of the Roman Empire. New York, The Modern Library.

Putnam, Emily James: The Lady. New York, G. P. Putnam's Sons, 1921, Chap. I (The Greek Lady), Chap. II (The Roman Lady).

Early Christian Era

The history of mankind now divides itself into two periods, one leading up to 1 A.D., the other following that date. Superficially, we would say that a new calendar was initiated at this time, but reasons far deeper than measure of time underlay what were revolutionary changes. It was a time comparable to the present, when great awakening follows in the wake of great human distress and political upheaval, when changes are made with only apparent suddenness, after centuries of preparation. Discerning minds of men like the Hebrew prophets, like Confucius, Buddha, Zoroaster, and the philosophers of Greece, had seen the futility of life if it could not yield a measure of satisfaction to all men. In spite of prophecy, religions, and philosophy, the predominant ideal of humanity remained that of subjugation of the weak by the strong. The Roman Empire represented the climax of this ideal, and Rome was now supreme over nearly all the peoples of the known world. Although nominally a republic, her emperor, Caesar Augustus (majestic), was an absolute ruler whose acts were believed to be authorized by the gods.

In many respects, conditions in this greatest empire duplicated those experienced by her predecessors in imperial powers. Hardy virtues of earlier times were disappearing. Taxation was oppressive. Religion had come to represent formal duties imposed upon worshipers who had other religions. Everywhere lands had passed into the possession of a few. A great chasm separated rich and poor, and slavery had lessened the value of life. The majority of people in the world knew that they could get nowhere. The minority, wherever it was possible, set examples of wasteful extravagance, callousness of heart, idleness. In Rome, so many slaves now did all kinds of work that work seemed to her citizens the occupation of a slave class, and they chose idleness in preference to work. While there was more wealth in the world than had yet been known, the need of distributing it fairly enough to maintain human dignity had not been foreseen.

CHRIST, THE REDEEMER

The administrative genius of the Roman people was occupied in the effort to organize under a central government the many parts that went to make up this cosmopolitan empire. They must have cohesion and give promise of protection if it were to continue as an empire. Any unity which Rome achieved, in the end gave added force to an incipient movement that was to give to humanity a new purpose. The questioning of idealists who had been seeking the good life for several centuries would be answered by a Child of Destiny who was born about this time in Bethlehem, a town of Palestine. Life was preparing the *Christ*, or *Redeemer of Mankind* to understand hardship. He grew to manhood among people accustomed to both poverty and toil. Son of a carpenter, the boy followed his father's occupation, and had reached the age of thirty before much was known of Him. His native land was a crossroads of trade which gave opportunity for observation of many kinds of people, and for learning about those who dwelt in countries far away. The greater part of humanity appeared to be in the grip of misery, the cause of which seemed to Him to lie in greed and injustice. Men overvalued power and put too much emphasis on the acquisition of wealth. Something could be done to make life worth while to the masses if higher ideals could be put before them and before those who, perhaps unwittingly, oppressed them. Life would be better if class barriers, which after all were artificial, were done away with, if cruelty were changed into kindliness, if peace and service replaced war and servitude.

The new Redeemer began to show the possibility of a world ruled by love, to advocate the responsibility of each individual for the general welfare, to urge a common faith in one Father God. By thus awakening in men the sense of their brotherhood as children of one family, He sought to do away with distinctions of race, position, and creed which raised walls of misunderstanding among them.

Hate of enemies, long looked upon as a virtue, He wished to transform into brotherly love. He hoped to send forth, even to the farthest corners of the great world, teachers whom He himself would prepare to influence all humanity toward a unity which it had lost. Among His teachings, the following contained seeds of social revolution:[1]

1. "Whosoever shall do the will of my Father who is in heaven, he is my brother and sister and mother." Matthew XII: 50. (Distinctions of race, creed, and social status which had been built by men were without foundation.)

2. "Thou shalt love thy neighbor as thyself." Matthew XIX: 19. (Selfish interests should cease to dominate men.)

3. "Love your enemies, do good to them that hate you." Luke VI: 27. (Hating was a virtue cultivated when men spent the greater part of the time at war with one another.)

4. "Suffer little children, and forbid them not, to come unto me: for to such belongeth the kingdom of Heaven." Matthew XIX: 14. (Infanticide was common. Neither marriage nor children were in favor.)

5. "Lay not up for yourselves treasures upon the earth where moth and rust doth consume, and where thieves break through and steal, but lay up for yourselves treasures in heaven." Matthew VI: 19–20. (Acquisition and hoarding of wealth was the ideal of man.)

6. "Blessed are the peacemakers, for they shall be called the sons of God." Matthew V: 9. (War had come to be man's chief occupation. Its results had been proved evil. Peace would bring good.)

7. "If thou wouldst be perfect, go, sell that which thou hast, and give to the poor, and thou shalt have treasure in heaven." Matthew XIX: 21. (This teaching, in many instances, was followed by early Christians.)

8. "Whatsoever ye would that men should do unto you, do ye even so unto them." Matthew VII: 12. (The Golden Rule.)

9. "Inasmuch as ye have done it unto one of the least of these, ye have done it unto Me." Matthew XXV: 40. (Pity was not a common characteristic of men in ancient times. They worshipped strength. This new outlook helped women, children, the poor and the sick.)

10. "Even as the Son of man came not to be ministered unto, but to minister, and to give His life as ransom for many." Matthew XX: 28. (Dignity in work, beauty in service.)

11. "For I was hungry, and ye gave me to eat; I was thirsty, and ye gave me to drink; I was a stranger, and ye took me in; naked, and ye clothed me; I was sick and ye visited me; I was in prison, and ye came unto me." Matthew XXV: 35–36. (Stimulus to charity, medicine, nursing, and work among prisoners.)

[1] From American Standard Revised Version of the Bible. Courtesy of The International Council of Religious Education.

12. "Let not your heart be troubled, believe in God, believe also in Me. In My
Father's house are many mansions. . . . I go to prepare a place for you . . .
and if I go and prepare a place for you, I come again, and will receive you
unto Myself, that where I am, there ye may be also." John XIV: 1–3.
(Promise of a future life, happier than the earthly one.)

The story of the Good Samaritan was one which turned particular
attention toward the sick poor, and by so doing also affected nursing,
medicine, and charity. It was a plea for sympathy, individual effort,
and generosity in providing shelter and care. It was to receive its
answer in the development of orders of women workers, in hospitals, monasteries, and in the gifts of those who have made possible
so many undertakings in the interest of social welfare through the
ages since.

"A certain man was going down from Jerusalem to Jericho; and
he fell among robbers, who both stripped him and beat him, and
departed, leaving him half dead. And by chance a certain priest was
going down that way: and when he saw him, he passed by on the
other side. And in like manner a Levite also, when he came to the
place, and saw him, passed by on the other side. But a certain
Samaritan, as he journeyed, came where he was: and when he saw
him, he was moved to compassion, and came to him, and bound up
his wounds, pouring on them oil and wine; and he set him on his
own beast, and brought him to an inn, and took care of him. And
on the morrow he took out two shillings, and gave them to the host,
and said, 'Take care of him; and whatsoever thou spendest more,
I, when I come back again, will repay thee.' Which of these three,
thinkest, thou, proved neighbor unto him that fell among the
robbers?"[2]

Jesus himself worked first among the poor who readily became
adherents of one who brought to them a comfort that they needed
sorely. They felt themselves rescued from an isolation which had
enveloped them gradually, and their self-respect rose as the accepted inequality was shown to be unreal. Their enthusiasm and
honest effort to live according to the principles that He explained
to them so affected the social life about them that men and women
of wealth and education were attracted to the group.

[2] Luke X: 30–36. American Standard Revised Version of the Bible. Courtesy
of The International Council of Religious Education.

For a long time Christians knew no meeting place but the homes of fellow Christians. From the beginning of His work, their Leader made use of group discussion in planning for effective organization of a living temple to replace the too formalized temple of the time. The new temple was to be the center of a movement for the people and by the people. It was to demonstrate all over the world the goodly life through everyday practice, by individual believers, of principles for which it stood. Its policy was to be one of participation by the membership in all activities, even to preaching.

The work of Jesus, in the beginning, was confined to Palestine. In order to ensure its continued advance, He selected twelve leaders from the early disciples, or followers, and these He instructed in methods of procedure to be followed in organization of churches and in teaching. They were known as "apostles," and freedom to devote themselves wholly to the work, and to travel as new fields opened up, was a requisite of their appointment. As time went on, we find the number of apostles increased to meet the need. Men from many walks of life were to be found among them—teachers, physicians, lawyers, and others of means and education. They carried the message of Christianity east and west through the known world, they recorded the history of the movement, and they gave clarity and permanence to its principles by setting them down in writing.

SAUL OF TARSUS

In the group which became eventually apostles of Christianity, one stands out among the great men of all time. A contemporary of Jesus, and almost the same age, *Paul*, or *Saul*, as he was known also, was a Jew born in Tarsus, a town on the Asiatic coast of the Mediterranean, not far from the city of Antioch in Syria which early became a center of Christian activity. We find him as a young man assisting in the persecution of a preacher of the new religion at Jerusalem. So deeply does Paul resent the intrusion of Christianity into the life of Palestine, that he secures permission to travel to Damascus with the purpose of preventing its further spread by imprisoning all who embrace it there. On the way he encounters a vision which appears to him in such blazing light that he is blinded, and with difficulty completes his journey.

Report of the presence in their city of a man reputed to have been harsh in his persecution of their brethren in Jerusalem spread rapidly among Christians of Damascus. One of them was divinely prompted to visit him. As they talked together, Paul's sight was restored miraculously. He hastened to become a Christian, too. From that time until his death about 62 A.D., he was able to make use of many talents and a rich enthusiasm which were invaluable to a young organization struggling to maintain a foothold. He worked amid a confusion of beliefs in a discontented world, and always in opposition to those who resisted change. An excellent education under Greek influence had prepared him for his task of teaching ever-changing groups. His management of an extensive field proved to be able and systematic, and his powerful preaching showed him qualified to catch and transmit the spirit of the Master.

St. Paul was especially well fitted for the work of a missionary in foreign fields. His energy was great, and travel apparently delighted him. Danger he could meet with calm strength, his personal comfort he could overlook. While cooperating with the other apostles in establishment of general policies, he was capable of making decisions of his own when necessary, and to the advantage of the church. Undaunted by imprisonment or persecution, he taught in Palestine and Asia Minor, in the principal cities of Greece, and, finally, in Rome. His journeys took him through the islands of the Mediterranean and adjacent seas, and it was his hope that he might carry the work into Spain.

St. Paul has been recognized as the chief exponent of progressive Christianity among the Gentiles of "people of all nations" to whom Jesus aimed to have His message carried. He went back and forth among them, revisiting churches when necessary, collecting and transmitting to the parent church funds for its maintenance and for alms. It was his wish that Christians set aside on the first day of every week what they could spare for the church. In addition to searching out constantly new opportunities for preaching, strengthening weak groups and starting new ones, St. Paul was a prolific writer. Many books of the New Testament owe their authorship to him. In the Acts of the Apostles, a book credited to a companion worker, *St. Luke*, "the beloved physician," the adventures and trials of St. Paul are recorded. In the Epistles, written by himself to his bishops or to churches under his supervision, he plans church organ-

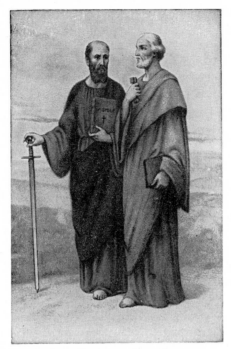

SAINT PETER AND SAINT PAUL
(Maison Bouasse-Lebel, Dauverne and Co., Paris.)

ization, sets forth ideals of living, admonishes, exhorts, or praises, as the need may be.

St. Paul's Attitude Toward Women   This great preacher is said to have had an indirect influence in lowering the status of woman. Although St. Paul helped her by deprecating divorce and upholding monogamy, it must be admitted that he looked upon woman with some degree of the ancient belief in her power as a temptress of man. He may have been fearful, too, of misunderstandings incident upon her undertaking of work side by side with men when tradition outside of Rome confined her so exclusively to the home. Besides, he took his own work with extreme seriousness, and he wished for the same attitude on the part of others.

We find St. Paul demanding that women be silent in church, that they wear veils, that their dress be of studied plainness. At the same time, he does not fail to speak highly of *Phoebe*, who as a deaconess in Greece, had been, as he says, "a helper of many, and of myself also." To Phoebe, who preceded him in Rome on legal business of her own, he entrusted his letter to the Romans. This was a precious missive, containing, as it did, the presentment of his gospel as well as of his intention of carrying it to the Gentiles. Much work and thought had gone into the preparation of his message, for it might be met with antagonism. The proud and callous city admitted his right to teach there if he wished to do so, but it was in Rome that he met martyrdom, at a date which, however, did not overtake him until he had accomplished two years of fruitful work in the heart of that empire which controlled practically all the nations that he hoped to reach.

Organization of Church   Systematic development of organization and capacity for leadership enabled the Christian movement to survive the early loss of its Founder, and the decimation of its ranks through long succeeding periods of persecution. Each little church of Christ emerged, ultimately, under supervision of a priest, presbyter, or elder. Bishops were placed in charge of designated groups of churches. A general council was in control, and met at stated intervals in different places. New offices were created as expediency required. We do not hear of *deacons* until after the crucifixion of Jesus, when His Apostle, *Peter*, who later became first Bishop of Rome, was carrying on notably successful work in the city of Jerusalem. Peter's own compelling influence had been augmented by the astounding ability displayed by his preacher assistants in the use of language. As the number of converts rose rapidly to five thousand souls, the difficulty of rendering necessary aid to many poor people increased. Seven men were appointed to assist the apostles. The name "deacon" was given them later because it meant "a servant." No duty was too menial for deacons to undertake. One of their chief concerns became that of distributing among the needy the property handed over to the apostles in the early days of the church by those who literally "gave up all" to follow the Christ.

EARLY CHRISTIAN ORDERS OF WOMEN
DEACONESSES

In a democratic mission for which women had shown active sympathy since the time of its inception, it was to be expected that functions would disclose themselves which they alone would fill. The *deaconess* came into being, and devoted herself to the needs of woman converts. The church required her to be unmarried or a widow but once. Like the deacon, she was also ordained to service, and worked on an equal basis with him as a church official. Friendliness to all expressed the ideal of both deacons and deaconesses. The majority of early Christians were poor, and, in response to a sympathy to which they were not accustomed, confided many needs. As the diaconate developed its own system, and the work increased, an outlet was provided for supervised, effective charity on the part of rich and well-to-do persons who desired to share in Christian activities.

To the social work and nursing done by these servants of the early church, the beginning of concerted private effort in the cause of charity owes its beginning. Deacons and deaconesses carried the church into the home in a very practical way. They prayed with some, gave food and money to others, and coped as best they could with sickness and those other social ills arising from poverty which sympathetic contact with the family in its own environment disclosed. Doubtless, their nursing was but a carrying over of that mixture of magic, empiric remedies, and home treatments which women of the time used for their families. We know of no new methods in nursing to be introduced over a long, long period, but organized visiting nursing outside of obstetrical nursing and social service had their functions interpreted by these men and women who accepted the office of servant in the churches of Christ.

Phoebe, a Greek lady of importance, whom we have mentioned as the bearer of St. Paul's Epistle to the Romans, is first mentioned among the women selected for deaconess service. On account of this and of the work which she did in nursing the sick poor in their homes, she has been awarded the dual honor of being known as *the world's first deaconess and first visiting nurse.* Visiting nursing soon became a major part of the work of deaconesses, who assumed responsibility for it throughout the eastern, as well as the western world. The Christian church had made possible the care of many more people than had ever before received medical or nursing care. A nursing service was brought to the home which has continued ever since. In bringing these accomplishments about, it had opened up an occupation to women, especially to those who, being unmarried, had held no definite place in society. Many other fields of endeavor were to claim the interests of this group as centuries rolled by, but the Deaconess Order, in spite of its periods of decline, has never died out wholly since the first century.

WIDOWS AND VIRGINS

Two other formal organizations of women, known respectively as *Widows* and *Virgins*, were developed. Women had held a place in the religion of most countries as Priestesses of the Temple. It was, therefore, not without precedent that they should occupy positions in the Christian church. Indeed, their loyal interest made them welcome. They provided lodging, food, and encouragement for the earliest leaders of Christianity. Their homes were the first church meeting places. They offered themselves for service with enthusiasm for the performance of all manner of tasks arising from the Christian assumption of work among the poor.

The Order of Widows was formed very early. Members had not been married, necessarily. The title "Widow" was sometimes used as designation of respect for age. If the widow had been married, it was required that she be the widow of one husband only, and she must vow her intention of not marrying again. St. Paul, in the fifth chapter of his First Epistle to Timothy, has explained the qualifications which made widows acceptable. Piety and a character above reproach are first essentials. Freedom from home responsibilities which would interfere with service is another. The age requirement he sets at sixty, although it is said to have been reduced later to forty, and, later still, to an even lower level. "She that giveth herself to pleasure," he says, "is dead while she liveth."[3] The widow must have a reputation for piety, be devoted in hospitality to strangers and saints, and anxious to relieve the afflicted. This zealous missionary, who seems to have had his work made difficult by many of the failings so often imputed to youth in social or health work today, asks his church to refuse younger widows. Too anxious to marry are they, and inclined to idle also. Besides, they indulge in gossip, carrying tales from one house to another, and they talk too much! The church cannot be bothered with them. Paul recommends that, in their case, marriage be encouraged.

[3] First Epistle of Paul to Timothy V: 6.

In spite of restrictions such as the above, Widows allied themselves with the church in considerable numbers. They did a good deal of work of the same nature as that done by Deaconesses, but they were not ordained.

An Order of Virgins was created when Christians began to interpret virginity as essential to purity of life. Women were consecrated to service in this, its third group of workers, to which men also are said to have belonged for a time. Virgins ranked in equality with the clergy, next to whom they sat in church gatherings. Ascetics as they were, society in the Christian groups of their time set them apart, and awarded them great honor for austerity of life—that crown of good works which they had chosen as an offering to God. Their chief duty seems to have been to assist with distribution of alms.

The three Orders of women which have just been discussed shared certain characteristics in common. All were enrolled for church service. Marriage automatically separated all from their groups. In the beginning, all wore the customary dress of women of the time, although distinctive garb is thought to have been adopted soon. All lived in their own homes. If they needed it, all were entitled to receive an allowance from the church, for, in its earliest days, when converts literally gave up all to follow Christ, they disposed of their property among the needy or handed it over to the church for distribution.

In the middle of the third century, the Christian church in the City of Rome abolished Deaconesses and gave over to Widows the work of visiting the sick. Elsewhere, the Order of Deaconesses attained its peak of success by the beginning of the fifth century. Its general abolition was destined to come within little more than another century, but, in spite of it, Deaconesses did not cease their work in some areas in Europe, and in the East. The traditional devotion of the Order to the care of the poor and the sick had won for them a place in public esteem which was cherished in memory wherever its workers had been withdrawn. Widows and Virgins, eventually, were absorbed into community life and became *Nuns* (*non nuptae*, not married).

Under conditions which permitted the use of their own initiative, women were likely to make greater progress. The eagerness with which they entered the social and religious activities of the church probably, in part, bespoke a need. A warring world made many widows, while it kept thin the ranks of marriageable men. There had been times, too, when popularity of bachelorhood had given concern to imperial authorities. The dependent woman could not but know that she was an unwelcome expense, and she was denied self-expression. If she was religious, the nunnery offered her a measure of independence and, in time, it became her outlet and her refuge also. Its protection secured her from the physical danger surrounding a woman who tried to live alone; the supervision of a woman helped to avoid that criticism of conduct to which she had been subjected from the first, and enveloping monastic walls facilitated her separation from worldly temptation at a time when virginity was fast coming to be looked upon as the supreme virtue.

Throughout the development of the primitive Christian church, women, as we have seen, took an active part. The names of many have come down to us through the Bible and other sources of history. In the beginning, they belonged to the poorer class of society, because it was among these people that the Christian movement found its first adherents. It was essentially a movement, like the present-day one of socialism, that worked from the bottom up. Christ, however, addressed himself to all classes of women. The qualities of character which He upheld were qualities which men associated with mothers, wives, and sisters, and women discovered in Christianity opportunities for strengthening them in new activities. We can well imagine the enthusiasm with which they applied themselves to these when we remember that, up to this time, the majority of women had known none but home duties. They gave their sons to be preachers, they sewed for the poor, they unceasingly gave of their hospitality to Christian travelers, and they served the church as Deaconesses, Widows or Virgins, and later as nuns.

PERSECUTION OF CHRISTIANS

Christianity, as a young religion, grew within an old one. For some time the Christian churches were allowed to develop without interference. Outside of an imperial requirement of certain religious observances from all subjects, Rome was tolerant of people who helped her with the vexing problem of satisfying her poor. The city itself had residents of many religions and bore a cosmopolitan atmosphere. Followers of the new religion were accepted much as the modern Salvation Army was accepted in its beginnings, with mild indulgence and some curiosity. They were excused from army service because of what seemed, to the average man of the time, to be an erratic belief in peace, but when attention was drawn to their refusal to admit the divinity of the emperor, or to sacrifice to any but one God, persecution began. At first, it expressed itself in a withdrawing of privileges like that of using public baths. As time went on, Christians were stoned, beaten, imprisoned, tortured, or put to death. The church finally was crushed into secrecy, but the misery of Christians only intensified the virtues of pity, gentleness, and charity which they upheld. Men began to note the sincere piety and fine characters of many Christian wives and mothers. Writers of the time extolled the need of virtues such as theirs. Husbands followed wives into the church.

INFLUENCE OF CONSTANTINE THE GREAT

The unquenchable spirit of the martyrs halted the attention of many a pagan, but the attitude of the Roman government did not change until the early part of the fourth century. The worst persecution that it had yet planned had failed to exterminate Christianity, and the death of its imperial instigator left the way open for new tactics. Slowly it had become apparent to Romans that these persistent Christians, wherever they dwelt, promoted peace and unity. Peace and unity had come to be very much desired and equally difficult to attain in an empire composed of people of varying religions and ways of life. Suddenly, it seemed, after the worst of her many persecutions, the empire under *Constantine the Great* discarded its efforts to uproot a faith which might prove to be a useful agent. Christianity was adopted as the official religion of the Roman State in 324 A.D.

Later Constantine became a convert himself, and, by so doing, not only became the first Christian emperor of Rome, but also relinquished claim to authority of divine origin. By that time Christianity had penetrated the upper or patrician class of society throughout the Roman Empire. The basis of equality on which all were admitted to its privileges and shared in its work was a manifestation of Christian democracy which gave evidence of a nascent social order. In it were gathering the seeds of modern nursing. Monasticism, that other movement already initiated within Christianity itself, was destined to provide shelter for the young plants and nurture them as they grew.

ROMAN MATRONS

Strange to say, it is the gay and licentious city of Rome herself that has handed down to us the greatest number of illustrious names among patrician Christian women of the fourth and early fifth centuries. This is not surprising when we recall how well fitted was the Roman woman of the upper classes, by social life and traditional freedom of action, for the use of her initiative. Roman women had been interested in public affairs and had participated in them. Those who managed the houses of wealthy husbands successfully were women of proven executive ability and social poise. The triviality and also the coarseness of the pleasures of a degenerate society had filled many of them with disgust. In their affiliation with the cause of Christianity, they encountered the prejudice of friends and lived, often, in families which remained pagan. To the fact that they did not falter we owe considerable progress in organization of charity and care of the sick.

Marcella   Three of the great names among Christian matrons of patrician Rome are those of *Marcella*, *Fabiola*, and *Paula*. All were members of a group of women meeting at Marcella's home on the Aventine Hill, which soon became a center of Christian study and teaching for her friends. Much inspiration came to them through a great friend and teacher, *St. Jerome*, translator of the Bible from its original Hebrew and Greek into Latin. His version is known as the "Vulgate" version, from the fact that he made use of that form of Latin in common use among the people. Jerome's influence in broadcasting the teachings of Christianity and making it a world religion was, as a result of this contribution, next to that of St. Paul. With Marcella and Paula, especially, he read and discussed much of this work. Both were able to render intelligent assistance, and Paula was endowed with mental gifts of an unusually high order.

In time, Marcella made her luxurious home into a monastery for women, and throughout the remainder of her life she devoted herself to their instruction, to charitable work, and to prayer. Her companions, like herself, were possessed of education which fitted them to become good students of Hebrew and Greek, and the learning of her group attracted admiration. This woman who had thus become head of *the first monastery in Rome* was referred to as an authority when questions arose on scriptural passages which were difficult of explanation. She had also assisted St. Jerome in his translation of the Hebrew prophets. Her work was ended when, in 410 A.D., she suffered a brutal attack from invaders of the city who had expected to find valuable plunder in her house, and took revenge on her when met by disappointment. She is said to have taken refuge in a nearby church and, soon after, she died.

Fabiola   Fabiola, a young woman of storied beauty that caught the imagination of a famous artist, was the idolized daughter of a great Roman family. Eagerly she had entered into the gay social life of the Empire, but disappointment awaited her. Marriage united her to a worthless husband from whom she found it necessary to get a divorce. Then she married again a husband no better than the first, and, on becoming a Christian, realized that in accordance with her beliefs a marriage following divorce made her guilty of sin. After publicly acknowledging her wrong-doing, Fabiola renounced the world and threw herself wholeheartedly into charitable work. Her charm and enthusiasm distinguished her among fellow-workers.

The *first Christian hospital in Rome* was founded by Fabiola in her own palace. She is said to have sought out the poor and the sick in the streets and byways of her native city, and to have cared for them herself. We are further told that she had fortitude which others lacked when it was necessary to dress ugly wounds and sores. Toward the end of her life, Fabiola is reputed to have gathered together what was left of her fortune, and to have joined with the son-in-law of Paula in building a great hospice for strangers at Ostia, a seaport of Rome. She died beloved of Rome and leaving behind her a lasting tradition of beauty, youth, and social opportunity given willingly as sacrifice to the expression of a selfless love for human beings. Thousands of young women, equally endowed, have followed her example through the ages since.

Paula   Paula had a daughter named Eustochium who joined her mother in adoption of Christianity, and shared with her in expressing its ideals through charitable work. Together they studied with Marcella. Paula was descended from famous lines, and the possessor of a great fortune. Broken-hearted by the death of her husband, she prepared to devote herself to the care of the poor and the sick. Taking with her Eustochium, she set out for Palestine with the intention of living there for the remainder of her life. In the course of their pilgrimage, they visited many places connected with the history of the early church and, ultimately, settled in Bethlehem where Paula organized a monastery. In the neighborhood of this town, she built hospitals for the sick and hospices for pilgrims. In all of these the design and construction of buildings were, by her instructions, of the plainest type, for a practical foresight made her determine to save all the money possible for the work to be done in them.

For twenty years Paula managed the institutions that she had built and, following her death in 404 A.D., Eustochium conducted the monastery for fifteen years longer. A life of Paula owes its authorship to her friend and co-worker, St. Jerome. He expresses appreciation of her wisdom and charity, and comments on the number of poor who attended her funeral. His description of the work done by her and Eustochium explains the origin of a tradition of hard manual work as an expression of self-sacrifice in the cause of nursing the poor. "They trim lamps, light fires, sweep floors, clean vegetables, put heads of cabbage in the pot to boil, lay tables, hand cups, help to wash dishes, and run to and fro to wait on others."[4]

The assumption by the Christian Church of a duty toward the sick had so far been met in the way best suited to an organization made up, in the main, of the poor and the slave classes. The duty was interpreted as a cooperative volunteer service. When care in the patient's own home was impossible, or when he had no home, a place must be found for him that would cost him nothing. Sometimes this was a room in the home of the deaconess; sometimes a friend of hers gave the needed shelter. Many women offered nursing care as well and, as the wealthy affiliated themselves with Christianity, their elaborate homes frequently took the form of hospitals. Not a few rich women like the Roman matrons delighted in waiting upon the sick, and this favorite charity was often, as in the case of Fabiola, a form of penance.

[4] Saint Jerome: Letters. Nicene and Post-Nicene Fathers of the Christian Church. New York, The Christian Literature Company, 1893, Vol. VI.

DIAKONIA AND XENODOCHIA

The responsibility of nursing care of the sick poor in private homes or hospitals was so closely associated with the activities of the Deaconess Order that the name popularly applied to institutions developed in homes was "diakonia." While their use was continued for centuries, another type of institution was already forming, for, with increasing numbers, it was found that there was need for greater stability of organization and service than was possible in scattered diakonia. The new institution evolved slowly from the same ideals of hospitality and pity that prompted the diakonia. It began in the house of the Bishop of the church who, like many ministers of our day, was expected to make his home a place in which welcome awaited all who needed help. As a result, this officer of the church, at times, was pressed for space. Rooms for the sick or homeless were added to his house, or a separate building might be erected nearby. Already the purposes of the ancient xenodochium had been fulfilled, and its well-known name was borrowed by the Christians for an institution that soon gave promise of permanency.

By the third century, the Christian xenodochium was on the way to becoming the center of a well-rounded system of relief. The hospital took its place within this readaptation of the traveler's inn, as one of many departments. Established Orders of Deaconesses, Widows, and Virgins needed extension only, in order to supply it with nursing staffs. A considerable number of Bishops and Priests had been drawn, it is said, from the ranks of physicians, a fact which enhanced their value as directors of institutions caring for the sick.

As time went on, the mingling of classes consequent on the democratic ideal of Christianity brought about a better understanding of social conditions. It became clear that much more than shelter, spiritual consolation, or care during illness would be necessary if poverty were to be even alleviated. Work had to be dignified, and work also had to be found. As the ideal of brotherly love prompted the rich to free their slaves, many of these were homeless, and could not support themselves. Epidemics of disease which carried off millions, among them many who volunteered their services to the sick, left behind numerous orphans.

Society had created beggary by accepting alms as the remedy for dependence. The Church followed this tradition in its distribution of the money which came to it in steadily increasing volume. Charity could not yet be very wise, but experience gradually made plain that for many of the population of the world of that time, housing, funds, education, and a trade would be essential to general well-being. Concentration of charitable activities would be necessary. The xenodochium promised possibilities of expansion in function and concentration of effort and resources. An example of successful management of this form of institution on a scale large enough to meet all of its requirements was still needed.

The magnitude of many Christian xenodochia is made clear by the statement that Constantinople, in 347 A.D., had a daily bread line of three thousand persons dependent on the charity of Christians. Besides food, it is logical to suppose that alms, with medical and nursing care, were included in this work of relief. The church also undertook to assuage the distress of prisoners, a function which it had carried out through the whole period of martyrdom when Christians so often endured this form of punishment. Prison work had become an expression of the Christian spirit identified with the visit of the deaconess. It was a phase of her work which, centuries after her Order was lost sight of, would help to bring her again before a welcoming public, and lead eventually to the founding of modern nursing.

Xenodochium of St. Basil   The extent to which Christianity succeeded in this task of giving protection and help to all who were poor, afflicted, or distressed, is best understood by a study of one of its early accomplishments. About the middle of the fourth century, *St. Basil*, a Greek Bishop of Caesarea in Asia Minor, began to build up what was to be *the most famous of Christian xenodochia*. In its physical organization, the institution, when completed, resembled a city. It was developed on the edge of town and its many buildings were of good construction and furnished adequately. They included the traditional hospice or inn for travelers, clinical facilities for ambulatory patients, a hospital for those who needed bed care, houses for the aged, for the crippled, for orphans, infants, and foundlings. There were buildings in which lepers and those suffering from communicable diseases were segregated. Living quarters were provided for full housekeeping and industrial staffs, and there was accommodation also for a staff of "ductores" or guides who were sent out to find patients and bring or lead them to the hospital.

In addition to housing facilities, it was necessary for a xenodochium of that period to provide for almost complete self-maintenance of the group within it. All who wished to work there or find work elsewhere could make application through an employment bureau. All among inmates who could perform any kind of labor were put to work. Factories did not exist which would supply the multitude of human needs for everyday living alone. These, and all articles of specialized uses, had to be made on the premises. St. Basil's xenodochium contained work rooms, refectories, shoe and clothing shops, blacksmith shops, foundry, laundry, dairy, and any other facilities necessary to supply a small city with its needs.

St. Basil will be recognized readily as a good organizer. He was likewise a capable executive and a good talker. An excellent education, part of which was received in Athens, had prepared him for administrative work, and he is thought to have had some instruction in medicine. A rare example of Christian enthusiasm for all good works, he drew to him the admiration of rich and poor, pagan and Christian. A great deal of money was put into his keeping for carrying out his plans, and he was successful in obtaining from the government remission of taxes. For charitable institutions this became an established precedent, one that is still followed.

Through the triumph of St. Basil, the hospital found a place as an institution within another institution which it held for many centuries hence. In the stress of those centuries, and under the uncertain influence of stagnant medicine, such protection as the xenodochium offered was not only of extreme importance to hospital development and development of charity, but was a factor in disease control. Private hospitals of the type started by Fabiola and Paula were apt to be left without endowment which would assure their continuance after the death of the founders. They did not represent permanency. Temporary hospitals must have been necessary to meet emergencies resulting from frequent epidemics.

One of the most widely distributed plagues of early times occurred about the middle of the third century, and "raged without interruption in every province, every city, and almost every family, of the

Roman Empire. During some time five thousand persons died daily in Rome; and many towns that had escaped the hands of barbarians were entirely depopulated."[5]

STATUS OF MEDICINE AND NURSING

We have seen that a great increase in the number of people who received nursing care had been brought about by Christianity. Much of this care was given them in their own homes or in homes of those Christians who wished to express their charity by giving refuge to the sick poor. At the same time, there was a considerable increase in the number of institutions provided for hospitalization of those who needed it. Strangely enough, there occurred little or no corresponding advance in medicine. The dominant western civilization, which had acquired all the traditions of Hippocratic medicine, neither assimilated much of them itself nor took the trouble to send them elsewhere. No Roman successor of greater wisdom than the "Father of Medicine" appeared.

Various reasons have been advanced for this failure on the part of ambitious rulers to show a progressive attitude toward conferring on the Roman people and subject nations benefits in the way of medical care of which they stood in sore need. All were suffering the strain of exhaustion resulting from many wars, and Italy, in particular, was called upon to cope with communicable diseases introduced by foreign slaves, and by soldiers and traders. The mosquitoes of the Tiber marshes produced for Rome a malaria which drained the vitality of citizens of the capital. Everywhere, indifferent morals, idleness, and inadequate sustenance of an impoverished middle class and an indigent lower class served to weaken further a world that was growing old while still young. Encouragement and virility, both necessary to evoke and sustain intellectual or inventive initiative, were lacking.

Indirectly conducive to the failure to disseminate and advance Hippocratic teaching was the prevailing opportunity to have all work done by a slave class. This stigmatized work and brought it about that Greek physicians, the bearers of Hippocrates' message, were reduced to the position of slaves to their Roman conquerors,

[5] Gibbon, Edward: Decline and Fall of the Roman Empire. New York, The Modern Library, Vol. I, p. 244.

and were forced to practice without social recognition. The status of medicine was lowered. Perhaps the real basis of an approaching medical stagnation, however, lay in a primitive tendency of the Roman to place reliance on a form of magic which related all troubles to omens and portents. Quackery flourished among a people who honored success in fighting above intellectual attainment. It was to the surgeon who attended injured gladiators, and to the army surgeon, that Rome offered her best experience in practice.

As the centuries passed, an ever-increasing influence against adequate care of the body came from the Christian church, which was making lack of emphasis on physical things a virtue. The spiritual side of man and his future life were becoming all-important, while belief in the early reappearance of Jesus and the attending dissolution of earthly affairs strengthened the tendency to belittle the value of medical care. Carelessness in regard to personal hygiene was pronounced in the eastern part of the Empire, whereas Rome's interest in cleanliness and her provisions for its maintenance opposed, in the west, a neglect which might induce disease. This attitude deferred Roman understanding of Christian disregard for the body and, at the same time, hindered medicine.

Soranus and Dioscorides   As we have observed many times previously, nothing of real use to a dynamic world is permitted to stop moving. In spite of the above and other obstructions which tended to slow down to stagnation the stream of medical progress, here and there throughout the Empire some man, usually a Greek or a student from the great school of Alexandria, would pour into it his contribution of new ideas to stimulate the current. One of these, *Soranus of Ephesus*, won fame as an obstetrician, pediatrician, and gynecologist, and was the author of many practical medical treatises. One helped little children by exposing the stupefying mental results of whippings received from their school masters. Another offered studies of muscles, glands, and nerves. Methods of ligation and torsion of vessels owe their origin to this period, while a surgeon in the army, *Dioscorides*, devoted his spare time with such industry to the study of plants, that his descriptions were accepted "word for word"[6] for sixteen centuries. Two names, however, stand out above

[6] Garrison, Fielding H.: History of Medicine. Philadelphia, W. B. Saunders Co., 1929, p. 109.

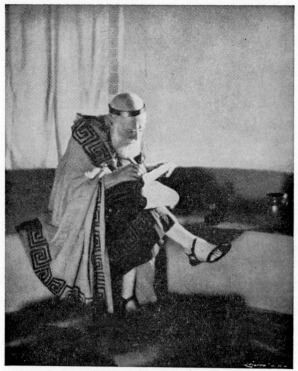

CELSUS (*circa* 25 B.C.–40 A.D.)
A present-day conception. (Courtesy of Davis & Geck, Inc.)

all others of the first five centuries for their influence on the future course of medicine, those of *Celsus* and *Galen*.

Celsus   Celsus was a Roman patrician of the first century who is best known for his writings, which included medical works. His great achievement was the rescue and preservation of knowledge of other men. To the painstaking ability of Celsus, generations living long after him acknowledged a debt for wisdom.

The clarity of his descriptions and the usefulness of his material have been admitted by the surgeon of modern times. The intricacies of procedure in amputation, surgery of plastic nature, hernias, venesection, cataract, and other operations are among the valuable contents of his collection. This consists of eight books on subjects concerned with medicine—the group entitled "De Re Medicina" (The Subject of Medicine). In Celsus' own time the compilation did not attract great attention. In a later time, men honored the author when they found in these books an answer to a great need. During the Revival of Learning in the fifteenth century, these books of Celsus were among the first to be printed.

Galen   Galen lived in the second century. Born at Pergamum in Asia Minor, he enjoyed the privilege of a good education which included work at the famous University of Alexandria. The knowledge of medicine which he acquired at Alexandria and through much travel was supplemented by independent investigation by means of dissection. As dissection of human bodies had again become illegal, Galen was forced to work principally on animals, but he became known as the "Founder of Experimental Physiology." He was also a popular teacher of anatomy. His work was done in the scientific spirit, and he restored Hippocratic medicine which had been hidden under a scum of pedantry. His great importance in determining the direction of the sluggish stream of medicine already referred to, is better understood when we know that "Galen's experiments on the physiology of the nervous, respiratory, and circulatory systems were the only real knowledge for seventeen centuries."[7]

Ultimately settling down in the city of Rome, he became physician to the gladiators. In this capacity, his experience with emergency and plastic surgery appears to have been extensive. His professional literary contribution accumulated to a considerable volume, and so popular were his works that, as late as the sixteenth century, they were still consulted as the chief medical authority. Through these interpretations of Hippocratic medicine, and the restoration of interest in scientific method which they brought about, Hippocrates and Galen, fortunately, gave direction to what medical thought and procedure continued throughout the Middle Ages. Negligible progress was made from Galen's time until the sixteenth century when modern scientific medicine began.

The brief study which we have made of the nursing done during the first four centuries after the birth of Jesus shows that it was largely in the hands of intelligent, educated, wealthy women of

[7] Garrison, Fielding H.: History of Medicine. Philadelphia, W. B. Saunders Co., 1929, p. 116.

noble birth. The emphasis which Christianity placed on pity made prominent the weak and suffering among mankind. It pointed to preservation of all, rather than to the maximum development of the fit. Infanticide it condemned, and because of the lessening of this common practice more children needed care, and more women survived among the population. Service to all in need took the place of military glory as an aim of life. Self-sacrifice on the part of the rich was idealized, and poverty looked to them for its alleviation.

THE FALL OF ROME IN 476 A. D.

In spite of many dissensions by which it was in time torn, Christian influence on the Roman Empire may be looked upon as steadily constructive. Other influences, for some of which we must refer as far back as the last century B.C., doomed to destruction whatever political integrity had been attained. The reign of Augustus Caesar (29 B.C.–14 A.D.) was the beginning of a considerable period during which Rome knew more peace, prosperity, and luxury than at any other time in her history. Romans were worn out with war. They were satisfied with the decision of the new Emperor to cease imperial expansion as soon as he had acquired a few remnants of lands which interfered with a boundary that seemed defensible with minimum of expense in money and man power. Augustus completed this task and confined Roman power within the following natural boundaries: The Danube and the Rhine rivers on the north, the Black Sea, the Euphrates river, and the Arabian Desert on the east, the Sahara Desert on the south, and the Atlantic Ocean on the west.

The world which Jesus entered had inherited an opportunity to relax into enjoyment of living. As happens during all periods of opportunity, some people took advantage of peace to extend their culture. The majority tended in another direction. A fashionable license and coarseness among the wealthy minority made the prevailing status of morals low, for lower classes were encouraged to follow their example. Disease made its inroads on physical vitality. Persistent malaria in the city of Rome kept citizens under par, and probably accounted, in some degree, for an increase in her vices. By recurring pestilence here and throughout the Empire, the general population was reduced by millions.

The worst menace, however, came from other sources. The constituent elements of the vast Empire felt no common interest in its successful administration. Protection of over two thousand miles of boundary proved to be very difficult. On the other side of this boundary lived people still in the tribal state—Jutes, Angles, Saxons, Alemans, Burgundians, Franks, Vandals, Sueves, Lombards, Visigoths, and Ostragoths. Huns and Alans, savage enemies of all, were straining forward from Asia toward southeastern Europe. The force of the general movement of people southward and westward made itself felt.

These people from the north were known as "barbarians" or "outsiders" to the Greeks and Romans. They represented a middle stage of culture between the primitive and the civilized. They were nature worshipers. Skins of wild beasts furnished their clothing in a rigid climate. They lived in fixed habitations, and the chief occupation of the men was fighting and hunting. Women performed the manual work of the settlements, and were subject to the rule of harsh husbands. None among these semisavage people could read or write. They made use of the cart, and must have known something of farming, for they repeatedly stole Roman tools. Some of the earlier arrivals were assimilated as they replaced Roman farm laborers who left the country for the city. Some became traders. Many of them were marauders, who plundered property and carried off captives whose fate was slavery if not redeemed by ransom. Romans themselves engaged in slave trade with these neighbors, and some Romans married barbarian wives, while a good many barbarians became Roman citizens. On the whole, there seems to have been in progress, for several hundred years, a comparatively peaceful penetration of foreign peoples.

By the fifth century whole tribes began to settle on Roman lands. Like the primitive pastoral people, they coveted the wealth of those who had attained civilization, and they were ready to fight for it. They were also pushed over the border by enemies behind them. Invasion followed invasion in such rapid succession that it was as if a flood had been let loose. Roman armies were unable to control the sudden influx. Greece was plundered, Gaul devastated, and the capital city of Rome was sacked, all about the same time. In 476 A.D. Rome fell, and within a year wild tribes controlled the whole western division of the Empire. Some Romans were able to migrate to the eastern capital set up in Constantinople. The majority had to stay where they were and submit to barbarian domination.

If the work of man for many centuries was not to be lost, there must be some force in civilization which would prove sufficiently strong to induce the invading hordes to discard barbarism. As we shall see, that force was in Christianity, and in the missionary and teaching spirit of its preachers lay the means of utilizing it. To the men and women who so shaped the affairs of monasteries that they could perform this service to mankind, the world gives tribute. They had to deal with unlettered, half-savage people of many gods and languages whom they must lead into the Christian fold, besides teaching them to read and write, to desire and to learn all the practical arts as well as the refinements of thought and action that are a part of civilized life.

Five centuries of Christian effort had provided them with a foundation on which to build efficient institutions through which these things might be accomplished. The sixth century found them with the Bible in the Vulgate form given to it by St. Jerome and his collaborators. It was in the everyday speech of the people. Great xenodochia had been built which could serve as models for commercial teaching, charity, and nursing care. The Orders of Widows and Virgins had been absorbed into monasteries. As nuns they would share in a new movement which would change the course of future history by making over the uncivilized. A time had come when the institution became a necessary protection. Life outside it was unsafe, and individual effort, or scattered organization of work in homes, could make little headway. Throughout Roman Europe, deaconesses sank into obscurity amid the general confusion. The church was beginning to assume guardianship over nursing, medicine, and charity, as well as of literature, science, and art.

SUMMARY, 1 TO 500 A.D.

The first five centuries of the Christian era witnessed the greatest glory of the Roman Empire, its weakening, and its collapse. Coincident with this decline and the final triumph of barbarism and confusion over settled government in western Europe, they saw the rise of a religious and social movement which held within it protecting forces for civilization. The world which Jesus entered was one in

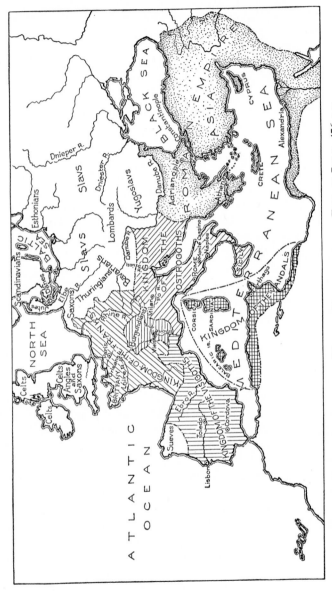

BARBARIAN KINGDOMS IN WESTERN EUROPE AFTER THE FALL OF ROME, 476 A.D.

which a minority of men enjoyed wealth and luxury while the mass of humanity was either poverty-stricken or in a state of slavery. Lands had passed into the control of the rich, and the middle class of men did not exist. A hundred years of successful war had produced exhaustion, misery, and corruption. No solace was to be found in formalized, official Paganism.

The Great Reformer brought to unhappy human beings a religion which, while it promised a better life after death, also taught a better way of living. It appealed for kindliness and brotherly love to replace hate and cruelty, and it advocated greater charity and a distribution of wealth. It dignified human life and labor. The first followers of Jesus were the poor, and a church was organized in which all could take active part. Assistant missionaries, called "apostles," were prepared for teaching. Additions to their group were made as necessary, and when the Leader of Christians was crucified, apostles carried on the work. Among these, St. Peter and St. Paul stand out in history as preachers and organizers in Asia Minor and in Europe, where St. Peter became first bishop of the capital city of Rome, and the antecedent of all popes. The fact that Christianity became a world religion is due, in large measure, to the work of St. Paul.

Women in this early church of Christ shared activities with men. In the beginning, none of them were separated from ordinary home life, but, in time, three Orders of women were developed. These were known, variously, as Deaconesses, Widows, and Virgins. Deaconesses were assisted by Widows, and among other duties nursed the poor, either in their homes or in diakonia. Organized nursing thus became an institution of society which has come down to our time, and the deaconess is looked upon as the forerunner of the modern nurse. *Phoebe, a friend of St. Paul's, is credited with being the first deaconess, and the first of all visiting nurses.*

Virgins had, as their chief activities, care of church vestments and assistance in distribution of alms. Eventually both Widows and Virgins became absorbed into monasteries as nuns. Deaconesses were never wholly lost although an organization such as theirs became difficult to maintain in the danger and confusion of later times, and in the face of changes taking place within the church itself. With some modification, their work is still carried on.

As Christianity spread it came into conflict with Paganism and with imperial authority which it refused to accept as divine. During more than two centuries many Christian martyrs suffered torture or were put to death. Constantine the Great, observant of its growing strength despite persecution, and recognizing its power for producing peace and unity among the people, made Christianity the official religion of the Roman Empire in 324 A.D.

Meanwhile, confusion in human affairs, oppressive taxation, persecution, sadness, or the desire for contemplation and study were driving men and women to abandon society for solitude. Monasticism did not meet with Roman favor, although it was an ancient institution elsewhere in the world. Early Christian monasteries knew only direst poverty but, as time went on, not only organization and management improved but rich gifts were received and rich people joined them. They grew in numbers, wealth, and power. Toward the end of the fourth century, the Church emerged from the secrecy forced upon it by persecution.

In the western part of the Empire, a considerable group of Rome's wealthy matrons became known for piety and charity. St. Jerome gave his tutelage to the group which included names now famous. The palatial home of *Marcella*, their leader, provided a meeting place where they could study the scriptures and engage in prayer. Eventually, it became the first monastery for women in Rome. *Paula* was a student versed in Greek and Hebrew who became an authority for students of Christianity. She assisted St. Jerome in his translation of the Bible into the form of Latin used by the common people of Rome, a version called for this reason the "Vulgate." Paula made a pilgrimage to Palestine where she remained and built a monastery and several hospices and hospitals. *Fabiola*, third of this trio, visited her and worked with her for two years, but her most notable activities were carried on in Rome. Here she brought into her palace the sick poor, and she herself gave them care. The hospital thus formed was called a "nosocomium" because it confined its work to care of the sick. It was the first Christian hospital in Rome. Fabiola also helped to found a great hospice near the port of Rome, besides giving time and wealth to many charities. So great was her popularity that people flocked to her funeral. So great was her beauty that it has been idealized by Henner, a French artist, who thus made it a perpetual possession of humanity, which is reproduced in the frontispiece of this book.

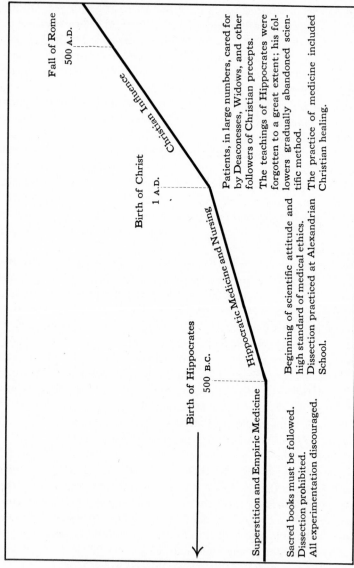

MEDICINE AND NURSING OF ANCIENT CIVILIZATIONS
5000 B.C.–500 A.D.

In a town of Asia Minor called Caesarea, the Christian Bishop, St. Basil, built up a xenodochium known as the "Basilias." So successful was this institution that it became the model for Christian xenodochia. It centralized church activities in an institution which provided homes and maintenance for thousands.

Any progress made in medicine during the period under consideration was due chiefly to the work of two men, Celsus and Galen. Celsus lived in the first century, and wrote an encyclopedia of medicine which preserved valuable knowledge. Galen, who lived in the second century, did much experimental physiology, and developed a system of medicine based on the clinical method of Hippocrates. He kept in sight the scientific ideal at a time when it was fading behind returning superstition. Until the Revival of Learning in the sixteenth century, Celsus and Galen were the chief sources of medical knowledge.

In 476 A.D., came the culmination of a progressive invasion of the Roman Empire by barbarians from the north and east. A sudden and tremendous influx of these "outsiders" overpowered frontier armies. Western Europe was thrown into confusion. The cultures produced through many centuries were endangered. Their protection became a chief function of the Christian church. The xenodochium and the monastery showed themselves to be necessary and worthy tools with which to work, and clergy and nuns took up the tremendous task of bringing millions of semisavage individuals to the civilized state. For a time, as we shall find, medicine found shelter in the church, and nursing became one of the chief occupations of women throughout many centuries.

TOPICS FOR DISCUSSION

1. Who was Emperor of Rome at the time of the birth of Jesus, and what factors were contributing to the unhappiness of the people?
2. Show how the teachings of Jesus contained the seeds of social revolution.
3. In order to ensure a world-wide spread of Christian teachings, what system of organization was adopted by early Christians?
4. Which apostle of Jesus became the first pope of Rome?

5. (*a*) What missionary preacher was largely responsible for carrying the teachings of Christianity to far-off places? (*b*) What was his influence on the position of women?

6. Who was entrusted with carrying the precious Epistle written by St. Paul to the Romans?

7. Who is known as the first deaconess and first visiting nurse, and why?

8. Describe the duties and responsibilities of early deacons and deaconesses.

9. (*a*) Make an outline of entrance requirements for each of the three Orders of women of the early Cnristian Church. (*b*) Members of which group are considered the forerunners of nurses?

10. What is known of nursing methods of the time?

11. (*a*) Show how visiting nursing came to have its beginnings with the Christian movement. (*b*) Which order of women engaged in this work?

12. Discuss, from the following standpoints, the Roman matrons who were converted to Christianity:

   (*a*) Characteristics typical of Roman women.

   (*b*) Social life compared with that of the majority of early Christians.

   (*c*) Their noted friend and teacher.

   (*d*) Attitude toward asceticism.

   (*e*) Their individual accomplishments.

13. What well-known artist made a painting of Fabiola, a copy of which appears as the frontispiece of this book?

14. If you had been a citizen of the Roman Empire during this period, what opportunity would there have been to be cared for during illness?

15. Show how institutional care of the sick gradually developed among Christians.

16. What is the quotation from St. Matthew VII which constitutes the Golden Rule of the Christians, and from St. Matthew XXV which shows their attitude toward prisoners?

17. If you had been a visitor at the Xenodochium of St. Basil at Caesarea, what kinds of social work would you have seen going on about you?

18. What do you know of the plagues of the third century, and how do you account for them?

19. (*a*) Add a dotted line to the chart on page 108 to indicate the *general trend* in the practice of medicine from 1 to 500 A.D. (*b*) What two men made contributions of lasting value?

20. What factors contributed to the general stagnation in medicine during this early Christian period?

21. Women of what class of society did the nursing during the first four centuries of the Christian era?

22. (*a*) What influences contributed to the break-up of the Roman Empire in 476 A.D. (*b*) What social institution was ready to assume guardianship of medicine, nursing, charity, and education, during the five hundred years of "Dark Ages" that were to follow?

REFERENCES

Asch, Sholem: The Apostle. New York, G. P. Putnam's Sons, 1943.

Bible.

Brown, Lewis: The World's Great Scriptures. New York, The Macmillan Co., 1946.

Dana, Charles L.: The Peaks of Medical History. New York, Paul B. Hoeber, Inc., 1936.

Dock and Nutting: A History of Nursing. New York, G. P. Putnam's Sons, 1907, Vol. I, Part II, Chaps. 1 and 2.

Fitch, Florence: One God; The Ways We Worship Him. New York, Lathrop, Lee, and Shepard Co., 1945. (Describes religious observances of Jews, Catholics, and Protestants. Many illustrations.)

Fosdick, Harry Emerson: The Man from Nazareth. New York, Harper and Brothers, 1949.

Friedlander, Ludwig: Roman Life and Manners. New York, E. P. Dutton & Co. and London, George Routledge & Sons.

Gibbon, Edward: The Decline and Fall of the Roman Empire (Giant edition.) New York, The Modern Library, Vol. I (180–476 A.D.).

Goodspeed, Edgar J.: Paul. Philadelphia and Toronto, The John C. Winston Co., 1947.

Heaps, Isabel W.: Five Marys. New York, Abingdon-Cokesbury Press, 1942.

Kirkland, Winifred: Discovering the Boy of Nazareth. New York, The Macmillan Company, 1944.

Members of School for Graduate Nurses, McGill University, Montreal, Canada: Vignettes from the History of Nursing, The Canadian Nurse, March, April, May, June, July, 1928.

Miller, Madeline S.: Footprints in Palestine. New York, Fleming H. Revell Co., 1936.

Reinach, Salomon: Orpheus, A History of Religions. New York, Liveright, Inc., 1930.

PART TWO

The Middle Ages

Circa 500 to 1500 A.D.

The Early Middle Ages

Society in Small Cooperative Units

Broadly speaking, the history of civilization divides itself into three great periods or eras—ancient, medieval, and modern. Within these lie lesser periods, but dissolution of the greatest state that man had yet been able to bring under one rule destroyed a composite Graeco-Roman civilization, the final product of those ancient cultures believed to have originated in Egypt. It was a civilization representing many centuries of human development throughout the world, and the process of building up a civilization to replace it consumed other centuries. An interval of about one thousand years between social destruction and social restoration has been named the *Medieval Period* in European development, or the *Middle Ages.*

This is a good place to remind ourselves that dividing lines between what we call *periods* in history can never be looked upon as hard and fast boundaries. One of these so-called periods begins within another through the activity of changing influences that grow imperceptibly and operate at times with sudden force. Periods fade out. They do not end precipitately, but there are times when events occur to hasten a change in the trend of affairs.

The early centuries of the Middle Ages in European history are collectively known as "the Dark Ages." In order to understand conditions prevailing immediately after the barbarian onslaught, we must try to imagine what it would be like to be ourselves surrounded by swarms of semisavage people who had descended upon our country, seized our property, and set about making crude homes for themselves right in our midst. No central government could interfere in our behalf, because there was none. The armies which we had become accustomed to looking upon as invincible in our support, no longer functioned. The officials who had done our thinking for us had disappeared and we would have to find our own way out of our difficulties. Meanwhile, robbers made life unsafe, and those who might have helped us with the administration of justice locally, found that Roman laws could not affect men governed by a variety of tribal law and custom.

Children could not go to school in the few places where schools existed, commerce was impossible, roads, aqueducts, sewers, and bridges, in great numbers, had been ruined. Destruction of utilities, combined with crowding, put public health in the same evil plight as business, education, and government. Romans who could do so met this situation by escaping to the eastern part of the Empire. Those whom circumstances forced to remain in the west found their problem one of wholesale adjustment, and settled down to slow working out of a social compromise which would enable barbarians and themselves to live together as citizens of a new world.

The fate of civilization rested upon health protection, a different form of government, the education of thousands of barbarians to civilized standards, and many changes in Roman outlook and attitudes. Time has shown that the Christian religion and its representative, the Church, accepted the burden of these tasks and carried them to fulfillment. The zeal which had helped this already highly organized religious enterprise to hold together kept it from becoming disorganized along with the political state. Its gospel of love for human beings found new reason for expression, and its leaders undertook to calm the excitement of people who had lost their sense of security and by common impulse were beginning to herd together in search of safety. Many turned to the *monasteries* which offered refuge, and peace as well. These institutions began a period of great expansion and, by enlarging their ideals as well as their physical scope, were able to hasten the return of order while they saved the institutions of religion, education, medicine, and nursing. In many instances, their own survival depended upon changing their outward character to that of fortified strongholds.

Also, secular units formed about strong men who helped individual members to establish a life routine by reviving, on great estates, an ancient governmental institution known as *feudalism*.

This was a type of patriarchal rule which provided men with homes for their families and with food and bodily protection, in return for their service as farmers and, in case of war, as soldiers. Rome had encouraged the growth of a land-owning class, and the number of great rural estates now increased. Their sites were preferably far from routes of travel, and, like the monasteries, they were frequently located in mountain fastnesses or in rich but remote valleys. The immediate problem of all groups was to arrange for adequate protection from attack and to make themselves self-sustaining. Interpretations of government within them was necessarily more or less individual, and dependent upon the chosen leader. Social poise and trade were gradually restored to a noticeable degree by 800 A.D.

Following upon the revival of commerce, a third type of protective unit known as a *guild* began to appear as, for the first time in history, workers organized for mutual benefit. In their protective character, these forerunners of modern labor unions were to become, eventually, the core of a great guild system which would regulate craftsmen and traders, manufacturers and commerce. Monasticism, feudalism, and guilds constitute pivots around which society learned to move during the Middle Ages, and, during the major part of that period of transition prior to 1000 A.D., the Church emerged as chief authority, with feudal government and guilds under its control. By a process of slow evolution, the Church, the feudal lord, and, later, the guild were forming small cooperative units of education, political, and economic organization about which could be developed a new civilization.

CHRISTIAN MONASTICISM

Monasticism, an expression of asceticism by groups of people living apart from the everyday world, is a system which we have found to be of very ancient origin and common to various religious beliefs. As a phase of Christianity it had developed to a considerable extent before the fourth century after Christ, when it received new stimulus from the enthusiasm of Marcella, Paula, Saint Jerome, and the altruistic group to which they belonged.

In physical aspect and internal management, the monastic establishment, up to this time, had varied with numbers of monks, their inclination or belief, or with climatic or pecuniary circumstances.

The primary purpose which it must serve was to house men who desired to live apart from the world and to promote their individual salvation, a purpose which did not change when Christianity brought into it the broader ideal of service to mankind. With the fall of Rome, Roman citizens of every class turned to the monastery for refuge, and barbarians, too, sought its help as they realized that an institution which resisted their destruction was also willing to show them kindness.

At first the old monasteries of Europe must have been greatly pressed. At first, also, there must have been much confusion as all these people tried to meet an emergency, and none had a settled place or function except those who had been monks. It must have taken time to develop system within and adequate protection from without. Some monasteries were strongly fortified; practically all of them were established in isolated spots which nature had made almost inaccessible, in swampy land, on mountain tops, in far-away valleys, or in deep forests. A tremendous amount of work was often done before these locations could be made habitable, and much more had to be done before suitable habitations were erected on them.

RISE OF BENEDICTINE MONASTERIES

To an Italian monk, history ascribes the credit for organization of many of these institutions, as well as for fixing the trend of monastic development for several centuries to come. In 529 A.D., this monk whom we now know as *St. Benedict of Nursia* was busily making use of stones from ruins of an ancient pagan temple to build a monastery for a few followers. The site was a rugged mountain top between Rome and Naples, and his neighbors were many of them pagan, some barbarian as well. Gradually, Benedict induced all to become Christians, and taught men who had been enemies to harmonize their customs and manners. An institution grew on Monte Cassino which was one of the most efficient of medieval protective monastic units, as well as a radiating center for monks whose numbers and success brought new hope and courage to other groups already hard at work trying to banish the barbarism which had deluged Europe.

Plan of Monastery Buildings and Grounds   Ultimately, many

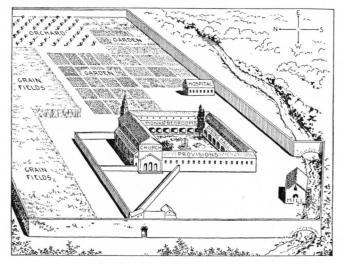

GENERAL PLAN OF A MONASTERY

(From Hayes, Moon and Wayland, "World History," by permission of The Macmillan Co., publishers.)

monasteries took on a characteristic arrangement. When a plot of ground of suitable size had been made ready and walled in with high stone walls, there slowly appeared upon its surface a church, a storehouse, dining room or refectory, and a row of cells or bedrooms for monks, all arranged about a square court. Beyond this group of buildings were fields of grain, orchards, barns, workshops, a mill beside running water, and such other buildings as the activities of the institution might require. Here also were a hospital and quarters for strangers. None could be turned away, and charity extended to the poor among them grew to great proportions. By the ninth century, the majority of monasteries maintained, in addition to such quarters, a school for children of the people who, as things settled down, began to live outside its walls.

The Benedictine Rule   During the development of Christian monasticism numerous rules or codes had regulated the daily life of monks and administration of institutional affairs. The Benedictine Rule was formulated to meet the needs of a new era. Manual labor, which Romans had relegated to slaves, had become a foremost necessity for all men. Christianization of barbarians could proceed only as their training in manual skills and in civilized ways of living kept pace with it. It was a time when every man had to earn the right to live, and all Benedictines worked. The abbot (L. *abbas*, father), whom they elected to be the head of their institution, worked side by side with his monks. Customary vows of poverty, chastity, and obedience were supplemented by a vow which made their service a life-long one. Rigorous asceticism was not required, personal worry was removed, healthful, busy, purposeful lives were devoted to development of personal piety, promotion of human welfare, and preparation for missionary work wherever the need might be greatest. Many monasteries were born of the motherhouse on Monte Cassino, and, in view of the upset lives of European rulers during today's social revolution, it is of interest to note that, in the centuries following its inception, twenty emperors and forty-seven kings abdicated to become Benedictine monks. Ten empresses and fifty queens, with many princesses and ladies of the court, became nuns.

The path of the monastic novice was not made easy. The Benedictine Rule made his novitiate a period in which he was to be tried out to determine his fitness for monastic life. Constantly under supervision, restrictions forbade him privileges accorded to those who had been accepted into the monastic organization. No one spoke to him without permission from the master who had charge of him, but he must rise to receive reproof from any monk who got permission from the master to administer it. Only by the master's permission could he again be seated, after making his apology.

Accepted monks were divided into three groups according to the length of their experience. Seniors, or "wisefolk," had passed fifty years as monks, a middle class twenty-four to fifty years, and juniors less than twenty-four years. Privileges and duties were arranged in accordance with these divisions, the hardest work falling upon the youngest group, who were enjoined to love the seniors who, in turn, were to know them as brothers. In addressing one another the use of names was not permitted. Grand rounds were made daily by the abbot, every evening the dormitories were visited, at midnight monks were awakened and called to prayer, and a general inspection of the whole plant was a periodic occurrence. It is not difficult to trace, in customs and organization, origins of traditions still followed in colleges, hospitals, and schools of nursing today.

A framework of routine set the pattern of each day for the Benedictines. Shortly after sunset prayers, all retired. At 1:30 or 2:00 A.M. in summer, and as late as 3:30 A.M. in winter, each awakened to a new day in which every hour would be occupied. Eight periods of devotion divided the hours before the next sunset. Between times, they worked, read, or studied, always on definite assignment. In winter time, when outdoor labor was minimized, one good meal was served daily; in summer when it was heavy, there were two meals. Comfort in dress was permitted, and the weight and texture of clothing could be changed to suit circumstances or climate. Should monks fall ill, adequate care was assured them, for an *infirmarian* saw to their nursing and supervised a special hospital in which they were housed until recovery. The hospital provided for strangers occupied a separate building. In the words of St. Benedict:

"Before all things and above all things care is to be had of the sick, that they may be served in the very deed as Christ himself, for He hath said, 'I was sick and ye visited Me,' and 'What ye have done unto one of these little ones, ye have done unto Me.' "

Experience and wisdom in meeting other problems common to group living are reflected in the Benedictine Rule. St. Benedict's solutions, which would be helpful to many an administrator today, embodied instructions to cover such topics as the following: qualifications for position of abbot; selection of heads of departments; reception and instruction of novices; division of work; an exchange system for kitchen utensils, clothing, and shoes; arrangements for revenue to maintain the monastic family; definitions of "good works" in communal life, of discipline, and of hospitality.

Agriculture, Arts and Crafts   Agriculture was necessarily a chief interest of monastic units of this time, and it was carried on with so much intelligence, and with such systematic recording and comparison of results by the Benedictines that their institutions took on the aspect of our present-day experimental stations. They performed a great public service by improving farm methods and reclaiming vast areas of previously useless land. It became the custom for monasteries to rent pieces of their property to tenants at nominal rates. Further income was derived from gifts, and, gradually, poverty was left behind and great wealth took its place. As people settled down in orderly groups, highways became safer and trade revived slowly. Travelers with goods to sell found their way to these distant retreats and improvised markets were opened for exchange of the products of monastic labor. Some tradesmen established permanent homes outside the wall, making the monastery the nucleus, eventually, of a rising town.

Inside the wall, meanwhile, arts and skills were becoming highly developed and specialized. Among monks and nuns could be found artists in architecture, music, and painting, expert silversmiths and goldsmiths, doctors and nurses skilled in the use of home remedies in sickness. Monastic hospitals cared for the major portion of the sick, while the activities necessary for their support outnumbered greatly those of the large municipal or county institutions of the present day, which are akin to them. The latter, however, draw upon innumerable organized industries, educational and other institutions outside of themselves that were not available to the self-subsistent groups of the Middle Ages.

Preservation of Knowledge   From its earliest days, the Christian monastery had known the influence of scholarly men and women. *Cassiodorus*, a patrician of literary taste and a contemporary of St. Benedict, is credited with introducing the copying of religious and classic manuscripts to the monks of a monastery that he founded. St. Benedict took up the idea, and these two brought to their fellow monasteries of the Middle Ages the privilege of preserving knowledge likely to have been lost in that disturbed era. From now on, the monastery more frequently included a library and, adjoining it, a room known as the "scriptorium" or writing room. The task of transcribing ancient writings from scrolls of parchment or papyrus to other and similar rolls, gave opportunity for artistic expression. The new parchments were often bordered with intricate designs, and letters were ornamented variously. Color, or gold, was introduced to relieve and brighten black and white. In times which anteceded printing or typewriting, all this tedious work was laboriously done by monks or nuns who worked in the chilly atmosphere of medieval buildings, and often, by the light of a candle.

As the manuscripts were passed from one monastery to another, they exerted a civilizing influence that surpassed their occupational

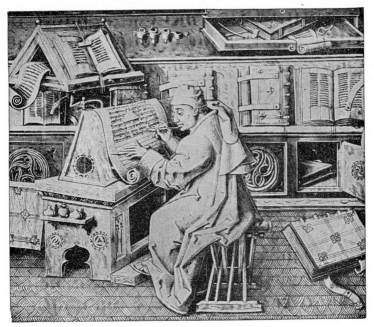

A MEDIEVAL SCRIBE AT WORK ON HIS MANUSCRIPT
(From "The Miracles of Our Lady," a fifteenth-century book.)

or artistic interest. The thought of great minds among the ancients was spread abroad, and eventually handed down to us. The books went to found libraries in which they were preserved with studious care for scholars of the future. They provided monks and nuns, who had to make immediate use of it, with some scientific knowledge regarding care of the sick. They were the groundwork of universities.

The ninth and tenth centuries saw decline in some quarters of this monastic prestige. Within the Church itself, there was dissatisfaction with institutions which continually acquired wealth and, with wealth, a greater ease of life and greater freedom to mingle with a society which was finding it possible to move about once more. Monastic severity of life was becoming less attractive, and relaxed as well. The remedy applied was an increased severity. However, a new Benedictine monastery at *Cluny* in France heralded a change of thought and a return to simple expression of Christian service. It also established a new tradition by making the various houses which branched out from this parent organization subject to its control. Its fruits appear in the late Middle Ages.

WOMEN OF MONASTICISM

We do not have to revert to the Middle Ages to learn that a world that has tumbled down is full of tragedy, and a world in process of rebuilding is full of opportunity for those possessed of foresight, preparation, and constructive talent. Romans who were attracted to monasticism after the debacle of 476 A.D., were men who were what the psychology of today would term "escapists." Individually, they sought forgetfulness in solitude; in running away from confusion they expected to find peace. As members of a group, however, they discovered in themselves capacities essential to a solution of social problems, and surrendered to a force which spurred them to creation of a civilization that would surpass that which had been destroyed.

The task drew women to share with men its difficulties and its satisfactions. Economic conditions were increasing a slowly developing discontent with those traditions which bound them to the fireside. Besides, for Roman women of the upper class, social ambition now had no outlet, the beginning political prestige of the aristocrat of her sex had faded in political confusion, the number of eligible husbands was not enough to go around when so many men were either impoverished or had withdrawn from the world. Anyway, marriage forced upon women for political reasons seldom had brought happiness. The public dole which had supported so many women of lower social status as wives of freemen had been withdrawn, leaving them helpless. For numberless others, social security had lain in their slavery. These were free now, but without home or occupation. To each group according to its need, the convent beckoned, as it offered self-expression in leadership or in occupation, the right to earn a home, or the benefit of alms.

Monastic houses for women grew in number with the prevailing need for protection and the progress of Christianity. Their founders were, commonly, women of influence. Many were allied with royal courts, some were daughters of powerful, converted barbarians, and often they had been accustomed to such luxury and were possessed of such education as were known in their time. Great properties were brought to the church, and numerous women became heads of great institutions. These women were known as *abbesses* or mothers. Frequently, abbesses assumed control of so-called "double monasteries" composed of men and women. In England, especially, this type was common, and a wall might be built through the middle of the church that the sight of one another might not divert the worshipers from their devotions, or a cemetery might separate their houses. Monks as well as nuns took the vow of obedience, and history honors the abbess for her success in handling what must have been a very difficult situation. Records also indicate her skill as an executive who developed orderly institutions. She was recognized as an equal by rulers and church authorities, and she managed business with financial acumen. She combined in herself the feudal lord and the churchman and shared the privileges of both. Often, she was a member of the Royal Council as an owner of land held direct from the king. The church gave her equality with the abbot. Some abbesses traveled extensively, some had literary talent, some were teachers or preachers. They enjoyed an unusual freedom of action during the earlier stage of social recovery, but their sun was already setting before the end of the tenth century.

Of the many abbesses who with their nun associates availed themselves of this new opportunity which Christianity offered women for usefulness to society, we shall mention only one who belonged to this period of the early Middle Ages—*Radegunde of Poitiers*. Radegunde (? –587), a barbarian queen, fled from a husband who, after many other cruelties, had just murdered her brother. Pursued by the king's knights, she managed to make her way to Poitiers where she took refuge in the Christian Church. Here, in sanctuary, none could harm her. She persuaded the bishop to consecrate her to religion and, becoming a nun, devoted life and property to a convent which she established. Here two hundred nuns assisted her in care of the poor and the sick. The leper's misery already had caught her sympathy, and, now that she was free to do so, she made him her especial charge.

Convent Dress   The abbess was not the only member of her community who enjoyed freedom of movement as travel became possible. Nuns of these early times were not wholly withdrawn from the world. Some of them lived at home; not all of them took vows. No distinctive dress was required, or, probably, thought of until circumstances arose which seemed to make it necessary. The monastic ideal of humility pointed to the use of plain, coarse materials in clothing, an ideal further encouraged by the poverty of many of the earliest convents. Convent women spun the wool and wove the cloth for their garments. A criticism made about the seventh century has survived the ages, and accuses nuns of paying too much attention to the making of fine clothes.

In the eighth century is heard a murmur regarding the freedom which permits English abbesses to leave the homeland and travel about the continent. To the same period belongs the following description of a sample of convent garb as thus far developed: "A vest of fine linen of a violet colour is worn, above it a scarlet tunic with a hood, sleeves striped with silk and trimmed with red fur; the locks on the forehead and temples are curled with a crisping iron, the dark head-veil is given up for white and coloured head-dresses which, with bows of ribbon sewn on, reach down to the ground; the nails, like those of a falcon or sparrow-hawk, are pared to resemble talons."[1]

In itself, the costume probably reflected only the fashion among aristocratic women of its time, and the wearers had but carried the ideas of their social set into convent life. Many of them, too, were not far removed from the barbaric state, and the asceticism which would appeal to a jaded Roman was yet beyond their understanding. The significance of the dress lies in the fact that its incongruity with monasticism attracted notice, and criticism of it prepared the way for that ultimate reform which ended in uniformity. This was still a long way off, for it is more than four hundred years later that we hear of a monk who recommended distinctive dress for religious women, and in the writings of an abbess find suggestion of a uniform headgear in the white turban with veil of red or purple worn by the nuns of her convents. Even they seem to have been free to choose the dress that accompanied veil and turban.

The veil as an adjunct of woman's dress has a long history. As a

[1] Quoted in "The Lady" by Emily James Putnam. New York and London, G. P. Putnam's Sons, 1921, p. 85.

means of keeping evil spirits away from brides, a relic of ancient custom which made a woman don it to distinguish her in her married state, and as part of convent dress, its symbolism has been that of humility, obedience, and service. After being accepted by all nations of the ancient world, it gradually came to mean that the bride, forsaking all others, guarded her charms for her husband. By the time of the Roman Empire, custom demanded that, while in public, ladies conceal their hair with veils or caps, and prescribed such distinguishing features as a red veil or veil with red stripes for the newly married woman. Veils of Turkish, Hindu, and Arabian women were to be removed only in the presence of their immediate families.

Within the walls of the church, Christian women veiled their heads. As the custom grew, added regulations in regard to the use of veils began to appear. According to social position, all women wore them, those of queens sweeping to the floor, those of plebeians reaching only to the waist. Among religious orders, where they came to be part of the prescribed habit, they are still worn, and, although veils of different types are accorded to nuns in the various stages of their service, the veil of probation of the novice is always white. In another form it is worn by nurses in many European countries, and by Red Cross workers everywhere. The cap of the modern nurse is a modification of it, and is even yet associated with humility and the rendering of service to mankind.

In spite of criticisms heaped upon them, as schools for the upper class of women, convents were earning that social prestige which they carried until replaced by the modern college. To have been educated in a convent meant that a woman had the influence of the refinement of her time, and acquired what was fashionable in manners and accomplishment.

FEUDALISM AND CHIVALRY

Modified by Christian ideals the ancient system known as *feudalism* began to take its place side by side with monasticism in western Europe. Imperial Rome had lent encouragement to the development of a class of gentlemen farmers who gradually acquired control of the major part of agricultural land. When the dissolution of the state left the greater part of the populace adrift, it was natural that these

Romans should seek protection from great landlords, many of whom had retired permanently to country life. It was natural, too, that powerful barbarians should set up similar estates, and that later barbarian kings should parcel out land to favorite subjects. Such a land grant was known as a "fief" or "feud" on the continent, while in England it went by the name of "manor."

Before 1000 A.D., there were scattered all over the continent of Europe cooperative farming units, isolated from each other and governed by individuals known as lords, knights, earls, counts, or barons. Kings nominally owned the land and these warrior lords held it in fief or feud. The central government of each kingdom was yet in its infancy and supported no standing army. The provision of a fighting force was left to the landlords, whose serfs abandoned the soil whenever called upon to do so. Abbots and abbesses, as heads of monastic organizations which often held lands in fief, had to meet the same obligation by maintaining similar forces of armed men, and monks at times were called upon to fight.

In general, soldiers comprised groups from three distinct classes— *knights, freehold tenants,* and *serfs* or *villeins.* Knights were members of the upper stratum of society, holding land in fief from the king. In the next stratum were freeholders who owned smaller pieces of land, and below these were the serfs or villeins who were assured of home, subsistence, and protection, but had only enough independence to place them in a stage between slavery and freedom to which feudalism had raised the masses. They were bound to the land, and when the land was sold they transferred their allegiance to the new owner. Each had a home in a village group, and an apportionment of a strip or several strips of land. When not engaged in fighting, in tilling the land reserved by the lord for himself, or in household duties at the castle, the serf was able to cultivate the little farm allotted to him.

Wherever he chose to live, the landlord built his home. In early feudal times it was a very simple dwelling patterned after the castella built by Romans for the use of officers on frontier service. Its purpose was to provide shelter and protection for the family of the lord, and a place of safe retreat for the families of his serfs who lived in the village outside its encircling wall. The location chosen for the castle was the most inaccessible spot on the manor, usually

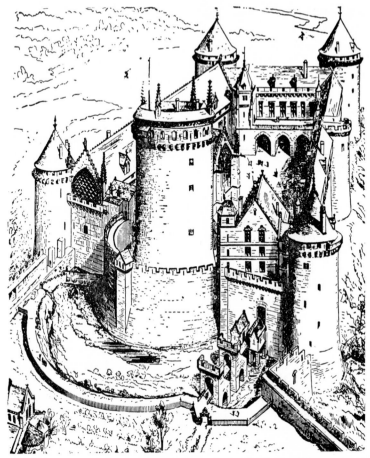

A CASTLE OF NORTHERN FRANCE BUILT IN THE THIRTEENTH CENTURY

A restoration by Viollet-le-Duc. (Gertrude Hartman, "Medieval Days and Ways," by permission of The Macmillan Company, publishers.)

high up on the edge of a rocky precipice from which could be had a view of the land from all sides. Castles in the early days of feudalism were of wood or stone, built with thick walls and surrounded by a water-filled ditch or moat, outside of which ran a second, strong, palisade-like wall. At intervals along this wall were towers for purposes of fortification. From the entrance on the second floor, a drawbridge to connect castle with mainland could be lowered or withdrawn at will.

The living quarters of the lord and his family in some respects resembled the ancient Roman home. Individual rooms, however, which ranged along the sides of the old atrium were absent from the castle. The common living room was called the *great hall*, and a chapel and two large rooms led off from it. The rooms were used as sleeping quarters, one for men, and the other for women and children. Neither group enjoyed any privacy. In the great hall, a huge fireplace gave warmth and served also as a cookstove. Here, too, was the bed of the lord and his lady, used by day as a couch. Around the walls were chests concealing household equipment, and serving also as seats. A dining table made of planking on trestles had seats of planking about it. Light entered the room through narrow slits cut in the deep walls, and covered with oiled cloth. The floor was carpeted with rushes, one layer on top of another as they were renewed but not changed.

Life in these first feudal castles was hazardous, and necessarily without luxury. The fine carvings, beautiful works of art, magnificent tapestries and elaborate furniture that we associate with great stone castles of many stories, belong to the latter part of the Middle Ages. Likewise, the lady of early days was far from being an idle, pleasure-loving beauty. Her lord loved war beyond everything, and barbarian tradition, like that of primitive Romans, pointed toward occupation for women. Her days were full of hard work. She had to be capable of supervising the establishment from one end to the other. She had to understand cooking, sewing, weaving, spinning, general farming. She had to bear and care for children, ride and hunt like a man, and command soldiers, or fight herself, if that was necessary. Her knowledge of home remedies for all kinds of illness had to be extensive, and she was called upon to nurse family guests, or villagers, as need arose. First aid and surgical emergencies were all in her day's work. She was doctor and nurse combined. In the absence of organized charity, the duty of providing for the poor devolved upon her also. Her very name indicated this responsibility, for "lady" is a word the derivation of which means "she who looks after the loaf," while "lord" means "loaf-giver." His frequent absences interfered with his assumption of this duty so much that his lady became well known as his representative in good works.

Isolation and circumstances which kept up social disturbance favored the independence of warring lords. Gradually they assumed the status of a privileged class, whose members were individually distinguished by feats of prowess. As generation after generation of bold fighting men added to the glory of a family, that family learned to have pride in its blood, and tried to stress to its children their obligation to maintain the record of achievement. Desirable marriages were arranged for girls and boys, sometimes in their infancy; boys were taught all the skills that would make them fearless soldiers. Fiefs and manors gradually became hereditary.

Very slim excuses underlay a long succession of petty conflicts which induced famine and disease through neglect of agriculture, and interfered with all attempts to bring about social recovery. The Church, which had always stood for justice and peace, took hold of the situation. A general feeling of need for systematic development in youth of ideals of soldierly conduct and ambitions gave it opportunity. Christian fathers helped to outline what became an accepted code for living the good life of their times, which ultimately went by the name of "chivalry" (from *caballus*, a horse—the ideal knight appears as a warrior on horseback). The system served the end of bringing the lordly class under the authority of the Church, while it infused their group with ideals of constructive living and refined manners. Service to God came before service to his earthly lord in the heart of every true knight. Elaborate ceremonies, in time, indicated the steps of his progress, and routine training took the place of home instruction.

By the end of the tenth century some progress had been made toward social recovery, but two privileged groups had arisen, represented by the monk and the feudal lord. The former was being weakened by ease as wealth was acquired and discipline was relaxed to favor prominent persons who wished to enter monastic life. The latter kept the continent in confusion through his determination to stick to the occupation he preferred, that of fighting. Agriculture suffered from the absence of his laborers; famine and disease accompanied the lack of nutrition that resulted from lack of food or from poor food. Farm animals became poor in quality and the bulk of meat was pork, fresh or salted. Few vegetables could be grown, for the women had all that they could do to keep other industries going. Some way had to be found to direct energies of the upper class into more useful channels, and the beginning of the latter half of the Middle Ages will find the soldier knight assuming a religious character and becoming a soldier monk, with a purpose that carries him far from his own land, for the rise of another religion threatened Christianity.

GUILDS

The third form of protective unit which aided recrystallization of society was to be seen in the *guild*, another institution derived from the past. In conformance with the needs of the time, it took on new characteristics, and became the first organization of workmen formed for the purpose of mutual benefit. This new form of guild united individuals not attached to monastic or feudal groups. It reached its height about the twelfth century, and in it lay the seed of the modern labor union, and of professional organizations as well.

When monasteries and manors had set up their orderly units of society and made it possible to bring about some revival of trade, they emerged somewhat from isolation. Markets grew up outside the manor as they had outside the monastery. Goods were peddled about the country and exchange of wares gradually increased. Great fairs for the display and exchange of goods came to be events of importance to both institutions. Merchants then formed *merchant guilds* or societies which protected members as they traveled roads now made even more dangerous by robber bands. Help was advanced to families if need arose. After a brief life, merchant guilds split up into *craft guilds*, each of which represented one type of skilled workmanship. *Religious guilds* also came into existence.

Craft guilds gave encouragement to good work by a system of inspection, as well as by dismissal from membership of the inadequate or careless. Guild leaders held the title of master which they won by producing a piece of work of outstanding excellence, or by spending several years under the direction of a master workman. Under the *master* worked *apprentices* and *journeymen*. Apprentices were youths whose fathers paid a fee for their admission to the privilege of learning a trade. They lived in the home of the master,

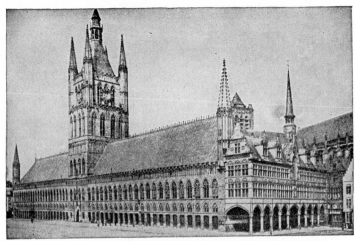

HALL OF THE CLOTHMAKERS' GUILD AT YPRES, BELGIUM
One of the most beautiful guildhalls in Europe. (Gertrude Hartman, "Medieval
Days and Ways," by permission of The Macmillan Company, publishers.)

worked at a specific craft for a period which was gradually lengthened to seven years, and received in return for their labor—which
grew continually more skilled—board, lodging, clothing, and more
or less character training. Discipline was usually very strict, and the
group was divided into seniors and juniors. It is a matter of record
that in one master's house, at meals no one but the senior could
speak without first having been spoken to by the master.

On completion of training, the apprentice became a journeyman.
The name is derived from a French word meaning "day" (journée),
and derives its use from the fact that the journeyman was free to
earn regular wages in employment by the day outside the master's
home. He frequently lived there, however, and paid his way by work
done between times. When he had passed his examination and had
enough money to set up his own establishment, he became a master.
The degree of Master of Arts, still awarded by universities, is a
survival of the system which gave him his title.

Regular assemblies became a characteristic of these guilds, and
rules were passed which aimed toward fair play among members
and advancement of crafts and wages. Because night work by candle
light was likely to be poorly done, it was forbidden. So also was

work on holidays or Sundays. Craft guilds cared for the old and feeble among their members, furnished funeral expenses, and pensioned widows. Sometimes they built hospitals for the sick, or endowed chapels in which masses were sung for deceased craftsmen.

Two dangers which proved definite evils in later times lay in the opportunity for securing preferment for certain crafts which organization opened up, and in the system of apprenticeship which the craft guild developed in order to train members for their work. The former ended in monopoly; the latter, introduced to fulfill a necessary function of education, led to exploitation that brought great hardship to youth, and that modern ideas and modern systems of education have not been able to fully exterminate.

In the guild apprenticeship lies the origin of a system which has characterized the management of our schools of nursing down to the present day. The director of nursing in the capacity of "Master" has led the instruction of her apprentices or student nurses who, in return, give care to patients. In some countries, nurses graduated from a school have been permitted to remain in its residence and give their services to the hospital when not employed in private duty outside it—true journeywomen.

ISLAM, A RIVAL OF CHRISTIANITY

Even while feudalism and monasticism built up little strongholds for the succor of distraught inhabitants of a disintegrating empire, a new barbarian invasion was preparing to advance upon Europe from the southeast. Far away from western centers of civilization, on the arid desert of Arabia, were thousands of nomadic people who, strangely enough, would be called upon by fate to play a part in the work of regeneration. They, also, lived in small protective units which we know as tribes. Tribal life obscured individuality, for each man and woman lived only for the good of the group, and the clan name was applied to all. Patriarchal chiefs, or sheiks, took the part of rulers. While nature indulged a love of freedom and the open spaces, she had made subsistence difficult for these tribes, and a settled manner of life impossible for most of them. Few and far between were the fertile spots in her sandy wastes which offered the fruit of date palms as food, and water as drink, for themselves and their horses and camels and flocks of sheep.

Oases became the cause of frequent dispute over right of occupancy or use, and petty warfare over property, or blood feuds exacting a life for a life were part of everyday existence. Distance, deep sand underfoot, and frequent sandstorms, forced the *Arabs*, as they were called, to resort to travel by camelback or horseback. Their riding of horses was unrivaled, and the animals that they bred were of an unusual hardiness, beauty, and swiftness. The merciless desert in which they lived made them enduring but merciless, too. Where heat and storm could suddenly leave men without food or home, they used their wits to snatch what came within their grasp, with no compassion for murdered men, or, under unusual stress, little sentiment for ties of blood. The following quotation from a poet of the seventh century explains the Arab's point of view:

> "You who admire the life of the city dwellers,
> What think you of us, the sons of the open desert?
> You may jog the streets on asses; we have our chargers,
> Clean-limbed, and our lances, strong and keen for plunder.
> When times are straitened, we raid the clans of Dabba;
> Then he whose time has come to die—he dies!
> Ay, it may happen to us to raid our brethren,
> When for our need no other foe comes handy."[2]

Outside of raising flocks of sheep and herds of camels, when they could do so, the principal business of these people, and their amusement as well, was the robbing of camel caravans of merchandise plying between cities and villages developed by their more civilized brethren, or by men of neighboring lands. The city of Mecca held a shrine to which they made pilgrimage for the worship of a sacred stone, black in color, and probably a meteorite, which had long held place in a cube-shaped temple known as the "Kaaba." In Mecca, too, and in Medina, great fairs were held which gave the desert dwellers opportunity to engage in trading. For four months each spring, a truce was called to warfare so that all might make the most of this excursion.

About 570 A.D., there was born in the city of Mecca a child of Arabia who was to be the first and only prophet of a new world religion. His father, one of a tribe of merchant men, gave him the name, *Mohammed*. The family was not rich, but the tribe to which

[2] Quoted in "Mediaeval Europe by Thompson and Johnson. New York, W. W. Norton & Co., Inc., 1937, p. 154.

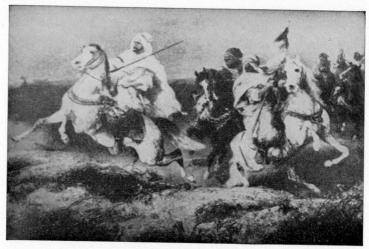

ARABS IN THE DESERT
(Courtesy of the Metropolitan Museum of Art.)

it belonged was possessed of considerable influence and power, and the son, who was orphaned early, is thought to have been trained to follow the caravan business in which its members were interested. As a young man, Mohammed was engaged by a rich widow of this tribe to manage a caravan for her, and so satisfactory was his work and so pleasing his personality that the widow became his wife. Her devotion to him led her to encourage rather than hinder a certain abstraction in religion which increased as time went on. It became his practice to withdraw frequently from the life about him and give himself up to meditation. He is thought to have sought to learn what he could about the religions of those who were not of his countrymen, and it was easy for a trading Arab to contact men of varied beliefs. The Byzantine Empire was Christian, and Constantinople was a principal commercial city. Egypt, Syria, Mesopotamia, and Palestine were penetrated in search of business. The Hebrew people, in particular, found caravan trade attractive and Jerusalem was the terminal of a trade route.

Later developments in Mohammed's life have led to the belief that he spent a good many years in such analysis of religions as was possible to one of his educational limitations, for these were considerable. Not until the age of forty did he begin to speak publicly on the subject dearest to him—a faith which would unite his countrymen and give them a better ordered life. When he did, indifference was his reward for trying to improve Arabia, and he finally left Mecca and took up his abode in Medina. Here, his success was not marked until he enlisted the interest of the wildest of Arab tribes known as "Bedouins." Mohammed's ideas appealed to Bedouins, especially as peace was so far from his ideal that it became their religious duty to force upon indifferent Mecca and commercial Medina a religion which their citizens had refused to accept. Desert Arabs were fighters, and Mohammed further sent them forth to fight a holy war, attacking throughout the world all infidels who refused to come into submission to the will of Allah, the God singled out by him from ancient Arabian deities for sole worship. "There is no God but Allah, and Mohammed is his prophet" ran the creed he offered. Mecca was conquered, and Medina, too. They went on into the Byzantine Empire, to Egypt, northwest Africa, to Spain and France, where at last their further progress was halted by the Christians a century after Mohammed's death.

Already, in 637 A.D., these Moslem zealots had laid hands on Jerusalem, thereby arousing among Christians the world over a horrified and helpless resentment. As Mecca was to the Arabs, so Jerusalem was to Christians a place of pilgrimage, the lodestar of Christendom. Nevertheless, Moslem mosques now arose for new worshipers, and a new religion held sway over this holy city for over four and a half centuries, although Arabs did not always rule.

Elements of the Religion What was this religion that could so speedily unite a disunited people, be spread so far as to make itself a dangerous rival of medieval Christianity, and be embraced today by twenty million followers? It is true that uncertainties of life in a desert which, periodically, failed to supply the barest necessities of food and drink, had already led numbers of nomadic residents of Arabia to seek better fortune in the Fertile Crescent to the north, and even in lands beyond it. To the smouldering discontent with hardship which was felt by those left behind, Mohammed had added the spark of religious enthusiasm. At his command they abandoned primitive gods and native animism, surging forth in thousands to spread the will of Allah, which his prophet interpreted for them.

Submission to this will was the core of the religion that Mohammed taught, and from this basic ideal it took its name "Islam" (surrender—to the will of Allah). Its followers called themselves "Moslems" (submitters).

The Koran Through Mohammed, the civil as well as the religious life of Moslems was directed. His teachings were written down, but not until thirty years after his death were they incorporated in the book known as the "Koran," now recognized as the Bible of Moslems. Following the precedent of Moses, Mohammed formulated rules for achievement of the good life. Gambling, lying, the charging of excessive rates of interest on borrowed money, wine-drinking, uncleanliness, and the eating of unclean food were sins to be shunned. Kindliness, honesty, hospitality, forgiveness of injury, almsgiving, cleanliness, and the eating of prescribed foods were virtues. No one could pray to Allah without first washing his hands. Sand would do for this purpose if there was no water to be had. Human beings anywhere might follow requirements as simple as those outlined for Moslems. No confusing array of gods had to be pleased. For one month out of each year believers were required to fast, and at five stated times each day they must address themselves directly to Allah in prayer. At these times they were required to prostrate themselves upon the ground but always with face turned toward Mecca. This city, which had been holy to Arabs and to their fathers, was still to be the shrine of pilgrimage, and as followers of Islam they might still kiss the black stone of the Kaaba. Indeed, under Allah's command, they were to make a pilgrimage to the shrine at least once in a lifetime.

Mohammedan Mosques Islam was a religion which could be practiced without temples, but simple platforms appeared soon in its history. To each of these a wall was attached, and so placed as to point the way to Mecca. Worshipers faced this wall in prayer. As time went on, platform and wall gave way to a building with domed roof which was known as a "mosque." The mosque itself might be adapted from a church built for followers of another religion. Nearby, one or more slender tower-like structures had their place, and were called "minarets" because they resembled lighthouses. A stairway inside of each of these led to a balcony or balconies high on the outside from which an official known as a *muezzin*, five times each day, called believers to pray to Allah:

"Allah is Almighty . . . Allah is Almighty . . . I witness that there is no other God but Allah . . . I witness that Mohammed is his prophet . . . Come to prayer . . . come to prayer . . . come to the house of praise, Allah is Almighty . . . Allah is Almighty . . . There is no God but Allah."[3]

The design of the interior was simple, the chief requirements being a recess facing Mecca and a pulpit from which a second official read the Koran. Mats or rugs covered the floor. These and other appointments varied greatly in richness, and much finely wrought silver and gold were sometimes used in lamps and ornaments.

Thus, in a brief space of time, and with minimum change in custom, a great revolution was brought about in the land of desert dwellers. Religion brought isolated and individual tribes together in common ways of thinking and living, and gave them a common aim. Islam was not hard to understand and fighting was much more intriguing than the difficult search for the barest kind of living which had heretofore been their lot. Conquest offered and brought them wealth. In a little over a century after the Bedouins undertook to spread Mohammed's teachings, not only had a Moslem empire sprung into being, but pilgrimage to Mecca of thousands of converts from many parts of the world was beginning to alter the face of society at large. Ideas were exchanged, people knew each other better, and an international language was found in Arabic, for translation of the Koran was not permitted and Moslems from everywhere must memorize it from their own reading.

All this serves to bring out a constructive quality not observed at first in militant Islam. Otherwise, empire building would not have been possible. As a matter of fact, Moslem military methods gave way, as time went on, to more peaceful ones such as the levy of taxes on those who clung to other faiths, and exemption from taxation of those who accepted Islam. The fearless riders of swift horses whose shining blades of Damascus steel had stricken terror into people of many lands doubtless realized the foolishness of destroying those things which made civilization different from the barren life

3 Lamb, Harold: The Flame of Islam. Reprinted by permission of Doubleday, Doran & Co., Garden City, New York. Page 11.

of the desert, and, in any case, time, association, and the responsibilities of rule develop tolerance. Besides, they were interested in what other people did, and with uncluttered minds absorbed readily all kinds of knowledge.

Medicine and Science under Islam   Eventually many of the sciences, and particularly that of medicine, entered into the debt of Islam. As people in the West tended to discard the teachings of Hippocrates and Galen and to revert to superstition, the responsibility for advancement of science shifted eastward. Moslems, Moors, Saracens, or Mohammedans, as they variously have been called, assumed the responsibility with eagerness. While Christian fathers held on to what they could of Galen, and labored to make barbarians ready to contribute their share to world progress, the Caliphs, who succeeded to leadership of Islam on the death of Mohammed in 632 A.D., began to find time and opportunity to encourage learning, including that associated with the practice of medicine. Hippocrates and Galen were translated into Arabic.

To this Islamic interest in learning, medicine owes a great deal. Physiology and hygiene were studied, and an extensive materia medica developed. Although Moslem belief in the uncleanliness of the dead forbade dissection, surgeons practiced, and learned to use hyoscyamus, cannabis indica and opium as anesthetics. Scholars from various countries profited by the opportunity offered them by Arabs. Great physicians were produced, the following Persians among them: *Rhazes* (860–932) who contributed material of lasting value on measles and smallpox, as well as an encyclopedia of medicine; *Hunayn*, an oculist who translated parts of Hippocrates and Galen, and *Avicenna* (980–1037) who wrote a "Canon of Medicine," in use for centuries after his death. In this medical treatise love has a place among the mental or cerebral diseases, where it finds company with insomnia, amnesia, mania, hydrophobia, and melancholia.

With advancing knowledge of medicine, great hospitals were built, probably after the Hindu model, and those of Bagdad and Cordova became famous. We hear of women working in them, but instruction seems not to have gone beyond bedmaking. In the following description is conveyed a sense of beauty as well as of a scope of institutional development which brought into combination in these Moslem hospitals, educational facilities, a technic of isolation for communicable diseases, dispensaries, and a system of care of the patient which overlooked neither the spiritual nor mental aspect and concerned itself with his capacity to earn a livelihood after discharge:

"It possessed four courts, each having a fountain in the center; lecture halls, wards for isolating certain diseases, and dispensaries for out-patients were also found. Among the most novel attractions was a hall where musicians played day and night and another where story-tellers were employed for the benefit of those who suffered from insomnia. Those religiously inclined could listen to the reading of the Koran, which went on day and night uninterruptedly in certain rooms. Each patient, upon being discharged from the hospital as cured, received some gold pieces that he might not be obliged to attempt hard labor at once."[4]

Status of Women under Islam   The position of the Moslem on the status of women is definitely stated in the Koran as follows:

"Men shall have the preeminence above women, because of those advantages wherein God hath caused the one of them to excel the other, and for that which they expend of their substance in maintaining their wives. The honest women are obedient, careful in the absence of their husbands, for that God preserveth them, by committing them to the care and protection of the men."

Certainly, neither desert life nor a warlike religion could offer much to woman outside her all too uncertain home. Commonly, education was denied her, and her husband chosen for her. Marriage was her duty, and fruitfulness her glory. If she proved faithless, she could be beaten. Polygamy to the limit of four wives was permissible, but no woman might have more than one husband at a time. Divorce was denied a wife, while her husband could secure it on slight grounds, and with the privilege of taking her back as often as twice after such separation.

On the other hand, Mohammed improved woman's position in some respects. He forbade infanticide, and made parents include daughters in the privilege of inheritance. It is even said that a few rich women were permitted to learn to read the Koran. Virtuous, obedient Moslem women shared with virtuous men the prospects of Paradise, and were given added happiness in the assurance of the prophet that death would endow all the old or homely among them with perpetual beauty. Nevertheless, woman's care during childbirth

4 Quoted in "Four Thousand Years of Pharmacy" by Charles H. LaWall, Philadelphia, J. B. Lippincott Co., 1927, p. 115.

and in case of gynecological disease remained as it had been, traditionally, in the hands of untaught midwives.

CHARLEMAGNE PROMOTES SOCIAL RECOVERY THROUGH EDUCATION

When people feel the need of support, they sink their individuality in cooperative groups. When the opportunity to recover independence arrives, they seize it, and declare their individual identity again. We have seen society in Europe left almost wholly without central government, and reverting for social security to feudalism, monasticism, and a system of guilds for those unprotected by either of these institutions. At the same time, the continent was splitting up into a number of kingdoms under barbarian rulers of various tribes, nominally under allegiance to the eastern division of the empire of old Rome. By the eighth century it was apparent that many weak kings far removed from the government responsible for their acts and policies, and many ambitious lords who did as they pleased, would never solve the problems following the barbarian seizure of the west. A strong central authority was the key to solution, and centralization meant grouping of kingdoms and the return of empire.

This imperial consolidation was the work of Charlemagne (Charles the Great), one of the outstanding figures in history, and sometimes called the "Hero of the Middle Ages." By 800 A.D., the whole territory from the Rhine to the Atlantic had been brought under his control, and a forceful and charming, but ignorant, barbarian Frank had become a new emperor in the West. Charlemagne began a series of reforms in administration which indicate his innate capacity for business as well as government, and his high conception of justice. In order to strengthen the monasteries which had lost some of their earlier virility through hurried growth and acceptance of novices of little or no education, he applied himself to the study of St. Benedict's famous Rule, and later ordered it to be introduced into all of these institutions.

Wholly untutored himself, Charlemagne took lessons in grammar and in writing. He learned to speak Latin and understand Greek, and is said to have slept with a tablet under his pillow that he might practice the formation of letters in script. His recognition of the influence of education in promoting civilization, however, led him to encourage the work of scholarly men. One of these, an English monk named *Alcuin*, became attached to the imperial court, and there started what has become famous as the "Palace School," and the center of revived interest in learning. The emperor himself became a student here, as also did the sons of many of his lords. Any children, rich or poor, whose ability was brought to his attention, were given the privilege of education with children of the official group. Teachers came chiefly from monasteries, for numerous scholars had been freeing themselves from the cloister to wander abroad.

The success of the Palace School, together with the stimulus of Charlemagne's encouragement, reflected itself in new intellectual development in monastic circles, where hurried growth and the reception of ignorant novices were lowering former standards. Many more of these institutions began to conduct schools for children in their neighborhood. Manuscripts were added to libraries, and a more legible form of writing introduced into the scriptoria where correct Latin also replaced the corrupted form used in many texts of the time. Here and there, throughout the land, men began to produce new literature as well as to preserve the old, and to translate into tribal dialects those books which would help to Christianize pagan peoples.

The period following the death of Charlemagne in 814, up to the end of the tenth century, was one of retrogression. Warfare among the lords and new barbarian invasions upset much of what had been accomplished in the way of social restoration in Europe since 500 A.D. The young Carolingian empire fell apart. Increased power passed into the hands of the lords as the people learned to rely upon their armies for protection. The huge fortified castle became typical of the later Middle Ages. Nevertheless, Charlemagne's educational and literary influence outlasted his political achievement. During the tenth century his method of spreading public enlightenment, through education of youth, was used in England by King *Alfred the Great*.

MEDICINE AND NURSING

The inundation of western Europe by barbarism which happened in the latter part of the fifth century brought to a standstill any scientific advance in medicine. Primitive people brought primitive beliefs and habits with them. They destroyed books, they upset public hygiene, and they made wretched the life of the man who wished to devote himself to learning. If they could do so, studious men of all professions fled to Constantinople where scholarship still throve and conditions of life were little disturbed. If they could not, they sought the peace to be found in monasteries.

In the West, monasteries and feudal estates could not immediately expand to their ultimate organization as social units. Meantime, even the provisions made by Romans for public hygiene through sewers, water systems, and public baths were ignored, and these utilities were destroyed or allowed to fall into disrepair. The teachings of Hippocrates and Galen were lost sight of, and talismans, incantations, amulets, charms, astrology, and primitive media from as many sources as there were races, were restored to favor in treatment of disease.

In monasteries, monks and nuns, confronted with the task of giving medical care to large numbers of sick people outside their cloisters, had to find a way to do it. Manuscripts which they secured were copied, used in teaching, and preserved, while books were compiled of recipes, plants useful as drugs, and commonly used home remedies. The foundations laid by Hippocrates and Galen were retrieved in part, but to the greater number of those in the monastic life, a lack of preparatory schooling made their works incomprehensible, and no further progress was made along scientific lines. The ascetic was busied with many things, and his chief interest lay, not in bodily welfare, but in religion and the safety of the soul.

It was inevitable that such scientific medicine as was acquired should be corrupted by the prevailing practices in the society of their time. Patients, then as now, had preconceptions as to treatment. In the passing centuries Roman, as well as more primitive superstitions, crept into it. Medicine became a corruption of science, superstition, and magic. Theology and philosophy absorbed the minds of learned men, and the century preceding the advent of Charlemagne passed into history as the darkest of the Middle Ages. A short-lived revival of medicine, due to his interest, did not stay its downward trend.

In the eastern division of the old Empire, interest in science was little disturbed by happenings in the West. Jewish students continued to carry medicine to various parts of the known world. Translation of medical writings into Arabic enabled Moslems to return medical lore to Europe by way of Spain. Medicine's further advancement under either Moslem or Christian influence was hindered by restrictions placed on human dissection. The follower of Christ saw in the body a temple for the spirit which would live again after death. The church as an organization feared the responsibility of medical practice by monks whose mistakes might induce loss of public confidence and thereby retard their real work of Christianizing pagans.

Little distinction was made between medicine and nursing. The novitiate served by both monk and nun anticipated the probationary period or, as it is now known, the preclinical course of modern schools of nursing. Nuns studied the same works as monks, and in the monastic institutions they treated or nursed women, while monks treated and nursed men, mainly according to household tradition. Both spurred themselves on by an ideal of hard work as Christian work, and, like St. Jerome, Paula, Fabiola, Marcella and other famous ascetics who shunned no task, however disagreeable, they expiated sin and experienced personal uplift in service to God through service to man.

Isolation of feudal manors and monastic groups, together with a general cessation of travel, kept these free for a time from recurrent outbreaks of pestilence. Skin diseases due to faulty diet, which minimized the use of vegetables and made salt meat, especially pork, a chief food, became prevalent and were often confused with leprosy. As far back as the time of Jesus, the leper had held the sympathy of Christians, partly on account of his pitiable condition, partly from associating him with that Lazarus whose sores were referred to by the Master. St. Basil had arranged for his segregation from other patients in the xenodochium. Lazarettos are mentioned in western church history during the sixth century and, as time went on, they increased with spread of the disease. Nevertheless, the pathetic figure of a human outcast, forced to warn men of his approach by means of horn or bell, was a familiar sight which touched the hearts of queens and knights who went out of their way to give him alms.

As a major portion of the population retreated into isolated protective units, the free-moving nurse deaconess of an earlier day found her field restricted. She was able to continue her work only here and there. The dangerous quality of life, when Rome's protection was gone, inevitably idealized the security of nursing in a nunnery for the medieval girl. She, who at one time might have served as a deaconess, became a nun. The monastery brought into the nursing field the young man also. Nun and monk became, preeminently, the nurses of western society during the early Middle Ages. With the advent of feudalism, the lady of the castle, aided by nursing lore handed down to her by her mother, rendered corresponding service to the sick on her lord's estate. She nursed or supervised the nursing of the sick in her family or among tenants and serfs.

In the guilds, private donation at first, and, afterwards, general funds raised among members, provided nursing for those who needed it. In time these funds also built and supported hospitals. The isolation of these and of the feudal groups necessarily threw, upon each, responsibility for care of its sick. The burden of public charity and the nursing of the poor were gradually turned over to monasteries, although three famous hospitals are known to have been built outside of monastic walls. These were the Hôtel Dieu of Lyons in 542, the Hôtel Dieu of Paris in 650, and the Santo Spirito of Rome in 717 A.D. One bright spot in the general darkness surrounding medical practice was the birth of the first school of medicine at *Salerno* in Italy where men, and women, too, were helping to inaugurate a return to truth.

SUMMARY OF EARLY MIDDLE AGES

The early Middle Ages (500–1000 A.D.) in western Europe were characterized by fixity of population in small, isolated units. Invasions of barbarians which had destroyed the functioning of central government, and necessitated the formation of these protective units into which individuals could be gathered, did not stop with the fall of Rome. As long as they continued, and until a new form of government could be established, the ordering of life became a function of three great systems growing out of this grouping—the monastic system, the feudal system, and later, the guild system. Guilds developed as war died out, trade revived, and industry offered opportunities for individuals to detach themselves from groups once more.

Civilization in the eastern part of the old Roman Empire went on without the interruption that barbarism brought to the west. Roman authorities moved the capital to Constantinople which, obviously, could be only a nominal center of government for the west. East and West went separate ways.

About 570 A.D., Mohammed, herald of a religion threatening to Christianity, was born. He grew up to organize the people of Arabia in a great crusade to convert the world to Islam. Having conquered Christians in Palestine and nearby lands, the Arab Moslems, as they called themselves, swept over the north coast of Africa, and into Spain and France. France drove them out, but Spain became Moslem territory, and remained so until the end of the Middle Ages. Absorption of new cultures was a Moslem trait, and they distributed what they learned. One way in which they improved the culture of Spain was by developing intellectual centers around great libraries. Here they brought the works of Hippocrates and Galen. Great hospitals, well organized and well managed, were built. Women worked in them, but chiefly as bedmakers.

In 800 A.D. came a brief return to empire when Charlemagne united a number of kingdoms and was declared emperor by the Pope. He made many improvements, the most lasting of which was his contribution to the spread of learning. Charlemagne established a school in his palace for his own children and those of officials, as well as for any others, rich or poor, who might be recommended to him. He also made the Benedictine Rule the rule for all monasteries and ordered the establishment of schools for neighbor children in all of these institutions.

During the period under consideration the progress of medicine in the West was persistently down hill, until the university of Salerno was established in Italy about the end of it. The practice of medicine followed the care of the sick into the monasteries, where unprepared monks and nuns whose real interest lay elsewhere did the best they could with a smattering of scientific medicine and collections of recipes for home remedies. The herbal garden became a part of every monastery and, unavoidably, many superstitions, both Roman and barbarian, crept into the care of the sick, until it was difficult to differentiate medicine from magic. Meanwhile, in the East, the Arabs combined Greek scientific medicine with their own which was largely pharmaceutical, and brought it back to Europe through Spain.

During the early Middle Ages, the position of woman was lower than it had been in Rome. The grouping of people in protective units, the barbarian tradition of giving her hard manual work to do, and the absence of organized charity forced her back into the home. She had to marry young, and without her consent, and her chief value to society lay in her breeding powers and her ability to manage a home. The loopholes of deaconess and other church work were denied the pious among them, and they made their escape into the convent. Here, the abbess achieved considerable distinction.

TOPICS FOR DISCUSSION

1. (*a*) Describe conditions at the beginning of the Dark Ages which made it necessary to seek the protection of an established institution. (*b*) To what cooperative units could appeal for help be made?
2. Compare the novice and the novitiate of medieval monasteries with the pre-clinical student and pre-clinical period of a school of nursing.
3. If you had entered a Benedictine monastery as a novice, to what types of activities would your attention have been drawn, and what would have been some of the ethical principles that you would have had to learn?
4. Compare the three stages of service following the novitiate with those following the pre-clinical period.
5. What was the attitude of St. Benedict toward care of the sick?
6. Describe the daily routine of the average monk of the early Middle Ages.
7. Discuss the women of monasticism from the following standpoints:
   (*a*) Social status
   (*b*) Ability and position of abbesses
   (*c*) Manner of dress
8. Explain the statement that the arts, education, religion, medicine, and nursing were preserved in the monasteries through the disturbed conditions of the Middle Ages.
9. How did the activities carried on in the scriptoria affect the practice of medicine and nursing?
10. Do you think that the nurse's cap has any relationship to the veil as a part of woman's dress?

11. If you had belonged to a peasant family on a medieval manor, to whom could you look for care during illness?
12. What was the origin of chivalry, and what purpose did it serve?
13. Show how continuous warfare carried on by feudal lords, led to malnutrition and disease.
14. Compare the guilds of the Middle Ages with labor unions and with professional organizations.
15. Do you see any similarity between the organization of the craft guild and that of nursing in a modern hospital?
16. How did the name of the degree of "Master of Arts" originate?
17. What circumstances led to the establishment of Islam as a rival religion to Christianity?
18. How did the conquest of great territory by Moslem invaders affect the prevailing practice of medicine and nursing?
19. What two barbarian kings, and in what way, contributed to the recovery of civilization after the barbarian invasions resulting in the Fall of the Roman Empire in 476 A.D.?
20. Discuss medicine and nursing of the early Middle Ages.
21. Why is our system of nursing education considered to be largely of the apprenticeship type?
22. Make your own adaptation of the first part of the chart on page 200 and add a dotted line for the general trend in medicine.

REFERENCES

An Outline of Christianity—The Builders of the Church. New York, Bethlehem Publishers, 1926, Vol. III, Book III, Chaps. 17–28 inc.

Blair, D. Oswald H.: The Rule of St. Benedict. St. Louis, Mo., B. Herder, 1907.

Davis, William Stearns: Life on a Mediaeval Barony. New York, Harper & Brothers, 1923.

Hartman, Gertrude: Mediaeval Days and Ways. New York, The Macmillan Co.. 1937.

Hayes, Moon, and Wayland: World History. New York, The Macmillan Co., 1941.

LaWall, Charles H.: Four Thousand Years of Pharmacy. Philadelphia, J. B. Lippincott Co., 1927.

Myers, P. Van Ness: General History. New York, Ginn & Co., 1927.

O'Connor, John B.: Monasticism and Civilization. New York, P. J. Kenedy & Sons, 1921.

Scott, Sir Walter: The Monastery. New York, Funk & Wagnalls Co., 1900.

Thompson, A. H.: English Monasteries. New York, G. P. Putnam's Sons, 1913.

Thompson and Johnson: Medieval Europe. New York, W. W. Norton & Co., Inc., 1937.

Wells, H. G.: Outline of History. Garden City, New York, Garden City Publishing Co., 1931.

Wishart, Alfred Wesley: Monks and Monasteries. Trenton, New Jersey, Brandt Press, 1902.

Zahm, J. A.: From Berlin to Bagdad and Babylon. New York and London, D. Appleton & Co., 1922.

VI

The Late Middle Ages

Society Becoming Mobile;
Detachment of Individuals

The opening of the eleventh century shows western Europe still holding the foreground of the world picture by virtue of difficulties besetting it after monasticism and feudalism had helped it to take its first steps toward the gateway of a new and better social order. Less obvious and more subtle than organized grouping had been the social process of race fusion by intermarriage which had been going on for five centuries. Barbarian women had proved to be an unexpected influence in furthering the cause of Christianity, for this religion appealed to them. Savage like their men, they accepted harsh treatment as a matter of course, and were able to retaliate in kind. This did not hinder the men from respecting them and idealizing in them a spirit finer than their own. This appreciation helped, for as women adopted Christian ideals and a change came over their manners, many of them were able to induce men to become Christians also. Whole kingdoms often followed in the footsteps of a queen who had led her king away from pagan gods. The primary steps in replacing paganism and barbaric modes of life by Christianity and civilization had been taken. It was still too early to expect more than a partial change in barbarian outlook.

Meanwhile, some of the enthusiasm of early pioneer days had vanished from the monasteries. Feudal lords had checked barbarian invasions, and now kept up a petty warfare among themselves as a matter of entertainment as well as a satisfaction for ambition. The whole land had been cut up into a picture puzzle of little kingdoms which increased confusion by their efforts to find themselves. Many people made laws, but there was no central power which could enforce them. The church remained the chief guiding influence, and Christians who were guilty of sin did penance or made pilgrimages when they could.

PILGRIMAGES TO PALESTINE

Pilgrimages or journeys undertaken to places associated with persons or things assuming a sacred character from their association with beliefs, had been a means of expressing zeal among adherents of all religions. Pilgrimages to Palestine, with its treasury of association with the life of Christ, had begun soon after His Ascension. We have seen Jerome and Paula and others of the fourth century making this pilgrimage and prolonging their stay in order to improve conditions for other travelers in this foreign land, by providing hospices as temporary dwelling places, and giving care in hospitals to those overtaken by illness.

The pilgrimage as a source of contact between peoples of the world, and an expression of devotion to an ideal of things greater than themselves, had been denied all but a few Christians in Europe. Its increase with the passing of the Early Middle Ages indicated a returning opportunity to travel and a restlessness that took hold of men and women as the narrow limits of life began to wear upon them. An influence greater than either of these lay in the general belief that the year 1000 A.D. would see the end of the world.

The beginning of the Late Middle Ages saw pilgrims in great numbers on their way to Palestine once more. Merchants of Italy already were reaping economic advantages of a midposition on travel routes, and we find that country providing comforts at her ports, and establishing an inspection of ships to prevent overcrowding. The pilgrim who had reached an Italian port, however, had probably met and overcome dangers to which fellow travelers had succumbed. Highways throughout Europe were not only few in number, but they were in poor repair and infested with robbers. A journey on foot was a hazardous adventure. A few scattered hospitals were insufficient to take care of many overtaken by sickness or failing strength. Pilgrims took no heed of condition of body or purse when they set out to find the Holy Land, and no organization took heed of them except the monastery.

The Truce of God   Food constituted another problem. Under necessity of supplying food which they could not carry with them, pilgrims stole what they could, and ruined cultivation where it existed. The line of travel was kept in constant ferment by disputes among themselves or with tradesmen or farmers. All of these things only helped to infect the knightly class with a spirit of adventure, all the more potent because conditions which had made the feudal lord a necessity were changing. The Church, too, had revived its determination to bring about peace in the land, and about 1000 A.D., it introduced the "Truce of God," a restraint on warlike activities which threatened with punishment all who failed to follow restrictions set down as follows:

"All Christians, friends and enemies, neighbors and strangers, shall keep true and lasting peace one with another from vespers on Wednesday to sunrise on Monday, so that during these four days and five nights, all persons may have peace, and, trusting in this peace, may go about their business without fear of their enemies.

"In addition you should observe the peace in regard to lands and animals and all things that can be possessed. If anyone takes from another an animal, a coin, or a garment during the days of the Truce, he shall be excommunicated unless he makes satisfaction."[1]

To escape troubles and to prevent boredom, the knight, whose chief occupation and favorite pastime thus suffered unwelcome limitation, turned his eyes toward Palestine and allied himself with pious pilgrims traveling thither. He used his martial accomplishments for their protection.

The requirements of the Truce of God were not always obeyed, but one of its early and visible results was better cultivation of the neglected and ravaged land, and some improvement in living conditions. Important, also, was the chance that even intermittent cessation of hostilities gave the Church to find means of bringing into the hearts of a great child-like family the desire for peace.

Education for Knighthood   An increasing stress on education for knighthood now becomes apparent, and ethical ideals modify more and more the military objectives of feudalism. In the eleventh century, the education of the boy of noble family begins at seven. At twelve years of age he takes an oath before the bishop to defend the

[1] Lamb, Harold: The Crusades: Iron Men and Saints. Garden City, New York, Doubleday, Doran & Co., 1930, p. 30.

weak, and to protect women of noble birth. Patiently a new conception of knighthood is developed, one in which ethical qualities combine with physical prowess in an ideal of glorious achievement which
places the worth of general welfare beyond that of selfish ambition.
Eventually the noble youth goes from stage to stage of growth.
Ceremonies ever-increasing in brilliance mark his progress, until, at
twenty-one, he attains the goal of knighthood, and begins a career
with another goal set for him, for,

> "A truly perfect, gentle knight" was found "to fear God and maintain the
> Christian religion; to serve the King faithfully and valorously; to protect the
> weak and defenceless; to refrain from the wanton giving of offence; to live for
> honour and glory, despising pecuniary reward; to fight for the general welfare of
> all; to obey those placed in authority; to guard the honour of the knightly order;
> to shun unfairness, meanness and deceit; to keep faith and speak the truth; to
> persevere to the end in all enterprises begun; to respect the honour of women; to
> refuse no challenge from an equal and never to turn back upon a foe."[2]

The stimulus toward service to others which this new form of
education was bringing to the knight, and the general slowing up of
military operations, turned his energies more and more to the adventure of making the pilgrimage to Palestine. More and more, too,
did the everyday pilgrim have need of his protection, for, with the
advent of more settled conditions, the general public was beginning
to follow man's roving instinct again. Reviving trade as well as
religious enthusiasm encouraged it. Feudal lords bewailed the loss
of escaping serfs whom the law freed if they could elude pursuit for
a year and a day. Monasteries felt a corresponding dwindling of
population, for those least fitted to stand the dullness of their seclusion began to leave them also. The incidents of sickness and accident
and the profits of robber bands increased with the traffic on highways, forest-bordered, and with long, lonely stretches between
settlements.

WILLIAM THE CONQUEROR

While feudal lords of central Europe were satisfying their restlessness by adventurous pilgrimage toward Palestine, one of their number in the northwest part of what we call *France* was getting ready

---

[2] Quoted in "Mediaeval Europe" by Thompson and Johnson, p. 324, from
"Chivalry" by Prestage. London, Kegan Paul, Trench, Trubner & Co., Ltd.,
1928, p. 24.

to make history of his own. A Duke of Normandy, restless too, looked across the channel with covetous eyes. In 1066, *William the Conqueror* made the southern part of the island of Britain his own. England profited by continental experiences, for William set about organizing it under central government based on a system of taxation under his own control.

About twenty years after his arrival, in a book which has come down in history as the "Domesday Book," officials of William the Conqueror presented the results of a great inventory of property throughout his kingdom which made it possible for him to levy on each landowner, according to his possessions, money tribute to the state. The parchment volumes of this interesting document are still treasured in England, and form the basis of much genealogical concern, for the custom had arisen among feudal lords of distinguishing their armor-clothed bodies from each other in battle by wearing, on shield and cloak, a coat-of-arms representing a family name. These names in the Domesday Book were the origin of surnames and the foundation of great families of today. To have the name of an ancestor in the Domesday Book is proof of English aristocracy.

Matilda, wife of William the Conqueror, is supposed, also, to have been a contributor to the store of history of the island through skill in a feminine art of her time. A tapestry, said to have been woven by her hands and those of her court ladies, portrays the story of William's departure from Normandy, his landing in England, and the battle of Hastings in which he defeated Harold, king of the Anglo-Saxons. Colored wools were used on linen in the weaving of it, and the entire piece, following the pattern of old parchment rolls, is long and narrow, thirty yards by twenty inches. It is famous among antiques as the "Bayeux tapestry," and may be seen today in the town of Bayeux, France.

THE CRUSADES (1096–1271)

The eleventh century opened with Arabia enjoying the prestige of world power. South and east of the Mediterranean, the lands belonged to Moslems, and Spain also had fallen into their possession. Since 637 A.D., they had held the city of Jerusalem. In Bagdad, city of wealth, beauty, and culture, men already knew how to make paper and to use the compass. They had found in India a system of numerals which greatly simplified addition, subtraction, and multiplication, and later gave stimulus to western mathematics. They understood higher mathematics themselves, and their medicine and pharmacy were well developed.

The original Moslem empire, however, had weakened itself by splitting up into three sections, each under the rule of a different caliph. In turn, it now found itself attacked by invaders from Turkestan—wild and savage people who seized its eastern division, and with it the Holy City of Christendom, Jerusalem. Although they adopted Islam, the Seljuk Turks, as the new rulers were called, did not show the same tolerance to Christians as had the other Moslems. As knowledge of pilgrim troubles leaked out, the world was stirred to hatred and fear of the Turks, and when they appeared in the neighborhood of Constantinople, threatening it with destruction, the emperor of the old eastern division of the Roman Empire sent out to the west a call for help.

A new zeal for religion had been stirred up throughout Europe, and in the papal seat at Rome was a forceful, charming man whose education combined the ideals of chivalry with the stern solemnity of the monastery of Cluny where he had formerly been a monk. Urban II answered the appeal of the East by calling an assembly of several thousand people at Clermont, in France. This, in part, is what he said to them:

"From the borders of Jerusalem and the city Constantinople ominous tidings have gone forth. Often, before now, have they come to my ears. An accursed race, emerging from the kingdom of the Persians, a barbarous people, estranged from God, has invaded the lands of the Christians in the east and has depopulated them by fire and steel and ravage. These invaders are Turks and Arabs.

"Even now the Turks are torturing Christians, binding them and filling them with arrows, or making them kneel, bending their heads, to try if their swordsmen can cut through their necks with a single blow of a naked sword. What shall I say of the ravishing of women? To speak of this is worse than to be silent. You, in France, have heard the murmur of agony on the border of Spain. The time may come when you will see your wives violated and your children driven before you as slaves, out of the land.

"Come forward to the defense of Christ. O ye who have carried on feuds, come to the war against the infidels. O ye who have been thieves, become soldiers. Fight a just war. Labor for everlasting reward, ye who were hirelings, serving for a few solidi.

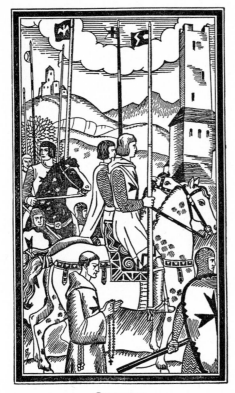

CRUSADERS

(From Reinach, Salomon: Orpheus—A History of Religions. New York, Live-right, Inc.)

"and more—whosoever shall offer himself to go upon this journey and shall make his vow to go, shall wear the sign of the cross on his head or breast."[3]

Urban's remarkable oratory moved the audience so that even before he had finished, they arose shouting. "Dieu lo vult!"—"God wills it." The pope then asked for volunteers, and to every man of these he issued a red cross which, as a soldier of Christ, he was to wear on his head or breast. "Dieu lo vult" suddenly became a battle-cry, and in 1096 the first of a long series of Crusades, or ex-

[3] Lamb, Harold: The Crusades: Iron Men and Saints. Garden City, New York, York, Doubleday, Doran & Co., 1930, pp. 39–41.

peditions of cross-bearers, set out for the Holy Land, to keep Jerusalem for Christians. In reference to mass movements of modern times, the crusading as well as the pilgrim movements of the eleventh century are comparable with the California Gold Rush of 1849, or with the World Wars I and II. Romance gave lustre to each venture, and a common aim united classes. Chivalry further enhanced the colorful march of medieval humanity. Troubadours sang songs. Lords and their knights rode the highways on splendid mounts, coats of mail jingled, and gay plumes floated from helmets glittering in company with shining shields and swords. More drab in attire, and often wearily, a motley throng of men, women, and children trudged on foot along the highway. Conditions of enfeebled health or age did not keep at home any who wanted to go. About all hovered sickness and death, but these were ignored for two reasons. Enthusiasm for the Christian religion had reached a peak, and men moved under the spell of a common spiritual impulse, their child-like hearts filled with child-like faith. At the same time, this unruly family of the Church had endured for five hundred years the repression of its native instinct for motion, and quickly discovered satisfaction in a general uncontrollable sweep toward the East.

ORDERS OF MILITARY NURSES

In an age when brigands infested forest-lined roads, and the sanitary precautions taken by Moses on a similar journey were unknown or overlooked, wounds and sickness soon became urgent in demands for attention. Crops failed as men abandoned the fields, or hungry Crusaders ruined them. The general nutrition was low, and multitudes in Europe and the East were exposed to contact with diseases for which they had no acquired immunity. Hundreds of thousands were dying on their way to Jerusalem. More hospitals and more nurses must be forthcoming. Existent xenodochia and monasteries were far apart and unable to fill the emergency in spite of heroic efforts to do so. Monasteries, too, declined in male population for many monks sought the activity of crusading experience.

Christianity and feudalism together worked out a solution of the problem. The Church promoted hospital construction, and cities and towns in time raised common funds to support city hospitals. Feudal knights assumed a large part of responsibility for relief of sickness and poverty in Europe as well as in Palestine. Nursing saw the introduction into its ranks of great numbers of men, for enormous institutions were founded and run by *military-monk* groups. Unavoidably, these brought into hospitals their military ideals. It was in Palestine that the influence of a change in hospital and nursing personnel was first introduced. This took place in two hospitals in Jerusalem, one for men, the other for women, that, as early as 1050, had been financed by private charity to meet the needs of pilgrims. They were named, respectively, the Hospital of St. John of Jerusalem, and the Hospital of St. Mary Magdalene.

Secular in the beginning, these hospitals took on a religious character, and became part of a monastery in which monks and nuns subscribing to the rule of St. Augustine did social work and nursing. So kindly was the spirit of these workers, who made no distinction between friends and enemies when help was needed, that sympathizers all over the world had already enriched their institutions with many gifts. Early in the twelfth century, necessity urged the monks of St. John of Jerusalem to serve the interests of Crusaders in an unusual way. Mounted on horseback, they began to ride out from the monastery to assist in battle with the Moslem. When the emergency passed they returned to continue with their work of nursing. In this dual role of warrior and nurse, they became known as *Knights Hospitallers.*

During the two centuries of warfare that comprise the Crusades, numerous orders of knights hospitallers met varying needs of the times, as rescuers of sick and wounded along the highways, in first-aid stations, or in hospitals. The order of *Knights Hospitallers of St. John of Jerusalem* remained the best known. A second famous order of hospitallers, founded late in the twelfth century, also had headquarters in Jerusalem, where a new hospital had risen about 1131 and been named the "Hospital of St. Mary of the Teuton." The monks who were nurses in this hospital formed the Order of the *Teutonic Knights Hospitallers.* A third and equally famous order of nursing monks confined its activities to the care of lepers, and derived its name, the Order of *Knights of St. Lazarus*, from the Lazarus mentioned in the New Testament as the object of Christ's sympathy.[4] Institutions known as "lazarettos" became fairly com-

4 St. Luke XVI: 19–31.

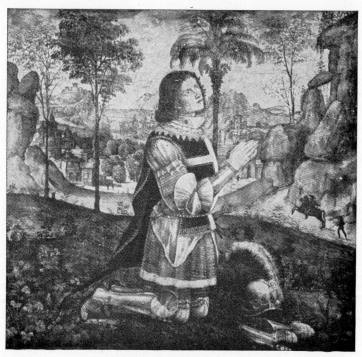

A KNIGHT HOSPITALLER OF ST. JOHN OF JERUSALEM

In armor with the tunic of the Order over his breastplate. Portrait in Chapel of St. John in Cathedral of Siena. (Painting by Alberto Aringhieri from Hume, Edgar Erskine: Medical Work of the Knights Hospitallers of Saint John of Jerusalem. The Johns Hopkins Press, Baltimore.)

mon. The hospitals now founded by the Knights Hospitallers of St. Lazarus took the same name. Many of their officers were lepers.

The soldier monk was to be for two centuries one of the outstanding figures in human society. His activities were by no means confined to Palestine, but orders originating there speedily spread over East and West. Orders of Hospitaller Sisters also developed in connection with some groups. Money, land, even principalities, often came under their control through bequests of grateful pilgrims or other sympathizers and great fortress-like hospitals began to arise wherever one of their branches was organized.

The youth of all Christian countries yearned for opportunity to

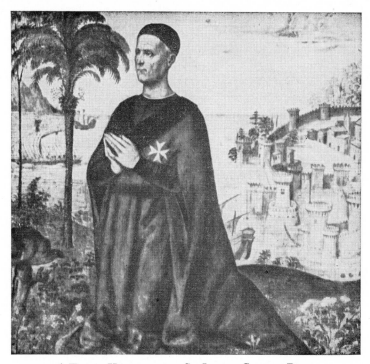

A KNIGHT HOSPITALLER OF ST. JOHN IN CONVENT DRESS

Portrait in Chapel of St. John in Cathedral of Siena. "In the background are seen the fortifications at Rhodes and some of the Hospitallers' galleys." (Painting by Alberto Aringhieri from Hume, Edgar Erskine: Medical Work of the Knights Hospitallers of Saint John of Jerusalem. The Johns Hopkins Press, Baltimore.)

join in work that appealed to youth's admiration of a uniform, its love of the adventurous, the chivalrous, of that ascetic sacrificing of self for the good of others which expressed the soul of religion in a time when religious spirit dominated men. Perhaps the earliest outward sign of military influence on hospitals and nursing was apparent in the spur which they gave to an ideal of uniformity in dress that had been gradually forming in monastic groups. Like all who joined the Crusaders, the various orders bore the cross of Christ. However, in order to differentiate themselves, they began to present variations in the form and color of the cross. Their choice of robes and cloaks further helped this necessary differentiation. The variety of these, and of their accessories, exerted the same spirited charm as does the variety in military or nursing uniforms today.

Each group was identified immediately as a participant in a cause of wide importance. Each had individuality and was able to take a definite place in a scheme for world good. When engaged in warfare, all knights hospitallers wore a regular coat of mail under the monastic habit. Members of the Order of St. John of Jerusalem wore the habit of their monastery, a red robe with a black cloak. In the beginning, the Sisters of St. Mary Magdalene wore a similar habit, but eventually abandoned the red robe for a black one. The cross of white linen which was appliquéd on each of these garments was one of eight points. We recognize in it the Maltese cross, for so it was named in after years when the Order of St. John of Jerusalem moved, subsequent to the fall of that city, to the Island of Malta in the Mediterranean. The Teutonic Knights Hospitallers wore a white cloak over a black habit, with black cross outlined in gold embroidery on the shoulder. The Order of Knights of St. Lazarus varied both habit and cross in different countries. The color of the original cross has been lost to us, but its form was distinguished by bars of equal length, with four slightly flaring ends.

A second military influence was the ideal of submergence of the individual, unquestioning obedience, opportunity for dominance by a few, and a hard business efficiency in management, which was substituted for the family spirit of early xenodochia or Benedictine monasteries. The hospital buildings themselves began to take on military and ecclesiastical characteristics in architecture, to be built for safety and strength, and to express a gloomy severity which has begun to disappear only during the last century.

This entrance of military discipline into monastic life has left its impress on schools of nursing. Through the military orders was inherited, too, a tradition of aristocracy in nursing started by the Roman matrons, and continuing through the early Middle Ages when queens and princesses so freely entered convent life. The greater the social distance between rich and poor, between nurse and patient, the greater the sacrifice involved, the greater the virtue. With interruptions this tradition also came down to our own day. No other occupation, except homekeeping, has entitled woman to the consideration won by the good nurse.

MEDIEVAL SOCIAL PROBLEMS

The thirteenth century began with stirrings of change. The Crusades, which had been under way for a century, had brought a progressive disintegration of those small protective units formed during the disturbance of western society by the injection into it of barbarism. With scattering of population and freeing of slaves, and often of serfs too, numbers of bewildered men were beginning to emerge as unprotected individuals. New conceptions of religious leadership and civil government were necessary as monastery and feudal fief declined, and greater power was centering about kings. The times demanded other social grouping with more freedom for expression. A sudden acceleration in growth of towns with strongly commercial ideals, a youthful independence, and the moral recklessness of "boom" were significant of this change in needs. So also were the guilds of craftsmen or of traders which were growing stronger.

For several centuries before the Crusades the inner life of many monasteries had been approaching a state of decay. Earlier days of hard work had earned its reward of wealth through increasing land values and gifts. No longer was it necessary for the abbot to go forth with his monks before sunrise to labor in the fields. A great missionary task had been accomplished, and pioneering days were far behind. As the democracy of St. Benedict gave way under a flood of riches, lay brothers did the heavy work. Monks abandoned manual toil for other pursuits, and abbots became politicians who enjoyed the privileges of great lords and vied with royalty in the pomp and luxury of their mode of life. Though scholarship managed to retain its place in some monasteries, an insufficient discrimination in selection of monks and nuns, as well as the cupidity of some among those who coveted wealth and power, often replaced industry and austerity with idleness and levity. As among our modern hospitals and schools of nursing, there were groups who maintained high standards, and there were others who brought criticism on the whole social institution to which they owed their origin. The dark spots were prominent against a background of centuries of glorious tradition.

Public opinion turned gradually against an institution which seemed to be lending itself to private rather than public ends, and people learned to criticize the Church which it represented. Efforts to reform abuses tended toward stricter discipline and attempts at reversion to the ascetic life. Some headway was made, but the times called for other means than revival of austerities within the monastery. There was lacking still an influence in the everyday life of the masses that would help to straighten out a world that had changed since the sixth century—a society even more confused in its needs than that which was left to find itself after the Fall of Rome.

Another medieval problem of great magnitude was the control of leprosy. During centuries in which people of the West had been gathered into immobile, compact groups separated by considerable distances, disease had been under a natural control. When they were set into motion by the Crusades and subsequent trade activity, both acute and chronic infections increased. Over and over, society was visited by epidemics which gained in severity, and, among chronic diseases, leprosy, or diseases mistaken for leprosy, became more and more widely diffused. Moses, fifteen hundred years before the beginning of the Christian era, had devised a technic of care and prevention for this long-lived scourge of men. The Knights of St. Lazarus were now taking it upon themselves to provide many more of their leper hospitals, but still the failure to cope with what had become an immense social problem was apparent.

A cruel policy of attempted segregation of the leper had come to be popular. He was a social outcast, with none of the rights of other men. Officially, he was dead, and the church read a burial service for him. He had no home, no belongings, no family, no way to earn a living. Denied the simplest comforts of life, he must beg his way without intruding the sorry spectacle of himself even on those who might help. Whenever he approached a human being, it was required that he ring a bell, sound a horn, or cry the warning word of "Unclean."

The leper's plight met sympathy here and there, and individuals of the noble or royal groups had done much for his relief. As a problem of public health, he continued to be a menace, and one which, in the thirteenth century, could not be met any more than other health problems could be met. Available medical knowledge was inside monasteries, and what was used of it had become so mixed with superstition and was so retarded by weakness in scientific leadership as to be ineffective. To liberate medicine and bring religion into the life of the people, the Church must now take into account altered social conditions demanding an adjustment to new social needs.

Two other social problems of acuteness hinging more or less on the problem of medical care were *infanticide* and the *orphaned or abandoned child*. The tragic number of adult deaths by war or disease left multitudes of children homeless. In addition, such conventions as existed in society gave way as they always do when people leave settled homes and, in great groups, suddenly become free lances. Moral laxity prevailed and was encouraged by long-continued war with its unfailing trail of illegitimate babies. Babies were often left on doorways or abandoned in alleys. Little children wandered about, homeless beggars. Parents lived in no fear of the law. Harsh times made orphans of thousands. The abandoned child of early and medieval times suffered cruelly. He could be picked up and sold for money, and so was at the mercy of slave-traders.

RISE OF MENDICANT ORDERS

During the Late Middle Ages, a unique development of the monastic idea finds expression in traveling religious missionary bodies pledged to literal poverty. The social security enjoyed by monks in rich institutions would be denied these men who knew no fixed abode, and had divided among the poor all that they might once have possessed. As exponents of Christian ideals they would not live apart from the world of men, but would troop barefoot through it. They would depend upon the uncertainties of begging for what they must eat, and the custom of begging would earn for them the name of *Mendicant Orders*.

It was recognized that if spiritual leaders were to have any success in spiritual guidance, there must be among them men who mingled with men, and recognized their spiritual adolescence. They must help them to help themselves. The asceticism of the Mendicants, therefore, was a sacrifice of personal desires and devotion of self to the good of others without retirement from the world. Church authorities sanctioned an innovation that strengthened the peoples' faith in Christianity by keeping before them the ideal of a Christ-like life.

Changing conditions brought forth, almost simultaneously, in

Spain and in Italy, two young social leaders who were to open the way to better things. Both would bring religion directly to the people by living among them as mendicant monks, and one would also stimulate a movement in the interests of public health as far as leprosy was concerned. They founded the Dominican and Franciscan Orders of the Church.

St. Dominic (1170–1221), of the noble family of Guzman whose castle stood in a village of Castile, gave up his plan of becoming a monk in a monastery. Famine in Spain and its resultant misery brought home to him the opportunity to serve anew the mass of poor men through revival of a closer contact. He set forth, hoping to restore to the fold of the Church those who had succumbed to distracting religious influences at work among them, and to convert others. Like-minded men, and women too, gathered about him and became known as *Dominicans*. These he sent abroad as traveling preachers, seeking to make Christianity the one religion through Christian teaching and example.

St. Francis of Assisi (1182–1226), on the other hand, belonged to that middle class just emerging from a society which had formerly known only two classes, nobility, and slaves or serfs. Francis' father was one of those merchants who profited by the trade revival accompanying the Crusades. The family accumulated some fortune in the business of selling cloth, velvet, and embroideries, and the son, when old enough, helped to manage the shop in the market place of a town called "Assisi" in central Italy. Legend tells of his being engaged in waiting on one of the customers when a beggar appeared, asking for alms. Etiquette required a salesman to stay with the first-comer, and the poor man left impatiently. As soon as he could, a kind-hearted boy was seen rushing off through the winding streets to find the beggar, and make up for his own sense of a failure to be kind by giving lavishly of charity. Other qualities besides his courtesy and generosity endeared Francis to neighbors in Assisi. He was one of those happy, unconventional youngsters who add cheer to small-town life. He had a good time with the young people, serenaded the girls, hunted amusement with the boys, led the fashions in gay clothes.

Like many another son of a father who works industriously to

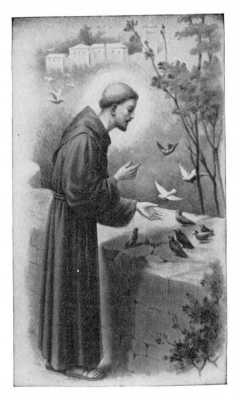

St. Francis of Assisi

(Krause, Gramer and Co., Germany.)

gather riches, his sense of money value was not well developed and neither did he settle down to the humdrum of business. At one time, we find St. Francis enthralled with the military side of life in a medieval fortified town whose boys were soldiers. Chivalry engrosses him and he learns to sing like a troubadour. Recurrent illness restrains him somewhat, but youthful irresponsibility finally brings open trouble with his father, who forbade him to ever again use the family name.

Then it was that St. Francis left home abruptly to live in the woods as a solitary, vowed to the service of God. The friendly boy, who loved flowers and trees as well as people, found it easy to be happy, singing with the birds, making friends of all the wild folk. St. Francis busied himself in repairing the local church, earning his meager necessities by doing any task that offered, and still found time to give devoted service to a small colony of lepers who lived nearby. As three years passed, the life of Jesus, literally followed, came to mean for him the life ideal. He felt himself fired with a determination to help all men to share with him the good life, and carry peace to other men of their unpeaceful age.

A merchant friend joined him, and then a church official. They decided to go forth among the people, and Francis unwittingly established an historic costume when he robed himself humbly in a rough, woolen peasant's tunic, and tied a piece of rope about his waist. The others with equal humility bound themselves to utter poverty and the service of the poor. Because there were so many lepers, miserable and neglected, and because, too, the task of caring for them was so completely disagreeable, they chose to identify themselves with the care of this group. Many lazarettos owed their establishment to the efforts of the *Brothers Minor* or Little Brothers, as Francis learned to call the members of the group which continued to gather about him. When they numbered twelve, all set out for Rome, where receipt of papal sanction gave the *Franciscan Order* a place in the church. Each of these men accepted his task of traveling from place to place preaching along the way, and doing the work of a religious revivalist, nurse, or social worker as he went.

The Dominican robe was of white wool surmounted by a black cape made with a hood which could be pulled over the head when necessary for warmth. This cape caused the brothers to be known, popularly, as *Black Friars*. The habit of the Franciscan was the same loose, rough, wool peasant robe with rope girdle which St. Francis himself had once donned on impulse. Its shade might be brownish or grayish, and the wearers were called *Gray Friars*. Gray Friars began to spread ever farther through the land. The Church found in them a new strength. Lepers were gathered up, surrounded by an encouraging sympathy, and sometimes cured. Whereas segregation without care had failed to curb the progress of leprosy, the Franciscans were able to contribute greatly to a public health movement which has ended in almost universal control.

The Second Order of St. Francis   While young Spaniards, young Italians, and all the other youths of medieval Europe were going away from home to join Crusades, military orders, or brotherhoods, were they leaving at home, and without opportunity to follow the traditional feminine occupations, all the equally ardent and attractive young women? Not all. Many types of women followed the trail toward Jerusalem, women everywhere became nurses in the ranks of the hospitallers, and women soon joined Dominicans as teachers, and Franciscans as nurses, although not permitted to be beggars. One young friend of St. Francis came also from Assisi. Beautiful, a lady of the noble class, and only seventeen, *Clarissa* waited with girlish eagerness for news of the work with lepers. Watchful parents had arranged a marriage for her, and they did not encourage an interest that might develop into the wish to be a nurse, but their daughter is said to have seen St. Francis now and then, and to have already made up her mind to leave the world to work for God.

In the awesome darkness of night in medieval Assisi, Clarissa ran away from home, and found her way to the little church that owed its restoration to her good friend's enthusiasm. He and his followers, by torchlight, were there lifting up their hearts in prayer. It must have been with fearfulness of consequences that they saw and welcomed Clarissa into their group, but St. Francis himself consecrated her at the altar, and himself cut off her long, beautiful hair to encourage her in humility. She threw aside her jewels with the expensive dress worn by girls of her rank, and wrapped herself, like the others, in a rope-bound robe of wool.

Then Clarissa was taken to the safety of a Benedictine convent in the neighborhood, where she remained under protection of the nuns until the Franciscans were able to establish her in an abbey of her own. It eventually stood by the home church which had seen her dedicate her life to a service of the poor that was to continue for forty difficult years. Huts adjoining this church were filled with lepers by the Brothers. Nursing care was provided by Clarissa and a group of Sisters who gathered about her. They received the name of *Poor Clares* or the second order of St. Francis. The begging of the Brothers Minor or Little Brothers supplied all with food. Mothers and fathers in Assisi must have mourned such general, seemingly overeager destruction by the younger generation of comfortable, outworn traditions, but youth discovered what the times had need of, and set out on the business of providing it.

RISE OF SECULAR ORDERS

The Third Order of St. Francis   Qualms of church authorities, now keenly alive to outspoken criticism, carried measures of monastic reform further and further in the direction of limitation of freedom. At the same time, inadequacy of the old tradition to meet new social requirements made inevitable the finding of other means to satisfy them. It is the way of society to discard what it has worn out if it will not be made over. While the Mendicant Orders were being welcomed, other groups of men and women interested in a religious life without seclusion began to be noticed.

As long as the bulk of charity, including the nursing of the sick, could be handled by feudal lords and ladies, or by scattered monastic or other church bodies, these nonmonastic groups had not been prominent. From the end of the eleventh century, however, they had been coming forward in different parts of Europe, and the term "secular orders," from now on, describes religious organizations of laymen or laywomen who took no perpetual vows, and might work under the church, or outside of its authority. Secular orders did not beg. Some of them were self-supporting, and provided for charity from a common fund. Their membership was composed of citizens who, frequently, did not leave either home or business to join any separate community. To a great extent, they identified themselves with nursing in hospitals or in private homes, and, in the latter aspect, their work reverted to that instituted by the once much beloved and now almost forgotten deaconess.

In Italy, the wave of religious interest among the laity became, on one occasion, a matter of embarrassment to St. Francis. In one of the towns through which he passed, everybody insisted on becoming a Little Brother or Sister. Anxious as he was to win workers, he could not accept them at the cost of home life, and with the consequence of childhood suffering. He therefore begged impulsive fathers and mothers to practice the principles of Christ-like living as they went about their customary tasks, thereby improving home and community relations. Then he formed among them a secular order, and

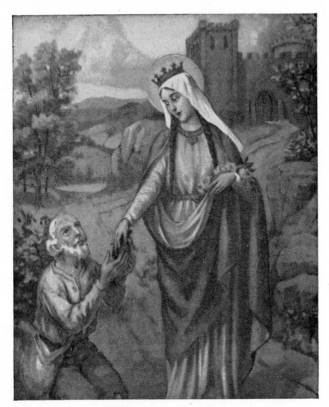

ST. ELIZABETH OF HUNGARY
("Miniature Stories of the Saints," Book Two, by Rev. Daniel A. Lord, S. J. [Catholic publications])

named it the *Order of Tertiaries* because it represented the third group in his following.

St. Elizabeth of Hungary   Throughout history, from now on, many famous names are to be found among the Tertiaries of St. Francis. One of the first to ally herself with the order, as it spread beyond the confines of its native Italy, was *St. Elizabeth* (1207–1231), a daughter of the royal house of Hungary. Beautiful and high-minded, this young woman had been reared in the tradition of good deeds, and among her family were some who shared the current interest in lepers. Fortunately, marriage at the age of fifteen made her the wife of a true knight who did not fail her in sympathy when she wished to ease the burdens of poor people about them. He helped her to build hospitals in his native Germany, and she went into peasant homes to assist when babies came, or to take food to the hungry.

The kindness of St. Elizabeth has inspired many of the legends of saintly women passed on to us by the underprivileged of medieval days who, in some respects, were victims of unusual suffering. Time lends variation to these, and the following is only one of several versions of a popular tale. The unearthly beauty of soul radiating from Elizabeth was miraculously revealed to her husband. Pulling aside her cloak one day, to see what she carried beneath it as she started out to visit his tenants, he beheld a basket of roses. Roses were out of season, and Elizabeth herself had filled the basket with food, and yet, there it was, overflowing with the lovely flowers which had blossomed to protect her from the possible pain of his displeasure. The chivalrous knight is said to have chosen one with reverence, that he might carry it through life as reminder of his wife's goodness.

Difficulties with relatives-in-law who criticized her charities as extravagance, an enforced separation from her children, the death of a beloved husband in a Crusade—all were personal trials which served to throw the interests of St. Elizabeth of Hungary more and more into nursing and social work. Twice every day, it was her custom to visit, in hospitals or in their homes, patients suffering from any malady, for she feared none. She gave baths, did surgical dressings, fed the helpless, and delighted, above all, in the care of children. The saddened young noblewoman earned for herself a place beside her friend, St. Francis of Assisi, and the early church deaconess as forerunner of the visiting and public health nurses of modern times.

The work of St. Elizabeth of Hungary and many of her friends or contemporaries serves to illustrate a growing interest in charitable work on the part of laywomen. Indirectly, it speaks of the introduction of welcome occupation into the lives of many women of the thirteenth century. During more than a hundred years of wars that continued to destroy many millions of men by disease as well as by the sword, the possibility of woman staying with her traditional business of home-keeping grew more and more dim. Western lands were shifting about; the most eligible of their marital prospects were in monasteries if not in battle, and the number of convents was inadequate to receive them did they choose this refuge. Just as they have done in later days, women set out to find new work.

Beguines   Coincident with development of secular orders in central Europe was to be observed an even more marked development farther west. About the time that St. Francis was born, Flanders (Belgium and parts of what we now call France and Holland) saw the establishment of a model community of independently organized laywomen of religious purpose. Within an enclosure just outside the city wall of Liège arose a church, and around it rows of little cottages began to pop up. Women called *Beguines* (be geens), members of an order dating back to the seventh century, came to live in them, and called the new establishment a "Beguinage." They kept house together, three or four to a cottage, and took simple vows of chastity and obedience. Society funds provided maintenance for the poorer among them, and the well-to-do supported themselves. Many Beguines preferred to remain with relatives in town, and residence in the Beguinage was not insisted upon. No one vowed poverty or gave up property, and all were free to marry, but no married member lived in community.

Busily, Beguines of Liège, with the help of the Bishop, set about finding jobs that would earn the way of an organization which must build up a common fund for upkeep of property, support of members, and charity. Sewing, lacemaking, the tending of children, teaching, and other tasks associated with woman's industry were undertaken. *Visiting nursing* in neighboring homes was started, and families able to pay for this service did so. When a hospital was added to their responsibilities, the Beguines nursed the patients who quickly filled it, and here, too, collected fees from those who could pay. Whole-hearted devotion to public service by thousands of women who joined this secular order at Liège and other centers brought its reward, and many gifts found their way into the treasury to provide for an ever-widening scope in work.

The fame of the Beguines spread about, and their cottage communities began to appear elsewhere in Flanders as well as in other lands. By the end of the thirteenth century there were two hundred thousand of these lay workers whose settlements were spread throughout great and little towns so that they might readily serve that portion of the public most in need of them. Small or large as the group of townspeople might be, they must be reached in days when transportation and communication, too, were so difficult that the nurse had to rely on being within easy walking distance. This made some Beguinages very small, and in large cities the number of them might run up to forty or fifty. The scattering of, and not the concentration of medical and nursing activities was the aim of the secular order of Beguines which reached its height of usefulness in the fourteenth century.

The strong tendency toward uniform, spectacular dress which characterized organizations of men or women during the late Middle Ages had its influence on the Beguinage. The pioneers of Liège usually wore gray, but all Beguines did not insist upon distinctive dresses while they carried on their work. Those who did were apt to choose color or pattern to suit their taste, and monastic features show their impress on headgear and cloaks reminiscent of the Knights or Lady Hospitallers.

Long ago the Belgian people learned to depend upon this secular order during national emergency, for Beguines on many occasions assumed obligations connected with distribution of food, clothing, and supplies, now included in the functions of Red Cross Societies. They have been ever ready to provide special nursing service when epidemic or disaster occasioned a need, and the two World Wars found them once more actively at work among soldiers. Their houses stand as memorials to a little group of high-minded, resourceful women who, in the later Middle Ages, opened an avenue to useful service for thousands of women who could not leave the world had they wished to do so.

GAINS AND LOSSES OF THE CRUSADERS

Three years after they left home, the first Crusaders were in possession of Jerusalem. The Cross, emblem of Christianity, supplanted the Crescent, emblem of success and progress to Islamic Turks. No peaceful methods had brought about the change, for we read that a celebration of the final event with prayers inside the Church of the Holy Sepulchre, which had been erected in the fourth century on a site supposed to mark the very scene of Christ's burial and resurrection, was rendered further satisfying outside by "riding their horses through the blood of slaughtered Moslems."[5]

Christians held their prize for nearly a century. In 1187 it was taken from them by *Saladin*, a cultured Moslem of Armenian birth who showed sufficient lenience to permit those who could afford to pay ransom and finance their journey, to return to Europe. Several thousand of his prisoners were freed. Pilgrims were no longer excluded from the Holy City, and something was done toward improving conditions for those who continued to make the journey.

European agitation did not subside in the face of defeat. Even little children banded together and started off on a Crusade of their own. In 1212 a large number of these set out in the direction of the sea which they expected to fall back at their approach, as it had once done for Moses. Many perished on the road. Many others were sold into slavery. Only a few of those who took part in the Children's Crusade ever returned. Among their elders, Crusade followed Crusade, although Jerusalem was never recaptured. The last part of the thirteenth century saw the end of these expeditions which, in their results, were a mixture of good and evil.

SOCIAL CHANGES ASSOCIATED WITH THE CRUSADES

Many changes were to be observed in western society after two hundred years of religious warfare. Some of these changes came through a natural growth of influences at work before the eleventh century, but others came directly as a result of the mingling of peoples and the contact of a young civilization with a mature one. Half barbaric Europeans of varied races learned a great deal about one another as they drew together in a common cause. Inevitably, all were touched by refining influences that emanated from eastern empire culture, which had known no set-back such as the western empire had suffered.

The magnificence of a great city like Constantinople amazed these sightseers when they passed through it, as much as the commercial efficiency of cities like Venice, Genoa, and Pisa. Naturally, they assimilated ideas of art, government, and business. In far eastern coun-

[5] Haynes, Moon, and Wayland: World History, p. 372. By permission of The Macmillan Company, New York, publishers.

tries they met people who knew many things that they did not know, and numbers of them lingered in Palestine to set up homes beside the Moslem and the Jew. Enforced neighborliness for several generations made it expedient for these to adopt some eastern customs in manners, clothing, and diet. There was experienced by such crusaders a tolerance for religious and racial differences that was at variance with the ideas that brought them to Palestine. There was even some intermarriage between east and west.

Buying and selling were inseparable from movement of peoples, and gave stimulation to commerce. Aside from necessities known at home, travelers learned to use and like new articles. The demand for luxuries spread, and luxuries soon became necessities. Western Europe wanted salt and spices, silks, fine muslins, luxurious rugs, and rare fruits, just as men want automobiles and all kinds of electrical conveniences today.

Shop-keepers, like the father of St. Francis, became rich men conscious of the independence that riches gave them. They began to stand out from that mass of men who had once left thinking to churchmen and feudal lords. As a group they were forming what soon became known as the "middle class." In the towns and cities which grew rapidly as these men pushed the development of industries, the middle class gradually learned to use its voice in government as well as in business. The guilds, protecting former peasants or serfs whom the new industrialists brought from the country to the town and employed as workmen, reached a high level of organization. The abbot of the monastery and the feudal lord both found that they were being shorn of considerable power by an urban group which was learning to look to a king as its guide in civil affairs.

As early as 1215 the doctrine of individualism, or the determination of standards for any social group by the individuals who comprise it, had developed to a considerable extent. It was strong enough to set the will of his people against the will of *John, King of England,* and force his signing of the Magna Charta. In this document he acknowledged certain rights as belonging to his subjects among nobility, church, and middle class, and in so doing abandoned any dream that might have possessed him of ruling as an absolute monarch.

Society was anxious to form new groups based on common traditions of race, language, and custom, and, while men were willing to give their loyalty to one man at the head of each of these groups, they intended to participate in the management of the group's affairs. National governments soon supplanted church and feudal government, and kings became responsible to the people. Individualism, nationalism, and democracy were features which entered western social development as a result of changes during the Crusades. They affected all institutions.

A series of free towns which controlled ports and shipping were developed along the Mediterranean as a result of increased trading and new demands for transportation. Trade routes were improved. Ships grew in size and were better built. Europeans learned the use of the eastern compass, and sailing charts became gradually available. The ancient custom of hugging the shore lines, and traveling only in seasons of favorable weather were fading in the light of new knowledge of ship management. The East taught western merchants improved methods of finance, and great banking systems grew. Successful business adjusted itself to a whole series of difficulties, while it stimulated the dreams of adventurous men who wished to follow to their source the things which Europe had learned to crave.

The western world, by the thirteenth century, had reached the rim of a great era of discovery. In 1271 two brothers of a Venetian family named Polo, who had already been to China, set out again. One of them took along his son, Marco Polo, a boy of seventeen who entered with spirit into all the adventures of a long and dangerous trip which culminated in residence among the Chinese for seventeen years. It was when a prisoner of war, shortly after returning to his native Venice, that Marco told to a fellow prisoner the well-known tales of his travels. The story was put into book form, and by its first-hand information of lands that she had dreamed of, gave added stimulus to the adventurous spirit of Europe. Two centuries later the book fell into the hands of Christopher Columbus.

CHIVALRY INFLUENCES THE POSITION OF WOMEN

In spite of the independence and position attained by a relatively small number of those who became abbesses, and the executive position often forced upon the feudal lady, women in general throughout the Middle Ages were becoming more and more servile in their attitude toward men. The freedom of action that we saw coming to the fore in ancient Rome slipped away. Both Christianity and feudalism helped to hasten its departure. However, from the time that knights became busied with Crusades, a spiritual influence representing a blending of ethics, etiquette, and romance began to soften the crudity of the times. France called it *chivalry*, and men called *troubadours* helped it along by singing about it. To castle halls or gardens, and to village greens, they brought music and lyrics of war and brave men, of spring and flowers, of beautiful, good, and gracious women who had the undying love of noble knights.

The woman of the Middle Ages, still a half-savage like her husband, began to realize as she listened to these songs that she might develop qualities to match those of the ideal in knighthood. Loveliness, the charm of courtesy, grace of motion, and beauty of dress became more important. She began to be her own saleswoman, and although for centuries after this she would still have to accept her lot of marriage without choice, the period of Crusades marks the beginning of something different for her. She learned the possibility of giving herself instead of being taken as a wife. She was led to a sense of romantic love with spiritual values which could give color and enchantment to marriage even if it remained for her an economic necessity.

Taken all in all, the woman of the Middle Ages had little chance for happiness. If she avoided marriage, and was religious, she sought a convent, or an indignant parent put her into one. If married, her home was likely to be in a constant turmoil of grief and uncertainty. To whatever class of society she belonged, she found hard work her lot, and often direst poverty. Always, one baby followed another in a procession cut short, usually, by her early death. For her care when they were born, she must accept the midwife in lieu of the physician. A husband's appreciation of his wife was based on the number of her sons. If she survived to bring them up, she was so ignorant of child hygiene and household sanitation that a brood of fifteen or more might diminish to two or three as she watched them die one after the other.

GREAT PLAGUES OF THE FOURTEENTH CENTURY

From the Fall of Rome through the early Middle Ages, the isolation of those units into which men banded for mutual protection had given almost complete defense against infections from outside the group. As these units slowly passed through a stage of disintegration, contagious diseases increased.

Travel and war brought people into contact with diseases for which they had acquired no immunity; and when, with industrial changes, families crowded together into towns, they had no knowledge of how to manage town life. Malnutrition increased the seriousness of a problem attendant upon urban growth as well as upon neglect of land and failure of crops. Epidemics became frequent, and on several occasions reached the pandemic stage.

If we stop for a moment to consider the elaborate machinery in use today for the control of communicable disease, it will not be difficult to understand how helpless the people of the Middle Ages were when it came upon them. The laboratory has become since then the scientific core of a great system of diagnosis, prevention, and treatment. An army of public health workers guards the public of today, and departments of public health see that protective laws are enforced. Travel between countries is subject to restrictions of quarantine. Tremendous effort is made to spread information regarding prevention and care. In spite of all this protection, epidemics are not unknown, and scientists know that their best efforts may be rendered ineffective by the fallibility of the human element.

The people of the Middle Ages had none of these protective forces about them. In the tenth century the only medical school in Europe was at Salerno, near Naples, and there were very few doctors. No medical corps accompanied the crusading expeditions that were organized throughout western Europe. There was no science of bacteriology, no serums, no vaccines, nothing was known of dangers in dust, house-flies, impure milk or water. Superstition decided the causes of disease, and charms, amulets, or conjuring of spirits were the means of preventing it. The poorest of sanitary conditions prevailed even in the country, and, in the towns, filth of all kinds was thrown into the streets to be trampled down in layer upon layer as the years passed. Houses were ill ventilated, poorly heated, and floors were covered with rushes which were seldom or never removed.

Even in the castles of the great, it is said to have been customary to leave dirty rushes under the fresh ones laid down from time to time. The moat around the castle furnished the most convenient medium for garbage disposal. In the palace of a king, the cook's helpers slept on the kitchen floor, using, most probably, the almost universal bed of straw. Animals, such as dogs or pigs, frequently shared the family living quarters. Pigs wandered around the streets, and there was a custom of attaching the stable for horse and cow to the rear of the home, which has not been abandoned even to the present day in some places.

Personal hygiene, in medieval times, was neglected as a matter of custom, even among those who could have afforded facilities for its practice; and men, women, and children lived in what today would be looked upon as conditions of utmost filth. Rich or poor, none conceived lice as dangerous pests, or even as any reflection on personal habit. All had them. Nobody bothered about rats. Famine often brought starvation to the poor. Blighted fields of rye grain crippled them through ergotism, and among those who could supply themselves with adequate food, there was immoderate eating of strangely prepared dishes.

The cooking of the time is said to have been based on ancient traditions handed down from Roman days, and there was little of simplicity about it. Many kinds of foods were combined in one dish, boiled, baked, or stewed to mushy consistency, and frequently served in a cover of paste that went by the appropriate name of "coffin." Food was usually eaten with the fingers, for forks were not generally known, although they were appearing. The common cup was indeed common.

A great variety of meat was served, and, for lack of refrigeration, it was often far from fresh. This was not noticed, for in cooking all the spices of the market were added to it. Altogether, although men and women lived under conditions necessitating much physical exercise, their diet alone would almost account for the shortness of their span of life, for food was very rich, highly seasoned, and consumed in great quantities. This inordinate eating, in combination with the fact that few escaped communicable disease whenever it appeared in their community, permitted slight resistance in the strong and almost none in the weak. It is little wonder, then, that terror seized upon any group of people among whom appeared a communicable malady of deadly virulence. Smallpox, bubonic plague, typhus, pulmonary tuberculosis, influenza, erysipelas, anthrax, trachoma, and leprosy were well known. The latter was often confused with scabies or psoriasis. Repeated outbreaks of mass hysteria and epidemic chorea led to the inclusion of epilepsy with communicable disease.

In 1348 appeared a terrible epidemic of what is said to have been bubonic plague, and was popularly known as the *Black Death* from the dark hemorrhagic spots which appeared under the skin of its victims. The disease had already passed through Asia and Africa before reaching Europe, and its fatalities are estimated to have totaled, in the end, one-fourth of the population of the earth. When it began its work in medieval Europe people either shut themselves up or fled before it. Families were disrupted and civil life was completely demoralized. The malady was in such acute form that victims seldom survived three days. Most of them died without medical attention or nursing. They were buried in great pits or thrown into the river or the ocean which returned diseased bodies with each tide.

In the fifteenth century, it is perhaps not surprising to learn that the populace of Europe, descendants of those who had undergone for centuries hardships like war, famine, and disease, should develop emotional disorders. These appeared in many forms, including excesses of cruelty, and climaxed in a *dancing mania* which spread throughout town and country. Everywhere, over the length and breadth of Europe, groups of people began to dance. Faster and faster they danced until they twitched and frothed at the mouth, and in the end dropped from exhaustion. St. Vitus was chosen as the patron saint of these wandering dancers, who left homes and kindred to follow one another. Their affliction has since been diagnosed as chorea.

About the same time, a virulent disease thought to have been influenza, and known to its time as *sweating sickness*, began in England and spread over the continent. Again great numbers died, and, in the light of present-day knowledge, the care received by many hastened the end. Belief was current that the patient must sweat continuously for twenty-four hours in order to have any chance of recovery. Windows and doors were carefully closed, the stove was kept going, feather beds and furs were piled upon him and, if these were to remain in place, sheets must be sewed to the bed. He was "stewed to death" as one writer puts it. Beside him sat attendants ordered to keep him awake that he might retain his senses, and these did their best, even to whipping him with a branch, or dropping vinegar into his eyes. "Once for all, the patient must not have his own way; what he would have you do for him, that must not be done."[6]

There were occasional physicians who disapproved of such treatment, and some who were not only more rational, but sensed irregular living and overeating as incidents affecting resistance. Some even advocated fresh air and fewer bedclothes. The undue weight of most people of medieval times stood in the way of their recovery from any of the acute diseases mentioned. Lacking dietetic science, and consuming excessive amounts of many foods, they suffered much from constipation, headaches, sourness of the stomach, and, undoubtedly in many cases, from an overworked heart.

SAINT CATHERINE OF SIENA; HOSPITAL NURSE AND VISITING NURSE

Two benefits may be traced to the miseries which tortured human beings in the late Middle Ages. The modern practice of quarantine grew out of experiments in restriction of travel which were made during the progress of the Black Death. There was a material increase, too, in the number of institutions for care of the sick, and in the number of volunteers who did nursing. These paved the way for that professional group which, eventually, would assume a share of responsibility for protection of the health of the public. One of the outstanding examples of the efficient volunteer in nursing at this period was a young Italian girl who has come to be known as *St. Catherine of Siena* (1347–1380). Siena is a town near Florence, and Catherine was one year old when the Black Death entered Europe. Unlike many other volunteer nurses who so far had gained fame in history, she was not of noble birth. Her parents were of the middle class, and only moderately well-to-do. Their daughter was brought up to help with housework in the modest home which sheltered a large family.

---

[6]Quoted in "Epidemics of the Middle Ages" by J. F. C. Hecker, p. 249. Trubner & Co., London, 1859.

Apparently the little Catherine grew to be a capable, willing girl with a decided bent toward asceticism. She formed the custom of flogging herself thrice daily, in expiation of her own sins and of those committed by all persons living or dead. Tired out with the labor of the day, she laid her head at night on a pillow of stone. Her spare time she spent in making visits to the sick in the town's hospital. Here, one of her first undertakings was bathing and dressing of a leper. Like many another young nurse who has since begun a career with a task equally distasteful, Catherine learned to be glad in the discovery that even the most difficult of patients turned over to her yielded to her patience and her earnest desire to be helpful. Nursing brought her great happiness, but it was natural that parents should find it hard to understand a daughter who did not choose to be just like the other young girls about her, and who set her mind on what seemed too serious things. They tried to dissuade her, but with tact and sweetness she won her way with parents, too. Back and forth, morning and evening for several years, she walked between her home and the quite distant hospital, until her lamp at night came to have for the sick poor of Siena very much the same significance as would attach itself to a lamp in the hands of another nurse when Florence Nightingale visited her soldier patients of the Crimea. Catherine of Siena made the hospital of La Scala a blessed place because of her presence there.

By the time she was twenty-four this unusual girl had succeeded in getting education enough to be able to read. She had to wait four years more to learn how to write, and then she was possessed of accomplishments rare among women in her day, and confined almost wholly to the upper classes. She became, too, a tertiary of the order of St. Dominic, and member of an organization of women within the order whose objections to her youth had to be overcome before they accepted her. Fortunately for Catherine at this time, any beauty which nature might have bestowed upon her head had been destroyed by illness. The ladies decided that her homeliness would be sufficient protection to allow of her going about the streets on errands of mercy, for they had volunteered to visit in homes of the poor, nursing cases of minor ailment, and seeing that acute cases, or those likely to be long drawn out, were taken to the hospital. The young woman whom they thus grudgingly admitted to their circle soon increased

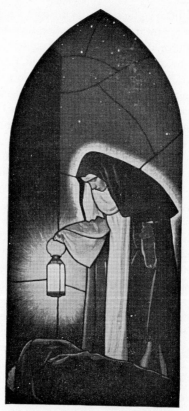

St. Catherine of Siena
A present-day conception. (Courtesy of Will Ross, Inc.)

its efficiency by organizing a corresponding body of men to provide a needed ambulance service. As volunteer stretcher bearers, this group carried sick and wounded to the hospital whether they found them at home or by the wayside.

In 1372, the plague reached Siena, and while it lasted St. Catherine no longer took time to go home, but worked day and night in La Scala hospital. Her few hours of rest were spent in a friend's house nearby. Even as the townspeople fled their city and hers, she was able to gather about her zealous helpers in response to courageous example. With them she nursed the sick, and, by selflessness, skill, and organizing ability won a great name throughout Italy. In later years, as they looked about for a way in which to honor her, citizens of Siena rebuilt the hospital of La Scala which still stands as her memorial. Passing centuries have seen them tend carefully the home in which she once lived, and her room, her lamp, and the stone pillow are there to remind the traveler of one of earth's gifted children whose talents were well used.

In divers ways, young Catherine, the mystic, was rendering service to her community as a citizen, and every day she became better acquainted with its life. Gradually she came to deplore the exhausting and unchristian prevalence of those long-continued feuds between families which made street quarrels and wounded men a feature of everyday life in the Italian town. So many of these did she contrive to settle that reputation drew her into political affairs of national or international moment, and her ability won for her such influence with the Pope that she succeeded in ending a prolonged strife within the Church itself.

Fame as a mediator had found St. Catherine, and fame as a writer, too, but it was as the nurse who gave of her best to the sick and the poor that she caught the public imagination, and inspired the sympathy of those men who have idealized her in art. The story of her devotion to an ideal, and the reward that attended her insistence on obtaining such education as was available, should lighten the task of any young nurse of today who must surmount similar difficulties of another age.

MEDICINE DURING THE LATE MIDDLE AGES

As the Middle Ages progressed, a returning fluidity of population from the seclusion of monasteries and feudal estates increased the danger from infectious diseases, and epidemics raged. Towns grew up, but sanitation remained in woeful state. The people were fear-ridden and, even as they submitted to disgusting forms of dosage and the most heroic of wrong treatment, they died by millions. The western world seemed in danger of losing forever all that heritage of medical science in its beginnings which had been derived from Greece. That it did not do so was due to the guardianship of three groups who preserved Hellenic medicine until the strangely mixed peoples of Europe were ready culturally to use it. These groups were

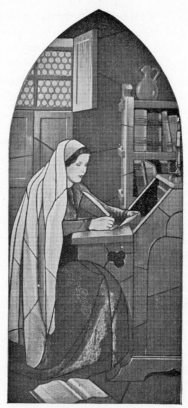

ST. HILDEGARDE
A present-day conception. (Courtesy of Will Ross, Inc.)

the monks and nuns of Christian monasteries, the progressive physicians of Constantinople, and those other physicians who entered
Spain with the invaders of the Moslem faith.

Medical Literature Preserved in Monasteries   The western
church, by copying and re-copying pieces of what classical learning
it could lay hands on, had taken Galen and Hippocrates into its
keeping. The manuscripts were in monastic libraries even if they
could not always be interpreted as the physician would interpret
them. There were always in the monasteries some men and women
who became experts in healing. Monks found their way to the Uni-

versity of Paris, and even before its time they were among students in Spain.

St. Hildegarde. In the twelfth century there appeared among the Benedictines in Germany an abbess, *St. Hildegarde* (1098–1179), who has been accorded an honorable place in medical and nursing history. Born into the nobility, Hildegarde was educated from the age of eight in a double monastery ruled by an abbot and situated near Bingen, a town on the Rhine. As a young woman, circumstances placed her in charge of the convent under the abbott's direction. She met the situation ably, and her superior intelligence was acknowledged by all about her, in the eleven years during which she occupied the position.

By the end of that time Hildegarde had grown impatient of restriction. She wished to be free to arrange her own life, and be free to devote more time to study. Gathering about her a group of noblewomen, she established a new convent, where she ruled as abbess for many years. Like other abbesses, Hildegarde was influential in Germany, and was able to foretell certain of its political developments. A student of many forms of learning, Hildegarde devoted herself especially to medicine, nursing, and natural science.

So skillful did she become in the practice of medicine that she went far beyond the men of her time, and was able to produce works which anticipated later scientific discoveries. People from far and wide sought her advice, and her cures were famous. By some they were attributed to miraculous power, by others they have been explained as the result of keen observation of the sick under her supervision in the convent, and life-long study. She was a strong believer in fresh air and the free use of water, wrote a number of books on medical subjects, and described jaundice, some worm diseases, lung diseases, and dysentery.

Byzantine Medicine   The eastern school of medical learning at Constantinople for many centuries served as a second custodian of that scientific medicine carried to it in early days by Greek schools, and whatever of it was brought later by scholars from Alexandria or Rome. Some of these Byzantine physicians remained permanently in Constantinople as teachers or copyists. Others, among whom were many of the Jewish race, carried what they learned to far-off lands. Some traveled to Arabia, some to Europe. Their services were sought by rulers and men of wealth, and, wherever they came together with other scholars, they aroused interest in Greek medicine.

Medicine and Moslem Invaders of Spain A third custodian of medicine was Arabia, to which country we have already followed it, and where we witnessed its translation into the Arabian language. In Arabic form, the works of Galen, interpreter of Hippocrates, were carried back to the west by Moslem invaders. Great cultural centers developed in the Spanish cities of Cordova and Toledo, where medical manuscripts were among the treasures of Arab libraries. Through students of Avicenna, Galen became the medical authority of Spain, and Spain a Mecca for students of medicine from other parts of Europe. Spanish Jews proved efficient translators of Arabic manuscripts into Latin, and Europe steadily approached conditions of social development favorable for the revival of science in medieval medicine.

By the time the medieval period was half over, and that period which we have called the Late Middle Ages was beginning, there had passed several hundred years of assimilation of barbarian neighbors by the Roman population. There was evidence, too, of the spread of new ideas as people gradually ceased to be shut off from one another in small social units. The influence of travel was toward new ways of thinking. Gradually, success came to the medical school in Salerno, Italy, and sick crusaders who made acquaintance with it as they passed through Italy became advertisers of its methods. Those who had experienced the care of eastern physicians joined with these in demanding better medical care when they returned home.

Rise of Universities A revival of interest in all learning was already becoming apparent, and learned men, many of them friars of St. Dominic or St. Francis, were being surrounded by groups of eager students. The consolidation in units of numbers of such groups was an innovation to which medieval scholars gave the name "university" (all turned together). In 1110 the University of Paris was started, in 1158 Bologna in Italy had another, in 1167 England organized the University of Oxford, from which a group migrated to start Cambridge, and in 1181 came Montpellier in France. By the fifteenth century, Italy had sixteen universities, and similar institutions were scattered all over Europe, and beyond it in England, Ireland, and Scotland. Medicine had become a branch of study widely pursued, and some of the great hospitals of the present day had been originated.

Status of Surgery   One serious drawback to scientific progress during the late Middle Ages existed in the objections to dissection held by those of both Moslem and Christian faiths. Another was the inferior position accorded to surgery by Avicenna who advocated use of the cautery wherever possible, and supervision by the physician of lay helpers when cutting was unavoidable. About the same time, it happened that the church was forbidding the wearing of beards by monks, and unwittingly there were introduced a popular mode for men and a new vocation. By the thirteenth century, barbers (FR. *barbitonsores*, or shavers of beards) are found organized as a Guild of Barber-Surgeons. By the fourteenth century, some of these were doing, in addition to barbering, bleeding, cupping, leeching, tooth extractions, and the treatment of surgical wounds. The physician held himself aloof from this group to which he relegated surgery, and while he gained for himself the protection of a license as well as the backing of universities, the surgeon remained unskilled and unrecognized for centuries. During this time, he struggled to overcome prejudices aroused in a public that suffered at the hands of ignorant barber-surgeons.

In 1453 A.D., Constantinople fell before the Turks, and this time fleeing citizens of a falling Roman Empire turned back to the west. They took Greek learning with them, and added their quota of medical knowledge to that of the monk and the nun, the Hebrew, and the Arab. Christians, Jews, Moslems—to these followers of three of the world's great religions, modern scientific medicine owes contributions toward restoration of that Greek foundation on which its superstructure rests. Although the first signs of returning consciousness after what has been called the "Age of Coma in Medicine" were thus apparent as early as the twelfth century, its full recovery was not seen until the nineteenth. It took all of that time to unearth scientific methods of thought, and to do away with slavish adherence to tradition. Superstition, we cannot deny, survives to the present day, in spite of everything.

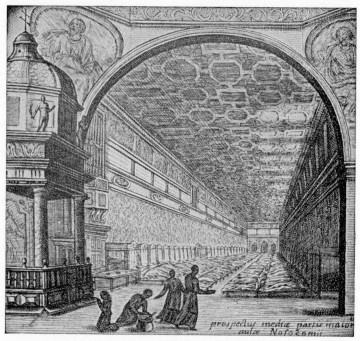

A WARD IN THE SANTO SPIRITO HOSPITAL OF ROME, SEVENTEENTH CENTURY
(Castiglioni, Arturo, M.D.: A History of Medicine. Alfred A. Knopf, New York.)

GROWTH OF HOSPITALS

Uncontrolled communicable disease, fluid population, and a hasty development of urban life have been noted previously as outstanding factors in the medical problem of the late Middle Ages. Solution seemed to focus on provision of increased facilities for segregation of lepers, and an adequate supply of beds in institutions that would be maintained, primarily, for care of the sick. Secular orders and private citizens made great public contributions as they supplied more and more lazarettos or hospitals, and volunteered a nursing service to cover them. When her people flocked townward in the wake of industry, the church, too, recognized the limitations of a system that left responsibility for medical care to isolated monasteries or crowded xenodochia.

In 1198 A.D., Pope Innocent III established in Rome what was intended to be a model institution designed for reception of the sick, and without those additional functions characteristic of its other charitable institutions. This was done by rebuilding the ancient hospice which was at the same time renamed, "Hospital of the Santo Spirito" (Holy Spirit). The secular order of Santo Spirito was asked to take charge of administration and nursing. Church executives or influential citizens who visited the Papacy on official business were invited to study the building and the plan of operation, and encouraged to organize similar institutions in towns from which they came.

The idea of city hospitals met with hearty cooperation, Germany adopting "Heilige Geist" as the equivalent in name, and France using the designation "Hôtel Dieu" (House of God), which we have seen applied earlier to two great institutions, one in Paris, the other in Lyons. In England, among others, there appeared the beginnings of three famous hospitals, St. Bartholomew's, Bethlehem (for the insane and better known as "Bedlam"), and that St. Thomas in which Florence Nightingale was to revolutionize nursing. Many major situations were relieved as individuals and the Church dispensed the charity of medieval times. The tendency, however, was in the direction of encouraging independence. Time proved the Santo Spirito Hospital in Rome to be the nucleus of a movement toward self-help through a more general participation in charity by the public. The English, and also the continental hospitals, early tended to pass over to city control, while xenodochia often adapted their organization to the newer need of hospital use only.

Meantime, some of those military orders which had originated in the emergency of pilgrimage and war made use of their accumulated wealth to meet an emergency obvious in times of peace, by furthering this stupendous development of hospitals. When seven hospitallers of the Order of St. John of Jerusalem escaped death in the final struggle to repossess the Holy City, they and their successors lived for a time on the island of Cyprus. Later, they were transferred to the island of Rhodes, and ruled there for two centuries. About the end of our present period, they came into possession of the island of Malta. Here, in the seaport town of Valetta, in 1575, they built a famous hospital.

This hospital of the Order of St. John at Valetta accommodated somewhat less than a thousand patients. One ward was a hall, five

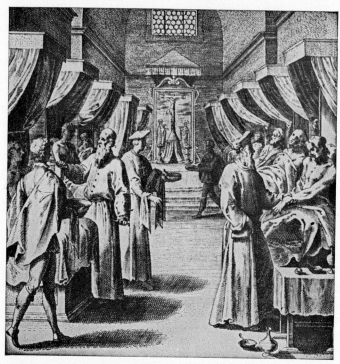

"KNIGHTS HOSPITALLERS MINISTERING TO PATIENTS IN THE GREAT WARD OF THE
SACRED INFIRMARY AT VALETTA, MALTA, IN THE SIXTEENTH CENTURY"
Woodcut from Statutes of the Order, 1584.

It will be noted that each patient has his separate bed which is fitted with curtains—replaced with mosquito nets in summer. There are bedside tables, on one
of which and nearby on the floor are several of the famous silver dishes from
which "Our Lords the Sick" were fed. (Hume, Edgar Erskine: Medical Work of
the Knights Hospitallers of Saint John of Jerusalem. The Johns Hopkins Press,
Baltimore.)

hundred feet long, thirty-four feet wide, and thirty feet high. Tapestry or wool hangings everywhere helped to take the chill from bare,
cold walls in winter time. Paintings enlivened them. To prevent drafts
and ensure privacy, each bed was enclosed in a tent-like curtain.
Wealth permitted luxuries, and the food service included bowls,
plates, and covers of solid silver, as well as a few forks—implements
just coming into use.

A well-perfected organization provided for department heads in charge of silver, linen, wine, diet, phlebotomy, buying, and accounts. Nursing, almsgiving, distribution of food to the poor, care of foundlings and of the insane were among institutional functions. Patients were segregated according to their status as pilgrims, as members of religious groups, or as belonging to the laity. Cases of slight indisposition were not placed with acute cases. Also isolated were cases of hemorrhage, lithotomy, and insanity, while mercurial inunctions were given in separate rooms provided for the purpose. A tailor's shop saw to the mending of clothing worn by indigents. A medical staff was assisted by a barber-surgeon who took charge of bleedings, the application of leeches, and blistering. Paid physicians instructed knights in anatomy and the care of the sick. Ten chaplains attended spiritual wants.

The architecture of this remarkable hospital repeated a tradition of the hospitallers in its fortress-like characteristics. Windows, small and narrow, were sunk deep and high in thick stone walls. The patient, even when not imprisoned within a tent of curtains, saw nothing of the world outside. He was also deprived of fresh air. This forbidding type of structure long influenced institutional building in Europe. Fortunately, other forms of architectural development made themselves apparent, too, during those centuries in which monasteries knew wealth, for men who abandoned their seclusion, or who were not monks, traveled abroad and saw the products of Moslem or Byzantine culture. Hospitals of the medieval period took on some of their architectural features.

New Gothic forms, such as were produced in magnificent cathedrals of the time, reappear in hospitals. Often the pattern was the palace of the wealthy or the cloister of the monastery. Especially in the south, gardens or colonnades gave patients access to the outdoors. In Spain, Moslem influence showed in lavish external ornament, while interiors here and elsewhere introduced much beauty in tiling. Often the hospital was a great ward built like a church, with lofty supporting arches, perhaps a gallery, and with an altar at the end which made it possible for the sick to be present at celebration of the mass. Then beds were commonly placed end to end along the side walls, that nothing might interfere with their seeing the holy place at all times.

The social problem of the abandoned child was met by these medieval hospitals. His welfare was among the considerations of those men and women who were eager to better conditions as social confusion cleared a little. Additional separate foundling hospitals were the result, while the reception and care of foundlings usually entered the program of any medieval hospital for the sick. From the twelfth century the crèche (cradle) became a feature of charitable work in the medieval city, and a cradle inside the portal of hospital or church was kept in readiness for the mother who wished to consign her babe to the care of others. Sometimes the children remained until grown, the boys learning trades, the girls being taught household duties, including spinning and weaving, and often provided with a dower by the hospital when they married.

NURSING OF THE LATE MIDDLE AGES

Looking back over the late medieval period as a phase in the development of nursing we find interesting changes, each due to an accompanying change in society; for nursing care, like any other service to the public, must adapt itself to ever-changing social needs.

From the great need of nurses to care for the sick and wounded during the Crusades, were derived those units of soldier nurses or Knights Hospitallers who nursed the sick only during intervals when they were not busy fighting. Great numbers of men became nurses, and the military ideal of order and discipline became apparent. There were women, too, who organized as auxiliary units of these orders, like the Sisters of the Hospital of St. Mary Magdalene and the Sisters of St. Lazarus. When the Crusades ended, the monasteries of military orders extended over the land from Palestine to England, their men and women nurses carrying on under the influence of the leper movement, and a novel war against disease. With the advent of the military order, a harsher element entered nursing. The vow of unquestioning obedience had long been incident to monastic organization, but monastic organization was on the family basis with abbot and abbess as father and mother. Emphasis was now placed on rank, and on deference to superior officers.

The many unsolved social problems of changing times, and especially the plight of those cast out as lepers, were causing criticism of conditions as they were, and awareness of need for bringing out among the people the simple faith and kindly service of the early followers of Jesus. This need was met by the Franciscan Mendicant Order, founded by St. Francis of Assisi.

Gradual disintegration of the protective units of the monastery and the feudal estate brought further changes. The new social need arising from redistribution of population and urban growth now brought nursing out of the institution and back into the home, where the deaconess first found need of it. The situation was met by the Beguines of Belgium, the Tertiaries of St. Francis, and other secular orders which included private duty nursing and visiting nursing with hospital activities.

In the late twelfth and early thirteenth centuries, as the city hospital, under civilian direction, came on the scene, a tendency to develop civilian nursing groups in hospitals accompanied the innovation. At the same time medicine was becoming differentiated from surgery and nursing. The newly organized medical schools were turning out men who had devoted much time to learning. Learning brought distinction to this group, while it gave them a new viewpoint on their work, and new methods. Procedures which had once occupied them were now given over to assistants, and became specialized in the hands of the barber-surgeon or the nurse.

All medieval monastic nursing was necessarily simple. It featured shelter, regular hours, simple food, pure drinking water, herbal medicine (mysterious often, but harmless), the washing of sores, the dressing of wounds, and a few simple nursing procedures. To these were added the mental solace of kindliness, music, and religion. The freedom with which alms were distributed helped to remove fear of return to a harsh world. Equipment, like procedures, had been accepted by tradition. Beds were large ones of wood, pillows or rings were covered with leather in lieu of rubber, and feathers, moss, or horsehair provided their filling. Long-handled warming-pans heated with hot coals or hot water anticipated the hot-water bottle. Catheters and enema bulbs had been in use even among ancient people. There were no thermometers, and nurses trusted mainly to their hands in determining temperature, although the bare foot seems to have been used as an extra precaution in testing water heated for the newborn baby's bath.

Sweet-smelling herbs, perfumes, or odors arising from burning of fragrant woods, and such things as orange peel, were favorite deodorizers which availed little in face of bad ventilation and a prevailing aversion to fresh air. The omnipresent fireplace made the hot shovel and hot coals readily available for carrying these about. Little oil lamps, such as we may yet see among relics of antiquity, were in use at night. Even the simplest procedures in bedside nursing were difficult and time-consuming for lack of conveniences which we take for granted. Among institutions for care of the sick then, as now, there were always some that were very good, and some that were very bad.

As time went on, exigencies arose to disturb whatever had been developed in nursing service. During and after the Crusades there were new social interests, changing social standards, periods of great poverty, recurrent epidemics, and an increasing disregard of health conservation on the part of the public. Tightening of restrictions in the life of monastic nurses hampered free development of nursing. The spirit of activity and newness in the post-Crusade air extended its influence to the monastery, and we find "accidia" (boredom) recognized as a malady of young monks, for which at least one abbot prescribed sitting on a special stone in the infirmary as treatment. There were not always enough nurses, and there was a change in their caliber as the later medieval monastery opened its doors to men and women who were the unfortunate product of a phase of low social morality, and low standards of home life and education.

With passing centuries, the sickbed came to hold more than one patient, and, at last, even as many as six. Medieval sensitiveness to bed crowding was not keen, for this was a home custom. The difficulties that it added to changing of linen for the sick are obvious. Patients were sometimes not only dirty but ill-fed. Indifference met the warning of any who dared to point out dangers in this crowding and poor nursing. The civilian hospital sometimes introduced women of low character to augment inadequate nursing staffs, thereby completing the range of medieval nurses from high-bred, intellectual men and women to the inferior.

Nursing had begun a decline which was to persist for a long, long time. Contemporary medicine, however, was in the ascendant, as capable physicians from medical schools were added to that scattered group of doctors, usually Jews or Saracens, and sometimes learned men from the school at Alexandria who had been handing medicine down from one to the other, throughout the Middle Ages. A revival of Greek science was beginning, and as universities arose everywhere to quicken medical interest in it, medicine and nursing separated.

Nevertheless, the tradition of early Christianity which made nursing the vocation of the finest type of individual persisted through the Middle Ages, and did not die with them. The early medieval monastery attracted the scholarly man and the highborn woman. Early monastic leaders in nursing had been men and women of intellect, their lives significant of culture, refinement, and democracy. Individual queens, like St. Radegunde and St. Elizabeth, princesses, ladies or knights, idealists of the middle class like St. Francis and St. Catherine of Siena, all contributed to establish a conception of the care of the sick as one of the finest expressions of interest in the common good. Henry II, king of England, established a lazaretto for women in Rouen, France, on condition that noble-women only should nurse the patients. As late as 1492 that Queen Isabella of Spain whose jewels went to finance the discovery of America was appearing in person on the field as she directed her own ambulance and nursing service. These names have been remembered. For one reason or another those who bore them stood out, but there were many, many others who worked with them to make strong and resistant the roots of a vocation that would not be publicly recognized for nearly four centuries.

Uniformity in Dress   There is observable during the progress of the Middle Ages a decided tendency toward uniformity in the dress of nurses. No uniform had been worn by the deaconess, and none distinguished the early nuns. The lady of the court or the castle who became a nurse continued to wear her fashionable clothes. Wool or linen was her common choice of material, but silk and velvet were not considered out of place, and the abbess dressed to accord with her feudal rank. The uniforms adopted by the military nursing orders encouraged uniformity in other nursing groups. In accord with its original purpose of making the wearer stand out from those around him, the medieval uniform was not inconspicuous. The idea of using color in uniform to harmonize with landscape or surroundings so that wearers are almost invisible or lose identity is of recent adoption.

As early as the ninth century, a distinctive dress had been recommended for monastics. During the Crusades it became quite common, and made its own appeal to church authorities who felt more and more the need of protecting that institution from public reaction to errors committed by some monks and nuns who felt safe in the obscurity of ordinary dress. As they were then developed, monastic uniforms or habits savored, naturally, of period fashions. These were growing gay and luxurious. Were the foundation of the habit black or brown, it followed that color would be used to offset dullness. Scarlet, bright blue, white, or purple was worn by men as well as by women. Robes took on the long, flowing lines favored in the east, and cloaks were freely bordered with ermine. In fact, the accessibility of all types of fur, combined with the chill of thick-walled stone buildings heated only in spots, encouraged its use, not only as trimming but as full lining.

Headdresses varied from the plain pointed hood or cowl of cloth, or the Roman veil assumed by the married woman on her bridal day as token of submission to her husband, to much more elaborate designs. The wimple, or folded piece of linen drawn up under the chin and tied on the head under a cap, veil, or hat, was common to civil society and monastery. As groups grew in number, details of uniform increased and changed with the effort to distinguish them from one another. The cross of Christianity, worn in common by all religious orders, took many forms.

When secular orders came into existence, choice of color in uniform veered to solid dull browns, grays, or blues, and some of the emphasis on its use was lost, outside of the Franciscan and Dominican orders. This was not only in harmony with the sadness of a miserable post-war period, but it accorded with a desire to abandon the cumbersome ceremony and the pomp of feudal times, and live simply on equality with those masses whose poverty brought such orders into being. The wealthy, isolated monastery turned to building of great cathedrals or a new interest in the Greek classics. The military spirit lived on in rule and regulation, but the gaiety of attire in which it had once embodied itself was gradually giving way before a rigid solemnity that was settling down upon religion.

SUMMARY OF LATE MIDDLE AGES

The late Middle Ages (1000–1500 A.D.) witnessed a new mobility of population with accompanying detachment of individuals from isolated units. The population was set into motion by religious expeditions called *Crusades*, the object of which was to rescue the Holy Land of Christians from Moslem rule. These brought many hospitals into being, and introduced great numbers of male nurses who, in military nursing, undertook the care of sick and wounded Crusaders. Ultimately, these supplemented the work of established monasteries all over the west as well as in Palestine.

By this time the pioneer work of Christianizing pagans and teaching them the arts of civilization had been accomplished. Church organizations had grown rich and powerful, and manual labor or a simple life were not essential to their existence. There was public criticism which pointed at the failure of the church to exemplify the teachings of Christ. This criticism was met by making monastic rules more strict. Then came St. Francis of Assisi (1182–1226) to relieve the situation by taking religion and nursing out among the people. Mendicant or begging orders were formed which owned no property, were composed of men and women who gave their possessions to the poor, and literally followed the Christ. The first order of Franciscans was called *Friars Minor* (little brothers), and later St. Francis founded a second order of *Poor Clares* or Franciscan nuns who helped his friars to nurse and feed lepers. The latter were segregated in a multitude of little huts or hospitals, and their removal from society aided materially in banishment of leprosy as a plague.

St. Francis founded a third order called *Tertiaries*, which was secular, for it was composed of citizens in their homes who pledged themselves to help society by charitable works, individually or as group projects. A tendency to avoid ecclesiastical precedent and rule was shown in a development of other secular orders. Prominent among these were the *Beguines* of Belgium whose members took no vow of poverty, and one of obedience and chastity only for the period in which they remained in community life. They were free to live in their own homes and to leave the order if they chose to do so. The Beguines did much private, hospital, and visiting nursing in Belgium where they originated, and also in France, Switzerland, and Germany.

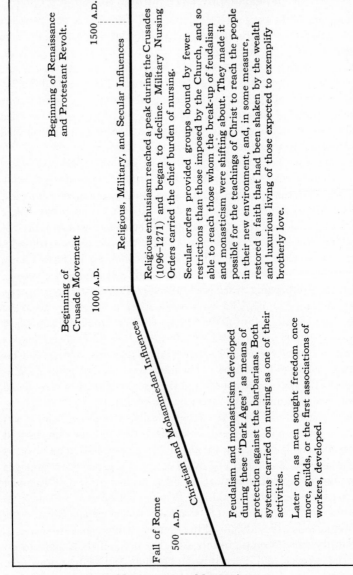

Beginning of Renaissance
and Protestant Revolt.

1500 A.D.

Beginning of
Crusade Movement

1000 A.D.

Fall of Rome

500 A.D.

Religious, Military, and Secular Influences

Christian and Mohammedan Influences

Religious enthusiasm reached a peak during the Crusades (1096–1271) and began to decline. Military Nursing Orders carried the chief burden of nursing.

Secular orders provided groups bound by fewer restrictions than those imposed by the Church, and so able to reach those whom the break-up of feudalism and monasticism were shifting about. They made it possible for the teachings of Christ to reach the people in their new environment, and, in some measure, restored a faith that had been shaken by the wealth and luxurious living of those expected to exemplify brotherly love.

Feudalism and monasticism developed during these "Dark Ages" as means of protection against the barbarians. Both systems carried on nursing as one of their activities.

Later on, as men sought freedom once more, guilds, or the first associations of workers, developed.

NURSING OF THE MIDDLE AGES
500–1500 A.D.

The Crusades ended without making Christians rulers of Jerusalem, but with other fruitful results. The people of Europe were thrilled with desire for adventure and eager to know more about the world. Ideas were exchanged with other peoples, trade grew lively, and as traders made fortunes and industry increased to supply them with wares, a great new *middle class* developed which lived in towns. Unfortunately, diseases were transferred as well as ideas and great plagues occurred, the most serious of which, occurring in 1348, carried off many millions of people. Weaklings, especially as represented by a great leper population, were destroyed.

Downtrodden labor became more independent through scarcity of workers. Plague experiences taught something about health protection through quarantine, and a little about disinfection, but, physically, the western world was dirtier than ever; mentally it had been roused to an activity not possible in the narrowness of restricted groups. Changes began to come swiftly. The way was being paved for a renaissance or re-birth of literary culture and art.

Later, medieval nurses served in and out of monasteries and were drawn from all ranks of society. They were active in war and also as institutional, private duty, and visiting nurses. When new interests developed, those belonging to the upper social strata became interested in new things. Monastic groups were becoming more and more bound by restrictions; inferior lay women were placed in the field, and nursing declined. Hours of work were long and nurses had to assume a staggering burden of domestic duties, for the precedent of free labor established by the monastery stood in the way of departmental distribution of work and of any adequate staffing. While physicians profited through an expansion of universities and medical schools, conditions under which they worked brought nurses, intellectually, to a standstill. A routine of nursing care was handed down from one to another, and that was all.

TOPICS FOR DISCUSSION

1. While a large part of the population of western Europe was shut up in monasteries and feudal estates, what changes were going on outside which made themselves evident after several centuries?

2. (*a*) What is the purpose of a pilgrimage, and why were so many

undertaken during the late Middle Ages? (*b*) What do you think of the wisdom of the "Truce of God"? (*c*) Do you know of any other type of pilgrimage than that of Christians to Jerusalem?

3. What were the objectives of the series of wars known as the "Crusades"?

4. What organization corresponded to our army nurse corps in providing nursing care to sick and wounded soldiers of the Crusades?

5. (*a*) How did the military nursing orders differ from the usual orders of knights and monks? (*b*) What new influences did they bring into nursing?

6. Name a number of the social problems confronting people of the Middle Ages?

7. What were the causes of public criticism which led people to welcome the development of Mendicant Orders?

8. (*a*) How did the Mendicant Orders founded by St. Dominic and St. Francis differ from other established orders of the Church? (*b*) What three orders were ultimately founded by St. Francis? (*c*) Are any of these in existence and active today?

9. What influence did the military nursing orders and mendicant orders have on the type of dress worn by those who did nursing?

10. What third type of nursing order, representing a wide departure from the usual restrictions of the church, was founded and became active during the latter part of the Middle Ages?

11. What famous nurse of this period became a member of the secular order of Tertiaries of St. Francis, and why might she be considered one of the first visiting nurses?

12. What other secular order became famous, and what type of nursing service was rendered by it?

13. (*a*) Were the Crusades a success or a failure in regard to regaining Jerusalem from the Moslems? (*b*) What social changes resulted from the vast movement of population in an easterly direction?

14. Give reasons for the fact that the late Middle Ages are considered to be the period of beginning of romantic love.

15. Compare provisions for safeguarding the public health during the Middle Ages with those of your community today.

16. Describe the great epidemics that swept over Europe during the fourteenth century.

17. Tell what you know of St. Catherine as a hospital nurse and a visiting nurse during an epidemic of Black Death in her home town of Siena.

18. By what three groups was Hellenic medicine preserved during the difficulties of the Middle Ages?

19. What contributions to the practice of medicine and nursing of the time were made by St. Hildegarde?

20. Discuss the advantages and disadvantages of being a patient in the Hospital of St. John at Valetta.

21. (a) What circumstances led to the development of city hospitals? (b) What provision was made for nursing care in them?

22. (a) Tell what you know of the nursing of the late Middle Ages. (b) Give reasons for the fact that nursing entered a long period of decline.

23. Why was contemporary medicine in the ascendency?

24. Give an account of the origin of uniform costumes for those engaged in nursing.

25. (a) Through reference reading in the encyclopedia and elsewhere, show under what circumstances the word, "Saint," is authorized to be used before the name of an historical character. (b) How many nursing saints can you name, and with what special type of work is each associated?

26. (a) What illustrations can you find that show the general tendency of architecture of the time, including that of hospitals? (b) Compare their emphasis on beauty with that on provision for carrying out principles of hygiene.

27. (a) Can any form of society be expected to remain stationary? (b) Discuss the necessity for ability to face changes and make a good adjustment.

28. Complete your own adaptation of the chart on page 200, adding a dotted line for the general trend in medicine.

29. What names can you add to your outline map of Europe?

REFERENCES

Bossard, J. H. S.: Problems of Social Well-being. New York and London, Harper & Brothers, 1927, Chap. 26.

Briffault, Robert: The Days of Ignorance. New York, Chas. Scribner's Sons, 1935.

Chesterton, G. K.: St. Francis of Assisi. New York, Geo. H. Doran Co., 1924.

Dana, Charles L.: The Peaks of Medical History. New York, Paul B. Hoeber, 1928.

Dock and Nutting: A History of Nursing. New York and London, G. P. Putnam's Sons, 1907, Vol. I, Part II, Chaps. 3–9.

Farrow, John: Damien the Leper. New York, Sheed & Ward, 1927.

Haggard, Howard W.: The Doctor in History. New Haven, Yale University Press,, 1934.

Hume, Edgar Erskine: Medical Work of the Knights Hospitallers of Saint John of Jerusalem. Baltimore, The Johns Hopkins Press, 1940.

Hutton, Edward: St. Francis of Assisi. New York, Longmans, Green and Co., 1950.

Jorgensen, Johannes: St. Francis of Assisi. New York, Longmans, Green and Co., reprint of 1912 edition.

Lamb, Harold: The Crusades: Iron Men and Saints. Garden City, New York, Doubleday, Doran & Co., 1930.

———: The Flame of Islam. Garden City, New York, Doubleday, Doran & Co., 1931.

Major, Charles: When Knighthood Was in Flower. New York, Grosset & Dunlap, 1907.

Mead, William Edward: The English Medieval Feast. Boston and New York, Houghton Mifflin Co., 1931.

Peattie, Donald: A Cup of Sky (St. Francis of Assisi). Boston, Houghton Mifflin Co., 1950.

Prestage, Edgar: Chivalry. London, Kegan Paul, Trench, Trubner & Co., Ltd., 1928.

Putnam, E. J.: The Lady. New York and London, G. P. Putnam's Sons, 1921, pp. 106–157.

Quennell, Marjorie and C. H. B.: A History of Everyday Things in England (1066–1799) (4 volumes). New York, Chas. Scribner's Sons, 1922–35.

Rayner, Edwin: Famous Cathedrals and Their Stories. New York, Grosset & Dunlap, 1935.

Riesman, David: The Story of Medicine in the Middle Ages. New York, Paul B. Hoeber, Inc., 1935.

Schimberg, Albert P.: The Larks of Umbria (St. Francis). Milwaukee, Wisconsin, Bruce Publishing Co., 1942.

Scott, Sir Walter: Ivanhoe (description of tournament).

Stubbs and Bligh: Sixty Centuries of Health and Physick. London, S. Low Marston and Co., 1931.

Tobey, James A.: Riders of the Plagues. New York, Chas. Scribner's Sons, 1930.

PART THREE

The Modern Era: Scientific, Economic, and Social Evolution

Beginning Circa 1500 A.D.

Renaissance, Reformation, and a Decline in Nursing

1500-1860 A.D.

When the year 1500 dawned on the western world, men were thinking of many new things. The spirit of revolutionary change filled the air as it had five and also ten hundred years before, and as it does today. The world had suddenly become very much enlarged by land or sea trade with the Orient and the discovery of America. Old ways of doing things would not work under new conditions. The individual was just making it known that he had had enough of cooperative living. A secular spirit, arising in commercial towns, had invaded the Church. People were ready to discard the old ideas, and even now were seeking some new form of the old religion that had been a mainstay in darker times. Kings by this time ruled supreme, each little nation speaking a different language, and developing different customs from the neighbors round about.

THE RENAISSANCE

By 1577 *Sir Francis Drake* had found his way around the world, his ship only one among many that had been bringing home to Europe and Britain tales of wealth beyond the seas in India, China, the East Indies, and above all, in America. Ambitious business men and nations saw profit in permanent trade with this new land, and power in its colonization. The compass, with ships of better build, had already improved transportation, and expedition after expedition was equipped and sent on its way. Gunpowder changed fighting methods, and increased kingly power by weakening feudal lords. Castles could now be blown up, and guns required new skills. Mailed knights on horseback and the old glories of chivalry gave place to the man from any class who asked pay for his fighting in a "standing" army, tax supported. Gunpowder affected surgery and nursing also, for it brought new types of wounds and new difficulties from infection.

The recent invention of the printing art was putting books into the hands of many thousands of people, and spreading ideas with strange rapidity. Before printing was invented, books had been written by hand, and copied by hand—a long, laborious task which grew more costly as time became more valuable. An astounding machine made it possible to turn out briefly great numbers of books, each one of which would have occupied a skilled copyist for at least half a year. The Bible which even in its Latin form had been read up to now chiefly by monks or other scholars, became before long the object of intensive study by the general public. The art of printing also gave to students of literature access to the works of their ancestors.

THE CLASSIC REVIVAL

A classical revival first showed itself in Italy, where wealth derived from an advantageous trading position during the Crusades had brought a leisure that came more slowly to other countries. As each country in its turn found opportunity to develop literary and artistic groups, it built these around remnants of classical literature and art, for there was little else available. Caesar, Cicero, Virgil, Aristotle, and Homer made their entrance to European and British curricula. Children were baptized with Greek and Roman names. People ferreted out forgotten manuscripts, and began to look with new eyes on old works of art. They copied the ancients, becoming more and more worldly under their pagan influence. The emphasis placed by medieval forbears on the virtues of self-sacrifice and self-denial was cast aside. They questioned everything, "debunked" existing ideals just as people have done in this century, exacted accuracy, and even doubted the Church. The new state of mind reflected itself in the general attitude toward charitable works, and, in particular, on medicine and nursing. It put its impress on literature, painting, sculpture, and architecture.

In the realm of literature, the Renaissance stimulated men, and women too, to classical scholarship. As writers, they followed classical formality in style. Leading trends of thought during these times were shown here and there. *Machiavelli* (1469–1527), an Italian, advocated despotic power for the ruler. *Erasmus* (1469–1536), the wandering scholar of Holland, encouraged education while he derided medieval ideals and superstitions. The Englishman, *Sir Thomas More* (1478–1553), dared to frame a "Utopia" just as men of our day dream and write of the abundant life for all. *Martin Luther* (1483–1546), in Germany, translated the Bible into his own language, and led a revolt against contemporary Christianity which ended in a division of the church into Protestant and Catholic sections. *Cervantes* (1547–1616), a Spaniard, made fun of feudalism and chivalry in "Don Quixote," *William Shakespeare* (1564–1616) drew upon life rather than upon the classics for his philosophy, and *John Milton* (1608–1674) gave to the world his "Paradise Lost," and in other works argued for political and religious freedom, with a free press for utterance of public opinion. These are a very few of the names which stand out in a period of brilliant intellectual activity and reorganization of human values.

In the field of art a corresponding awakening was taking place among the painters, architects, and sculptors. Its wealth and natural beauty made an artistic center of the city of Florence, one day to be the birthplace of Florence Nightingale, whose fame as a restorer of the nursing art would equal that of the painters, sculptors, and architects gathered there. Florence was ruled by bankers of the family of Medici, who took pride in helping men to make it more and more beautiful. *Luca della Robbia* (1399–1482), a native son, designed and made a wonderful choir gallery for its cathedral. On this he carved life-like children making music in varied ways as they responded to the call of the one hundred and fiftieth psalm:

"Praise ye the Lord.
Praise Him with the sound of the trumpet; praise Him with the psaltery and the harp.
Praise Him with the timbrel and dance; praise Him with stringed instruments and organs.
Praise Him upon the loud cymbals; praise Him upon the high-sounding cymbals
Let everything that hath breath praise the Lord."

If we take time to reflect that the printing press was just coming into use, and that reading was an accomplishment possessed by only a few, it becomes evident that these expressions of art were necessary for transfer of biblical teachings to the people. At the same time, art no longer made religion its first expression, as religion no longer was the whole life of the people. Courts patronized the arts, aristocracies flattered artists, and increasing wealth made it possible for the delights of art to penetrate the middle class.

A school for artists developed in Florence. Each master had his following, and pupils served on the apprentice plan. There were innovations in artistic method. The easel was introduced for convenience in working on a piece of canvas which took the place of the plastered wall on which it had been customary to paint frescoes. This required a new kind of paint mixed with oil, and painters must learn secrets of mixing as well as of applying it to the canvas. Besides tools through which they might express themselves, masters of this and other Italian schools of painting during the Renaissance gave their pupils new ideals of scientific accuracy in the representation of people and things, and helped them to solve problems of perspective, light, and color. Anatomy and natural science were made complementary to art.

Two students in the school of Florentine art stand out as geniuses. *Michelangelo* (1475–1564) and *Léonardo da Vinci* (1453–1519) were architects, sculptors, engineers, and painters. Both took part in supervising the building of the greatest of churches, St. Peter's at Rome. For four years Michelangelo painted frescoes in the Sistine Chapel of the adjoining Vatican, palace of the Popes. As these were on the ceiling, he was forced to work hours at a time, lying on his back on a high scaffold. His task and his position were so strenuous as to draw from an inspired workman the following:

"So weary I get lying on my back, looking upward, pains shoot through my head, my neck, my eyes. In truth, I am getting so that I cannot read except when I am lying upon my back and holding my paper over my head."[1]

Leonardo da Vinci painted the "Last Supper" on a wall of the refectory in a monastery at Milan, and he with like intensity worked from dawn to dark, forgetting to eat. In this masterpiece, Jesus is

[1] Hartman, Gertrude: Medieval Days and Ways, 1937. Quoted on p. 276. By permission of The Macmillan Company, publishers.

shown seated with his twelve disciples at a long table. Marvelous variations in expression on the faces reflect the individual reaction to the words that have just been heard: "One of you will betray me." Da Vinci's "Mona Lisa," a portrait of a lady which should hang in the Louvre at Paris, is of such life-like beauty that too ardent admirers have, now and then, stolen it. The last suspect, however, is said to have returned it because the plumpness of the hands eventually wore upon him.

Botticelli (1447–1515) made delightful representations of Greek gods and goddesses. One of the best known among these is "Spring" in which appear Venus, Cupid, and the Three Graces. *Raphael* (1483–1520), another student of Florence and among the "moderns" of the sixteenth century, is best known for his Madonnas, most famous of which is the "Sistine Madonna." The great *Titian* (1477–1576) led a second group of students in Venice. The Venetian school was noted for its mastery of color, as the school at Florence was noted for form and grace of line.

A school arising somewhat later in Flanders produced *Rubens* (1577–1640) and *Van Dyck* (1599–1641). Spaniards were led by *Velásquez* (1599–1660), and the Dutch by *Rembrandt* (1606–1669). The English did not evolve their own school of painting until the time of *Sir Joshua Reynolds* (1723–1792) who painted the well-known "St. Cecilia," and *Sir Thomas Gainsborough* (1727–1788) who painted the "Blue Boy" and the "Duchess of Devonshire."

"Blue Boy" and "Duchess of Devonshire," however, were significant of other changes going on in society. The former pictured the son of an ironmonger, the latter a member of the aristocracy. The times permitted a class of newly rich to dress its children in blue satin, with rich lace and plumed hats. These children lived in homes where fine portraits were no longer out of place. Their fathers and mothers had leisure to acquire appreciation of the arts and to enjoy the privileges which wealth once had given only to the class which the Duchess represents.

POLITICAL REVOLUTION

During the medieval period, the great family of the Mother Church had grown up. Strong men now ruled kingdoms which they felt they should be allowed to manage without parental interference, and by right of divine power in themselves. Under kings, a system of private ownership and private enterprise was taking shape. An era was beginning in which desire for wealth and the grasping of opportunity would hold chief place in men's minds. Individually, and as nations, they would seek power. Kings of nations were now testing out autocracy, the popularity of which England, already nearer to democracy than other countries, was able to disprove through Parliament and the ancient Magna Charta.

In France, the once all-powerful feudal lords soon found that they could get nowhere without royal favor. It became the fashion among them to take up residence near the royal person so that no opportunity for gaining this favor might be lost. As courtiers, they were flattering accessories, but often financially dependent. *Louis XIV* (1643–1715) used them and their ladies to build up around him such a royal court as overshadowed the colorful one of Queen Elizabeth of England. He made himself the center of a great machine representing power. Around him were thousands of richly dressed, often very attractive and clever men and women, all basking in a glory created from the labor of the French common people.

The marvel of Versailles, with its glittering gilt, its crystal and mirrors, its paintings and tapestries, was conjured into being. Gay pastimes found their way into its gorgeous drawing rooms. Grownups played at hide and seek in its mystery maze of boxwood hedge, or strolled about its flower gardens. A precedent of regal magnificence had been established that all the royal courts of Europe were to follow as best they could. Idleness reigned. By the time *Louis XVI* became king of France, the country was nearly bankrupt. His vain queen, *Marie Antoinette*, knew not what she did when she took up the thread of life that was handed to her. She loved Versailles, and gaiety, and luxury, and indulged herself to the limit. All her extravagances, great or small, every bit of foolishness or display went to make more bitter the hatred of those men and women who were getting ready to do away with it all.

The ambition of kings led to war, and the spirit of national competition was fostered in the people. Germany, Spain, England, and France kept Europe in uproar. From 1689 to 1763 nationalism was rampant. One great struggle followed another until the Seven Years' War (also known as the French and Indian War) beginning in 1754, put England foremost. In that struggle France lost Canada, which thereafter was an English colony. The poverty which followed the wars brought a discontent that flamed up in a series of equally great revolutions, the American Revolution (1775–1783), the French Revolution (1789–1795), the Latin-American Revolution (1800–1825). These reflected a popular reaction against the accepted theory of human inequality, and the insistence of the individualist of getting his rights. While the disturbance was not yet over, there arose from the angry masses a dictator who undertook to unify Europeans and manage their affairs for them. The Napoleonic wars began in 1797. They ended in 1815 when the Duke of Wellington, at the battle Waterloo, buried dictatorship for a time. At the beginning of the nineteenth century, England and democracy were in the lead.

INDUSTRIAL REVOLUTION

War and revolution thus attained a scope that affected the political aspect of two continents. Individuals of the time, as well as generations following them, were called upon to make many and difficult adjustments. These adjustments, however, were minor in comparison with those which would be the consequence of a revolution of a different kind that began even while armies fought and men were guillotined by other men who saw no other way to get certain considerations that they had learned to call "rights." This other revolution, beginning in England about 1750, upset long accustomed modes of life by changing modes of work. For this reason, it has been named the "Industrial Revolution," and with ever-increasing momentum it still goes on. A revolution in transportation has followed in its wake.

All countries of the world now experience the stress of its constant change, but England was the first to be affected. The raising of sheep and the manufacture of cloth from their wool had long been a chief employment of her people. Spinning and weaving were done in farmhouses, by slow hand processes. Machinery was now invented that speeded up production and lessened the number of people needed to make cloth. Ways were found to utilize power to run not only one but many machines, all at the same time, and factories were built where these could be placed. If the farmhouse family wished to earn a living it must move to the place where the factory stood. Its members would have to adjust to new ways of working, as well as to the confinement of life within the narrow limits of tenement flats and city streets. Guild principles of fairness would no longer control the price asked for the cloth they made, and wages would be kept at a minimum so that the owner of the factory might have a maximum profit.

The skill that it might have taken a life-time to acquire in order to turn out an especially fine article no longer had the same value. The machine could standardize quality. Before long, the independent master of apprentices bound to learn his craft from him in his little shop, and the farmer who held a strip of cultivable land, were forced to give up craft and land, and become laborers for rich men, or factory hands. These changes heralded corresponding ones in other industries. The efficiency idea took hold of agriculture and business. An era of invention opened, the number of manufacturing cities grew.

THE REFORMATION

The Reformation or Protestant Revolt, beginning in 1517, helped to precipitate the disaster toward which the vocation of nursing was headed. The Church had tried to overcome a waning tendency in that enthusiasm for religion which rose to a peak during the Crusades, but her efforts to restore a faith shaken by practices which she admitted, proved unsuccessful. There were those who insisted on finding their own way to a truthful expression of a simple Christian belief, and they had been gathering energy to assert themselves. Two outstanding groups of reformers, by this time, were at work—those who stayed with the Church, and those who were throwing in their lot with revolutionist *Martin Luther*, once a German mendicant monk, now leader of a separatist group called "Protestants" (those who protested). Whole countries began to emerge as distinctively conservative or protestant in their bent. Where there had been only one church, there were henceforth two, differentiated by the names, Protestant and Catholic.

Where the popular majority held to old beliefs, there were reformers who continued their efforts to cure abuses by slower methods than those of upheaval. Representative of this group was one *Ignatius Loyola*, a Spanish soldier who, in 1534, inspired the organization of an order of teaching clergy to attempt to reach a solution by utilizing the channel of education. The missionaries of his Society of Jesus, commonly known as *Jesuits*, were militant preachers, upholding orthodoxy, but they were also among the earliest of trained teachers, and equipped with an unusual thoroughness of method. Wherever they went, they won respect for scholarship, and took a leading place as educators, especially in institutions of the higher grades. In this time of stress the Catholic Church welcomed their support, which was augmented, shortly after, by the foundation of the *Order of St. Ursula* (patron saint of maidens), a woman's order dedicated to the education of girls. Many convent schools were founded by the Ursulines in Europe.

In 1545, a general council of church authorities was called at Trentino, in Italy, for the purpose of discussing ways and means of removing causes of criticism and clarifying the church position. This meeting lasted eighteen years, and so much was accomplished during that time that this *Council of Trent* has since been looked upon as one of the most famous and decisive of ecclesiastical gatherings. Doctrinal issues were re-stated, financial relationships discussed, and the position of the Catholic group thoroughly identified.

The two religious bodies, however, utterly failed to reach a middle ground of tolerance. Also, each country's ruler tried to make all of his people think and worship as he did. The result was an era of cruel hatreds, with a tremendous development of sects as an outlet for repressed individuality. Civil conflicts were induced and the climax was reached in an international conflict known as the "Thirty Years' War" (1618–1648). Political, economic, and religious issues were fought out, and a state of comparative religious tolerance was reached. To ensure themselves true freedom in religion, people had begun to leave the Old World for the New.

TRANSFER OF EUROPEAN CULTURE TO AMERICA

Not long before America was discovered, the spirit of adventure and the desire to Christianize heathen pervaded Europe, and led men to India, China, and Japan. Trade outposts were established and there was some fleeting religious influence. The most far-reaching result of her foreign contacts was the awakening of Europe to the advantages of commerce and increased power through wealth coming from the outside. Her real expansion began when a new continent

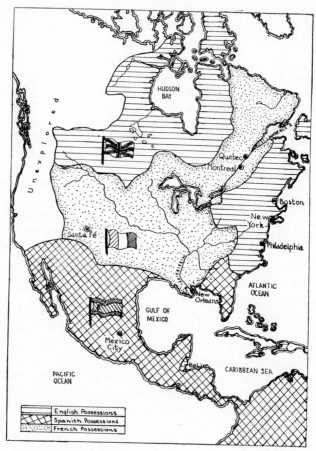

NEW ENGLAND, NEW FRANCE, AND NEW SPAIN

was discovered unexpectedly. By that time Spain, Portugal, and England stood ready and eager to grasp the hand of opportunity. France finished one of her wars and then followed them.

A New Spain, a New France, and a New England grew up on the other side of the Atlantic, and Portugal appropriated what is now Brazil. The northern continent, before three centuries had passed, was divided among European nations in almost transverse sections. The southern section belonged to Spain, the middle one to France, and lands in the far north with Newfoundland and a strip of Atlantic coast were English. What is now California was away off across great deserts, rivers, and high mountains, and was the most remote spot on the face of the earth to people who thought of such a country at all. This area, the land directly north of it, and Alaska, were all of North America that remained unclaimed.

If Spanish or French, the pioneer in America was of the Catholic Church, and, usually, a man who loved adventure which, if he was a friar or priest, he combined with zealous Christianization of the Indian. The English colonist was a Protestant, as determined to set up a permanent home for himself and family in a land where he looked for religious freedom. Each national group brought national customs with it, and hoped to set in motion the transference of European culture to America. Old ideas and new ones, superstition and wisdom, monasticism and Puritanism—all established themselves in new soil. The spirit of the sixteenth century Renaissance, however, came too. Those to whom its transmission was entrusted were human beings, capable of evil as well as good, and the difficulties which they encountered caused some setback in its fruitage.

Of all the nations speculating in colonization, Spain appears to have been, easily, the most lucky in her beginnings. In Mexico and Panama, she walked into a land already possessing a high degree of civilization as well as mines of fabulous wealth and stores of mined gold. She could begin shipping fortunes to the homeland at once, and she did. Many of her noble adventurers found a way to personal fortune and set up homes in a land which offered freedom for initiative. They established a university, a medical school, and a magnificent hospital in Mexico City. They introduced Spanish art, dressed with the richness of famed grandees, and made life gay for every one with music and dancing, ribbons, gilt, and bright colors. Gay-plumed cavaliers made love to beautiful señoritas.

French neighbors of triumphant New Spain brought gaiety with them, too, but did not find so ready an opportunity for wealth, power, or ease. Both climate and Indians were less friendly, and the extraction of wealth was more difficult. Some of them ruled tracts of land as lords of miniature feudal manors, or "seignories" as they were called. Only a few French women dared to leave their beloved France and build up a social life in more austere surroundings. On the banks of the St. Lawrence may still be seen the remnants of tall poplars brought from France to line the road to her home and relieve the homesickness of one of these. Like the Spaniards, however, Frenchmen were not at all averse to assimilation with the people about them. French-Indian populations soon matched the Spanish-Indian combination that was the first of many mixtures to enter the American melting pot.

The influence of the Englishman was different, and lasted longer in the life of America. His religion was simple, and often harsh in its expression. Sabbath observance was strict. He was not averse to owning slaves, and advocated the virtue of work with all his might. He brought his wife with him from England, and his ideal was a good home—a better one, if possible, than he had left in the "old country." His attitude was the basis of ideals of wealth and never-ending strenuousness in its pursuit, and this same attitude, until recently, characterized his descendants. Theirs was a substantial type of character that wore well and fitted them to meet the heavy odds against them. Northern Indians were fiercer. Northern climate was harsher, and the rocky New England soil produced food grudgingly, and held no gold. The amusements of a people who were taught not to seek relaxation were few and simple. All evils befalling them were the "will of God," and happiness after the miseries of life were over was the far-off reward of virtue.

The Protestant Church led the intellectual life of New England as the Catholic Church led that of New Spain and New France. All citizens on occasions took on additional functions of farmer, lawyer, physician, or political adviser. Graduates of European, English, or Scotch universities, they brought books into and stamped their ideals on the colonies, and frequently were authors of its earliest literature. It is to their credit that the time was not long until those who labored with them had the advantage of schools for their children.

The life of the American pioneer, to whatever nation he owed allegiance, remained under the influence of Europe. Separation did not free him from the burden of her political troubles or cut the currents of her thought. The ships which made their way so slowly and with so much hazard across a great ocean, did what the radio does today. They supplied a means of transmitting both good and evil. They encouraged men or reduced them to despair with the news which they brought, kept their vanity alive with fashions in manners and clothes, amused them with society's gossip, or inoculated them with the virus of national hysteria. Wars fought at home by colonizing nations had to be fought, too, in America. At the same time, a great era of manufacturing development, beginning in England and manifesting itself on the continent, was causing a rapid evolution in modes of living. America, whose trade was partly responsible for this, felt, inevitably, the influence of changing trends in her own industrial organization, as well as in the lives of her people.

MEDICINE OF THE RENAISSANCE

As in the fields of art and literature, so in the field of medicine came a rebirth of the science of a classical past, with new viewpoints, new methods, and outstanding men to exploit them. Throughout the Middle Ages scientific thinking had given way before the unscientific, and Galen, eventually, had shared the earlier fate of Hippocrates. Superstition and quackery superseded both, and both had been almost forgotten. Knowledge of the anatomy of the human body was very meager, and surgery had come to be looked down upon. For several centuries, however, there had been evidence of returning scientific interest in the study of Aristotle, master of all learning. In some monasteries, as in the universities, many a patient plodder made ready for a new day. *The sixteenth century Renaissance included medicine.*

Numerous names now became prominent where no name had equaled that of Hippocrates for two thousand years. Old theories were disproved. The new era announced itself through *Paracelsus* (1493–1541), a German educated in Italy who threw to the winds all the time-worn medical tradition, did his own thinking, and urged others to do the same. His progressive spirit reinvigorated the practice of internal medicine. He introduced new drugs, among which was mercury as a cure for syphilis; he improved treatment, and shared with those of his time the deductions which he was able to draw from a wide experience.

The work of bringing the fundamental science of anatomy into medicine fell to *Andreas Vesalius* (1514–1564), a German who studied in Paris, and whose belief in the need for dissection led him to do it in secret, and in defiance of law. Vesalius' part in progress was that of proving that Galen's theory was based on animal, rather than on human anatomy. His own book, "De Fabrica Humanis Corporis" is the foundation of present-day anatomy. One of Vesalius' favorite pupils was *Gabriele Fallopio* (1523–1562) who went further than his master, describing among other of the minute organs the ovaries and the Fallopian tubes.

The life of *Ambroise Paré* (1510–1590), another radical, was bound up with the advancement of surgery to a position of greater dignity. In youth, he was apprenticed to a barber, and later was accepted into the Guild of Barber Surgeons. It was he who brought back to use the ligature for bleeding vessels due to gunshot wounds, which his contemporaries treated with boiling oil. He stood also for less interference with nature than was customary, and the inscription on a monument which France erected to his memory explains this attitude in his own words: "Je le pansay, Dieu le guarit" (I dressed him, God cured him).

About this time the raising of social and professional distinctions between barbers and surgeons had manifested itself in England and on the continent. Requirements were being set for preparation to practice. The physician was a man with university accomplishments, while the surgeon was a skilled craftsman. More and more restrictions were placed on the work of the barber, although complete separation of his function from that of the surgeon did not take place for some time. When it did, the red and white spiral decoration signifying the blood and bandage incidental to phlebotomy remained the emblem of the barber who once had this piece of surgery delegated to him.

In the seventeenth century *William Harvey* (1578–1657), an Englishman, gave impetus to the study of physiology when he discovered the system of blood circulation with the heart acting as a central pump. By many of his time, his only reward was ridicule and receipt of the appellation, the "Circulator." *Athanasius Kircher* (1602–1680), a Jesuit monk, used a microscope and connected microorganisms with contagion. *Anton van Leeuwenhoek* (1632–1723) made improvement of the microscope his contribution, and wrote many scientific treatises of value to medicine on microscopic life and plant histology.

While science was securing its foothold in a field where quacks flourished, her adherents tended to become argumentative and scholastic, and to lose sight of the patient in speculation about the source of life and health. In reaction to this tendency, an Englishman, *Thomas Sydenham* (1624–1689), stressed the ancient Hippocratic practice of observing symptoms with great minuteness and recording them accurately, and was able to revive the clinical point of view. He also influenced the trend of medicine by his detailed description of prevalent diseases, by advocating fresh air to replace the stuffiness of sick rooms, and by simplifying prescriptions and abandoning disgusting ingredients generally relied upon.

Treatment of the insane was notable chiefly for its inhumanity up to the latter part of the eighteenth century. In England, at that time, a Quaker by the name of *William Tuke* introduced more understanding methods in a retreat or sanitarium which he himself established. In France, *Philippe Pinel* followed a Belgian example in abandoning the use of restraining chains, and also instituted other humane reforms.

In 1798 *Edward Jenner*, an Englishman, discovered a satisfactory method of vaccination against smallpox, a possibility of avoiding one of the many epidemics which had long harassed mankind. In spite of its proved efficiency, however, it has been avoided stubbornly by a considerable portion of the public even down to our own day.

Innovations like these serve to illustrate a trend in medical thought indicating eagerness on the part of enlightened men to discard old ideas for new ones. Scientific machinery remained incomplete, however, and superstition still ruled the practice of the average physician as it did also the beliefs of the public. While here and there men hit on cures which withstood the tests of later science, others were giving out theories which did not withstand them. Meanwhile, both doctor and layman retained faith in the power of individuals to work on one another for good or evil, and in two instances, at least, the seventeenth century saw this faith gain emphasis.

Great importance was now given to the ceremony of the King's Touch, which offered the victim of scrofula a promise of cure if a royal ruler laid his hand upon him. For this reason, scrofula was known as the "King's Evil." The modern dictionary defines it as "Tuberculosis of the lymphatic glands, and sometimes of bones and joint surfaces, with slowly suppurating abscesses and fistulous passages, the inflamed structures being subject to a cheesy degeneration." The superstition growing up around it is supposed to have originated about the time of the Crusades, and to have been intensified, as time went on, by influences drawing medieval society toward belief in the divine power of kings. It degenerated into the use of touch-pieces of medals touched by the king's hand, and worn about the neck of the scrofulous person.

In opposition to the beneficence of the King's Touch, stood out the harmful influence of the evil spirit, and imagination endowed this spirit with the form of an old woman, and name of "witch." In the absence of any better explanation of its source, people of the seventeenth century placed ever more responsibility upon this worker of evil when disease appeared. Their helplessness expressed itself, at last, in a form of mania which discovered such evil spirits in neighbors, especially any who showed peculiarities in personality, and their destruction was demanded. Thousands of innocent victims of public apprehension, often mildly insane, were put to death in one way or another. The favorite method was that of hanging and the mania spread to America where it ended in the scandal which gave fame to Salem, Massachusetts.

MEDICINE IN AMERICA

Far off in America, dangerous and isolated country that it then was, the health of explorers or immigrants had had no such guidance as was needed. Dominican or Franciscan friars, or Jesuit priests accompanied Spanish expeditions and, usually, were possessed of some medical skill. Nuns as well as clergy went with the French and supplied the luxury of nursing care. Most ships carried one of the inferior type of surgeons who might be fortunate in possessing the medical equipment gained by an apprenticeship. The English colonist companies appointed company physicians, but the professional medical practitioner seldom stayed in the colonies more than a year, for it was unusual if he possessed the pioneering enthusiasm required to endure their hardships.

The result was that colonial medicine, especially in New England, found itself in the hands of any man who possessed education, once the capable mother of a household felt the case beyond her skill. Clergy, school teachers, and political leaders alike shared responsibility as sources of advice. Some of them had studied a little medicine, others depended on the few books of home medicine then available, and all mixed their intelligence with prevailing European or Indian superstition, and much prayer.

"Of medicine the Puritans knew little and practiced less. They swallowed doses of weird and repelling concoctions, wore charms and amulets, found comfort and relief in internal and external remedies that could have had no possible influence upon the cause of the trouble, and when all else failed they fell back upon the mercy and will of God. Surgery was a matter of tooth-pulling and bone-setting, and though post-mortems were performed, we have no knowledge of the skill of the practitioner. The healing art, as well as nursing and midwifery, was frequently in the hands of women. . . . The men who practiced physic were generally homebred, making the greater part of their living at farming or agriculture. Some were ministers as well as physicians. . . . There were a number of regularly trained doctors—though not a physician had more than a smattering of medicine."[2]

Disease lurked always in the white man's neighborhood. His earliest houses were ramshackle shelters lacking in sanitary protection, and with poor water supply. Yellow fever proved a deadly stranger. Measles, scarlet fever, smallpox, and diphtheria were often epidemic, and typhoid was especially prone to appear whenever the snow melted. Indian contacts of white communities succumbed readily to their diseases. The Pilgrim and the Puritan continually mourned the dead in whose memory they erected the thousands of headstones that seem to be lined up inescapably before New England. The names and ages inscribed thereon offer a perpetual reminder of the inadequacy of care received by mothers and their children in the early days of a country that was to attain international prestige in the practice of medicine.

As time passed, living conditions improved. Fine homes often came to replace the poorly ventilated, badly drained shelters, as men grew prosperous, and it is these homes of the second growth that

2 Andrews, Charles M.: The Fathers of New England. The Chronicles of America. Copyright Yale University Press, New Haven, Vol. VI, p. 82.

we are accustomed to associate with the colonial period. Still the colonies had few doctors, and profiteering quacks sometimes had to be punished.

Medical Apprentices   Opportunities for medical education were limited to personal instruction by individual physicians. Sometimes a doctor handed down what he knew to a son; sometimes he accepted an apprentice. This apprentice might or might not be equipped with the bachelor's degree. The doctor permitted him to read his medical books, discussed points in medical practice with him, had him visit patients, and between times kept him busy with chores such as cleaning the office or grooming and feeding the horse. Just as in industry, the medical apprentice worked up slowly through a period of almost wholly practical training, usually lasting five or six years. Then, if he could afford it, the new doctor undertook a long, expensive trip to Britain or Europe where he studied in medical schools and observed procedures in hospitals. If this was beyond his purse, he went immediately into practice, and shared it often with men who had no training at all.

The apprenticeship method had advantages, for the aspirant to medical practice came into close contact with patients. These represented the master's private clientele, and usually dwelt far apart. The apprentice had to take much personal responsibility for their care and the improvement of their condition. Social distractions were not numerous, and the intimacy of private conference with the master illuminated texts and cases. As an educational system, apprenticeship depended too much for its results on the proper combination of instructor and apprentice, and offered no standard organized equipment of practice or theory to the latter. It did not protect the public from inefficiency. The apprentice lacked the dignity and added effectiveness of learning that derives from planned, intellectual development, and helps to distinguish a professional individual from one who has only training. In Europe, where the physician could study at a university, and the surgeon learned by apprenticeship the motions of a manual craft, it was this very difference that privileged one to belong to a group which did not acknowledge the other. In America, this distinction automatically disappeared under conditions requiring both functions to be filled by the same man.

Development of Medical Schools   The matter of medical education increased in importance with colonial development. The Revolutionary War and its aftermath exposed the inadequacy of medical protection, and stimulated provision for it. Departments in medicine, however, did not find a place in colleges and universities until after Harvard, the first American university, was over a hundred years old. Then they were organized in rapid succession, at the College of Philadelphia in 1765 (later a part of the University of Pennsylvania), at Harvard in 1783, at Dartmouth in 1798, and at Yale in 1810. The Middle West followed with its own schools, and there were commercial medical schools that sprang up as if by magic. Four hundred schools of medicine were founded before 1860, and many of them were responsible for inflicting very poorly educated doctors on the public. Little was done yet to regulate them, and there were short courses and easy ways of attaining the status of physician. Instruction was very frequently of poor quality, libraries were inadequate, there were no laboratories, and little or no opportunity for dissection. Often there was no connection with a university or even with a hospital.

The early colonies have been accused of narrow, gossipy tendencies in their social life. It was a tendency they could hardly have escaped, isolated as they were, and with a population scattered around in small groups having few facilities for moving about. The wisdom of mother lands was transferred slowly and intermittently. Doctors of that time must have been lonely men, deprived almost wholly of contact with those who were interested in medical work and progress. Nineteenth century America saw a great development of medical societies, organized on college, city, county, or state basis. The earliest were formed for discussion of common problems, and some reports of meetings were developed.

A group consciousness was being built up and a group pride sustained that made possible improvement of abuses in the medical practice and educational opportunities of America. By 1846 the time was ripe for concerted action, and a congress of physicians was held in New York. Certain improvements in medical schools were advocated, and in 1847 the *American Medical Association* came into being for the avowed purpose of advancing medicine and rendering service to humanity. Among its committees was one called the

"Committee on Medical Education." Medicine in the United States now had the strength of organization to back needed reforms, and to push plans for educational advancement along medical lines. A similarly progressive movement toward organization and better medical education was begun also in Canada.

Advances in Medicine   Individual effort toward improvement of medical procedure was not lacking. *Oliver Wendell Holmes*, Professor of Anatomy at Harvard University, was also a general practitioner of medicine who, from observation of maternity cases, arrived at an opinion that anticipated modern obstetrical asepsis. In 1843 he published it for his associates under the self-explanatory title, "On the Contagiousness of Puerperal Fever." Applause was not immediate; in fact, professional approval was withheld for the time being, and the idea ridiculed. Over in Europe, *Ignaz Semmelweis*, physician of Vienna, had managed in 1867, through practice of cleanliness, to reduce the death rate in a maternity ward from 10 per cent to a little over 1 per cent. He, too, published a paper under the title, "The Etiology, Nature, and Prophylaxis of Puerperal Fever," which European contemporaries likewise refused to accept. Not only did they make fun of their progressive colleague, but so persecuted him that he suffered a mental breakdown and died prematurely. In 1846 *Dr. Crawford Long* and *Dr. W. T. G. Morton* introduced the use of ether as a general anesthetic, a piece of initiative followed in England a year later by *Sir James Simpson* who made chloroform serve a like purpose.

American affairs, meanwhile, in spite of wars had moved swiftly on. Great projects of engineering and agricultural development were put through. Frontiers moved in a westerly direction, ever farther, until in 1849 the discovery of gold in California placed them on the shores of the Pacific. Vacancies in the field of labor, which pioneers of the west left behind them, were filled by immigrants. Millions of people changed their abode in a comparatively brief space of time. Always, medicine went with them, and always it passed through pioneer stages of development as they did. Always, it was a little further ahead when the pioneering began, until, eventually, it caught up with Europe. Men who acquired wealth in America as she developed trade, transportation, and material resources found pleasure in endowing universities after the manner of European princes.

PUBLIC HEALTH MOVEMENT: ERA OF SANITATION

Up to 1837, when Queen Victoria ascended the throne of England, government had not made health one of its responsibilities. Disease prevention was a rare dream. No one had grasped the principles of hygiene and sanitation. Epidemics continued as of old, and a few quarantine regulations which had grown out of the Crusades were the accepted and wholly inadequate medium of control. Boards of Health were unknown in spite of the fact that population now centered itself in cities. Garbage found its way to the street where pigs did their best to remove it. There were no city sewers, and city water supplies were drawn from dirty rivers or exposed wells.

Individually, the rich, the learned, the poor, and the ignorant were alike dirty in their habits. The significance of dirt on the person or dirt in the household was not recognized any more than that of dirt on the street or in the river. The connection of body discharges with disease was unknown but, with city crowding, smells had forced themselves on human consciousness. When they grew so bad that even perfumes failed to comfort the senses, fear followed disgust, and blame for sickness began to fall upon them. Not much was yet done to remove their cause. Personal cleanliness might have added much to comfort, at least, but it was a difficult thing to attain, and people got along happily without it. Private bathing facilities were far from adequate. The open fireplace furnished limited supplies of hot water. Cold water had to be carried, often from a considerable distance. The public bath was not accessible as in old Roman days. Clothing was heavy, hard to wash, and worn for long periods. No dry cleaning was used on the feminine apparel that often found itself handed down from one generation to another. Underwear, not to mention nightgowns and sheets, was a luxury hardly known. Straw provided beds for all who could not afford the monstrous wooden structures in use among the well-to-do. Fleas, rats, mice, and lice traveled with all grades of society.

Hairdressing fashions for women lent themselves especially well to the hygienic problem. The old simple style of braiding had disappeared. Fashion had long insisted upon complicated styles which ultimately had become so fearful and wonderful that sleep in any but an upright position was not possible. Once a month the heads were "opened," and hairdresses rebuilt. Much powder of varying shades might be introduced during the process, false hair was added to the wearer's own, and everything combined to make an unusually satisfactory medium for the growth of insects. Jewelled pins resembling the modern hatpin and used as "scratchers," had to be added to ensure some comfort. Eventually, some people resorted to shaving of the natural tresses. The men and women whom many of us proudly view as not very remote ancestors wore those powdered wigs as a preventive of miseries attending the inevitable presence of pediculi.

The time was very ripe for men interested in public welfare to begin to apply some of the laboratory achievement of the scientists who had been at work for what seems now to have been a long period. To *Sir Edwin Chadwick* (1800–1890), an English *lawyer*, is credited the initiation of a great sanitary era about 1830. A commission began to study the health of towns and cities, and the government assumed the role of promoter of national health. Emphasis was placed on disposal of sewage and garbage, and water purification. With decaying matter, many germs were disposed of, and health conditions began to improve. Many men and some women in various parts of the world came forward then to help by agitation to make legislation possible, to demonstrate statistical methods, to improve the quality of medical service, to study epidemics, and hunt out the sources of disease. Among these new sanitarians was *Sir Sidney Herbert* who, as Secretary of War when it broke out in the Crimea in 1854, was able to rely upon his friend *Miss Florence Nightingale* for an understanding interest in military hygiene, and intelligent cooperation in developing it as far as the scientific resources of her time, and military conservativeness, would permit. In America, *Lemuel Shattuck* (1793–1859), a socially minded *layman* with an interest in statistics, was digging the foundation for a corresponding movement to lead eventually to the founding of the United States Public Health Service.

WOMEN OF THE RENAISSANCE

The Renaissance was a period when Europe had time to think. Great wars and little wars were over for a time. Roman imperialism, feudalism, and church supremacy had all been lived through, and a young and energetic society combining many elements and influences had grown up sufficiently to take its place as a group of nations.

Men now wanted to be free, to live their own lives, to be individuals, and to be happy. An enlarging world increased their opportunity and satisfied those adventurous longings that had subconsciously actuated much of their fighting. Wealth with peace brought radical changes into everyday life. Women enjoyed new opportunities which added some impetus to that evolution toward social equality with men which medievalism had checked.

The passive role which women had had forced upon them began to change to a more active one as the privilege of learning was extended to them. They began to expect from men the gentle manners and devotion which decadent chivalry had introduced and shown desirable. There were other prominent figures, like Elizabeth of England and Mary of Scotland, whose position or beauty made it possible to exact these from courtiers and set standards for all men to follow in their approach to women. Chivalry was not allowed to die and the singing did not stop. There was much writing of poetry, romantic drama, and songs dedicated to the charms of women who were both beautiful and good.

There were now three social groups, upper class or aristocrats, middle class or bourgeois, and lower or industrial. The benefits of changing times were felt in corresponding order of sequence, and affected Italians earlier than people elsewhere. We are accustomed to associate the Renaissance with books and art, but books and art were prominent only among many other expressions of a new spirit. People began to change their surroundings. They longed for beauty, and they desired to live in pleasant places, now that they did not need to fortify their homes. Moats and drawbridges began to disappear. The houses now could have sunlight let in through windows; they could have their faces to the street, could provide loggias, balconies, or courts for outdoor living, and gardens. They could be built beyond the city wall. Wealthy men of the aristocratic and middle classes began to live in suburban luxury, and the desire for friendliness showed in the pleasure taken in entertaining. This attitude reflected itself on the position of wives and daughters of this group who must now, in the role of hostess, complete a picture of loveliness and charm.

Inspiration for the new life was drawn, naturally, from what people gathered from books and traditions of life in ancient Rome.

This was modified to suit the taste of another age. Much ornament softened the hard surface of walls and furniture. Women as well as men wore rich clothing and varied its pattern. The Italian woman of wealth made the classics a part of social life. This meant a new kind of education for girls as well as boys. The fashion of knowing Greek and Latin spread, and the fashion of talking in Latin made it a school-room subject with which little children must struggle. The beautiful Mary Stuart of Scotland included Latin oration in her accomplishments before she was fifteen, and her enemy, the imperious Elizabeth (1558–1603) had to learn her classics too. The entire leisure class of women, wherever the Renaissance was felt, soon learned to use a smattering of classics to add to their charm by bringing into relief the wisdom of men. Intellectual conversations became a fad and dwindled into smart repartee.

Classical influence further expressed itself in stiff formality of manners and artificiality of dress. Loose flowing robes were abandoned. Rich, heavily embroidered materials were used, and the small waist with the voluminous skirt brought the corset into woman's life. Exaggerations were inevitable. At the court of France, during the time of Marie Antoinette, fashion bulletins are said to have been issued every five days. Heads were dressed in monstrous styles. At one time a ship in full sail floated atop the head, at another the success of inoculation was celebrated by an intricate arrangement combining a serpent for smallpox, a wand for medicine, and an olive tree for accomplishment, its fruits living in the light of a new day, which is represented by a golden ball, the sun.

Men decked themselves in lace, satin, and velvet with accessories such as silk hose, handsome shoe buckles, and the daintiest of handkerchiefs. The use of snuff was a general affectation. Heavy clothing and constriction of the waist restrained the ladies from exercise, and helped to accentuate a later tendency in their admirers, and hence in their own custom, to emphasize uselessness and physical delicateness as charmingly feminine qualities. After the French Revolution the pendulum swung to extreme simplicity of dress, with extreme delicacy of politeness, and extreme daintiness of surroundings. By the nineteenth century the women chose to don soft muslin rather than rich, hard brocades. They wore pale pink or blue sashes and tied their hair with simple ribbons.

By the time of Florence Nightingale (1820–1910), women of the upper classes had become part of an aristocracy which disapproved of manual labor. They played with languages, knew some music, and often dabbled in painting. Their business was to please men, and men gladly used their wealth to make of them baby dolls, pious and adorable, but dutiful in the wifely sphere which was the accepted destiny of girls. A wave of romanticism, finding its expression in sentimental literature, surrounded their youth with an intriguing rosy glow subdued by formality that set women apart for worship. There were those among them who longed to use their intelligence more actively, and these unconventional ones found ways to do it. Meanwhile, they and their conventional sisters modestly covered themselves with very long, full skirts, to which were attached plain, tight waists softened by fichus. Their hairdress was severely plain, their most becoming background the drawing room, their entertainment the novel, their aim a husband. For pictorial purposes, their beauty was often enhanced by a flock of children about them, or by a precarious seat in a side-saddle, atop a high-stepping horse too thoroughbred to be annoyed by a long, flapping skirt.

EDUCATION OF WOMEN

The new educational opportunities of the period beginning with the Renaissance were confined, naturally, to women of the nobility and well-to-do families of the middle class. Convents were in a disrupted state. Teaching was done at home, at first by tutors and later by governesses. Sometimes learned fathers, like Mr. Nightingale, undertook to give additional instruction to their daughters. Among the Italians, an occasional woman won public recognition as orator, preacher, doctor, or the lawyer typified by Shakespeare's *Portia* in the "Merchant of Venice." In other parts of Europe, women remained in greater seclusion, grouping eventually to develop in France the *Salon*, in England the *Blue Stockings*. The Salon came into being in the upper circles of French society when clever women began to draw together in distinguished drawing rooms or salons, guests equally distinguished for intellectual, artistic, or political accomplishments, and for good manners. Its success was a partial acknowledgment of the desirability of learning in women, although French women used their wit and wisdom primarily to entertain pleasurably, and were careful to shine intellectually only enough to provoke the brilliance of men. Incidentally, they were successful in obtaining a powerful influence on general affairs.

In England, the Blue Stockings were a more distinctly middle class group who met in drawing rooms also, and, for motive, aspired to converse together in such a way as would bring mental improvement. They formed a sort of literary club which received its name from the apology of a gentleman guest who introduced himself to one of the evening gatherings by alluding to a lack of appropriateness in his dress which the member who invited him had promised they would excuse. The Blue Stockings were very precise, self-restrained, and proper. A tendency to pedantry and some weakness of domestic attributes to be noted among members led to the use of the club name as a slang expression standing for the unhappy combination of pseudo-learning and poor housekeeping. At both the Salon and the Blue Stocking meetings, there was much theorizing in regard to Platonic love which made of women mystical or spiritual beings and so tended to elevate their position. Both clubs helped to prepare the way for the quite democratic woman's club born in the nineteenth century, and now representative of a multitude of women's interests, as well as of all interests affecting national and international welfare.

These early attempts toward self-improvement were, by their nature, isolated. Formal education for women did not advance to any great extent for a long time. Always, a few ventured into intellectual fields because they had the independent urge to do so. Among them were some who dared to pioneer the rights of their sisters. On the whole, however, although the feminine status showed a tendency upward, and woman had reached some recognition as a being of intellectual capacity, she yet had no legal equality with men. Women were minors in the eyes of the law. They could not own property, and all business of a legal nature must be done through their husbands. Man's ideal of her was the loveliness and dependence of Juliet rather than the wisdom and fearlessness of Portia. Among the Puritans, up to the middle of the nineteenth century, the conception of womanly virtues combined modesty and chastity with no intellectual development.

The life of a good woman, as in the days of ancient Greece, was to be passed within the home. All her actions centered about her duty—duty to parents, to children, to husband. Self-effacement in service to them was to be her aim. The larger aims of duty in relation to citizenship and to world betterment she could not visualize. If she learned to read, she read pious books. If she could write, she confined herself chiefly to letters, and only occasionally appeared in print. No woman of any but the lower class worked outside the home without apology. Widows and maiden aunts existed in the households of their relatives.

In America, by the time the pioneering movement turned westward, the children of early settlers had grown up to a greater hardihood and self-reliance. The pioneer wife worked side by side with her husband, doing whatever came to her capable hands to be done. Less hampered by the traditions of older societies, she found it easier to adapt herself to the wilds, and as far as her individual conservatism permitted, she slipped away from conventionality and class distinction.

RISE OF FEMINISM

As early as the beginning of the seventeenth century there began to be heard from women, and from men here and there, brave statements in regard to the equality of women with men, and even broaching their right to an education. Little by little the voices became louder and the chorus of greater volume—great enough to drown out the voices of those who opposed it. While men took their places on either side, a group of courageous, persistent women, now famous for championship of their sex, earned for themselves the name of "feminists."

Feminists eventually stood for things which it took time and a struggle to get, including legal and academic privileges for women, a reform of marriage that would put it on a basis of preference rather than arrangement, and the right to vote and to hold office. They began by analyzing the respective sexes. Italian *Lucretia Marinelli* dared an essay on "The Excellencies of Women and the Errors of Men." There appeared in Holland a book called "The Learned Maid" by *Anna von Schurman*, which was read by Englishwomen in translation. England's feminist of this period, *Mary Astell*, wrote "A Serious Proposal to the Ladies." She advocated reform of marriage and a school for noblewomen whom she considered as well worth educating as their brothers.

As time went on, the Revolutionary War in America and the French Revolution made people very conscious of rights through which men could share more equably the good things of life. It was natural to begin to think and talk more forcibly about the rights of women. *Hannah More* (1745–1833), an Englishwoman whose success as a writer of poems assured her a hearing, wrote two volumes on "The Strictures on Female Education." In 1793 *Mary Wollstonecraft*, another Englishwoman, threw down the gauntlet by publishing a paper with the significant title, "Vindication of the Rights of Women." Of keen intellect herself, Miss Wollstonecraft had acquired education and entered the business world as translator for a publisher in London. Nineteenth century supporters of her ideas turned them into action.

The women of the Italian Renaissance, of the French Salon, and the women remembered in England as Blue Stockings had acquired the learning that they wanted, and enjoyed themselves while doing so. The crack in the door of opportunity for all women, through which they dared to peek, was pushed wider and wider by others behind them. Women learned to make use of intellectual endowment in schoolrooms as well as in drawing rooms. The position of governess in a family offered an outlet to many a girl of the middle class brought up close to the spreading culture of the time, and longing to relieve parents of the economic pinch that went with large families and small salaries. Quite a number of women, too, were talking on paper, becoming acknowledged authors on subjects varying from love to science. In novels or poems they expressed freely, if still in formal language, feelings long repressed, and gave rein to imagination. The influence on their sisters was great, and was an added spur toward freeing the individual. The fashion of diary-writing lent itself as a beneficent outlet for an intense consciousness of self.

The era following the close of the Napoleonic wars in 1815 was one of comparative peace in which nations were learning that revolutions could be prevented only by improving conditions for the ordinary man who went on insisting that he had a right to a better footing in society. Its social unrest, its economic and intellectual feverishness, its sudden release of inventive genius, and the great improvements made in communication and transportation were all reflected in the lives of women. In a steady stream they emerged from the seclusion forced upon them by dangers of the Middle Ages and subsequent religious conflicts. Many among the infants born about this time were to spend their lives in unusual activities. Some of them became world figures, always to be remembered because they made that world a better place in which to live. A brief résumé of this womanly achievement, as exemplified in England and America, where democracy had more rapid growth, will show its trends. Its chief source was in the middle class of society, and women of European countries participated only in less degree.

Fanny Burney (1752–1840) and *Jane Austen* (1775–1817) became writers who produced successful novels like the former's "Evelina" and the latter's "Pride and Prejudice," while novels were yet unapproved for reading. *Charlotte Brontë* (1816–1855) and her two sisters also essayed the literary field to relieve the family poverty. Poems and fiction, of which the still living "Jane Eyre" and "Wuthering Heights" are representative, came from their pens. *George Eliot* (1819–1880), friend of great men in her day, taught people to understand each other better in such books as "The Mill on the Floss."

The extension of suffrage was one of the moot questions of the time. Women rallied to advance their right to this privilege when they found that social reforms which they desired required voting power to push them. Some sponsored with equal vim a temperance movement. Prominent in the two groups were *Elizabeth Cady Stanton* (1815–1902), *Susan B. Anthony* (1820–1906), and *Frances E. Willard* (1839–1898).

Some women set about the improvement of educational opportunity. Numerous schools were founded and books written. *Emma C. Willard* (1787–1870) started a seminary for girls, while she found time also to write poems which include the popular "Rocked in the Cradle of the Deep." *Catherine Beecher* (1800–1878), sister of the famous preacher, Henry Ward Beecher, likewise established a seminary, and wrote under constructive titles such as "True Remedy for the Wrongs of Women" and "Letters to the People on Health and Happiness."

Philanthropy touched even more closely the lives of still another group of women. *Elizabeth Fry* (1780–1845) undertook the reform of prisons, a loathsome task. *Harriet Beecher Stowe*, sister of Catherine Beecher, wrote "Uncle Tom's Cabin" in the interests of Negro emancipation. *Julia Ward Howe* (1819–1910), whose husband shared her friendship with Florence Nightingale, became a preacher and lecturer interested in prison reform and world peace, and author of "The Battle Hymn of the Republic."

Three girls in the brilliant circle found their sphere among the sick and wounded. *Dorothea Lynde Dix* (1802–1887) devoted her life to the welfare of those afflicted with mental illness. *Florence Nightingale* (1820–1910) uncovered the disgrace of poor care of the sick in hospitals, and discovered a means of assuring good nursing through systematic education of selected young women as nurses. *Clara Barton* (1821–1912), who saw hospital service during the Civil War in America, directed her work and influence afterward toward organization of the American Red Cross Society. Into the midst of these ardent reformers, chiefly middle class women, came another woman, *Victoria*, queen of an Empire, friend of international good will and human betterment, exponent of temperate living. By the social standards which she set for them, she sustained their efforts in the "Victorian Age."

WOMEN OF THE INDUSTRIAL REVOLUTION

The women outside of these two groups—aristocracy and wealthy middle class—belonged to that great group whose husbands were craftsmen in the towns, or small farmers, or laborers. These women suffered much from the social evolution of their time. The Industrial Revolution brought strange, new problems into the life of the countrywoman. She who had managed her household, and directed the industries of spinning and weaving which usually went on within it, saw these industries moving away from her. Independence and social prestige were lost to her if she remained in the country. If she was young enough to be acceptable as a factory worker, she joined the wife of the craftsman in the new town, working side by side with her in the big factory. If she was too old to do this, she stayed in the country to watch a wretched poverty close in about her, as her handwork grew costly and people learned to prefer the machine-made goods.

Women who became factory hands fared as badly as the countrywoman, even if they were a little more independent as wage earners. They, their husbands, and even their children were swallowed up by the mechanistic processes that invention had set going. Fourteen hours a day of work that was being ever speeded up, left little energy or time for the demands of life. Homes must be made in rickety, unsanitary houses with no privacy for a family, no village green in the neighborhood where friends might gather, no opportunities for children's play, and only the barest subsistence for all, with food that lacked the healthful qualities of that which she had once grown in a garden.

As time passed, the hastily thrown together towns lost their newness, town life lost the thrill of newness too, and the degradation of human beings began to show. No nuns in nearby convents taught the children, no schools took their places for a long time after men had turned against the church and destroyed monasteries. More and more hopeless was the outlook as unthinking exploiters raked in unheard-of profits at the expense of a group that grew ever poorer. The townswoman, without education, lacking any real economic independence, toiling in never-ending drudgery, knew that her tired children were whipped sometimes to make them work too. Work in the factory was the child's lot as soon as he was big enough to do it. No laws prevented child labor; in fact, no legislation gave protection to any worker in industry for many years. Terrible accidents befell them while they learned to manage power machinery, for safety devices were lacking in the early days of industry, and weary, undernourished children and adults were ready victims. Medical and nursing care were unorganized, and no compensation plan existed. Unfitted for work, they lost their jobs and those who did not die often were forced to become street beggars.

The lower class woman lost morale in this atmosphere, and it is not very surprising that the public house attracted her as well as her man. She coarsened and grew hard. When the French Revolution broke out in answer to the insane extravagances of her sister, *Marie Antoinette*, and the court which surrounded her, women of this class betrayed an almost inhuman desire to get even with her and her kind. In fact, the vindictiveness of spirit with which they entered into this disturbance is not only an expression of the harm which industry unwittingly had wrought, but promise of a demand for rights for women as well as for men. Some women realized already that society owed them a share of that betterment in standards of living which had come to those closest to opportunity. The harshness of industrial adversity, affecting Englishwomen first, was spreading to women everywhere, and the harvest of an efficiency that overlooked the human being is being reaped in our own time.

A DECLINE IN NURSING

Disturbed political conditions, the Renaissance, the Protestant Revolt, the general low status of medicine, and the position of women all affected the nursing of the period between 1500 and 1860 A.D. The essential spirit of the Renaissance, intellectual enlightenment, could touch it only indirectly, since nursing was an art yet outside the intellectual or the esthetic realms, although sensitive to influences from both. Continued withdrawal from the church of vast numbers of tributary supporters who allied themselves with Protestants reduced the number of nurses in monastic institutions. A general lack of interest in monastic life lowered it further, and monastic suppression ushered in the climax of its decay. To Luther and other Protestant leaders, the existence of many thousands of offending monasteries seemed an obstacle to be met only by forcible removal.

A widespread movement toward suppression of monasteries brought about conditions similar to those produced in England by Henry VIII (1491–1547). Here was a sovereign who did not even trouble to change his religion, but took advantage of Protestant disaffection to free himself from papal authority. With covetous eyes fixed on monastic properties that represented one-fifth of his kingdom, he based his revolt on the petty excuse of church refusal to sanction his divorce. On the strength of reports made by a royal commission appointed to inspect them, he wantonly destroyed over six hundred monasteries. Beautiful old buildings were wrecked, their gaping wounds left for the gentle ivy to cover reverently. Precious vessels, art treasures, splendid windows—everything of value even to the ornamental utilities of hand-wrought iron and the lead on their roofs—was either ruined or taken away. Some of the wealth accrued from sales was diverted to new schools or colleges, some eventually found its way back to ancient establishments under new organizations, but the greater part went to court favorites.

The immediate result of monastic dissolution was that hospitals and inns were suddenly snatched away from a public dependent upon them for many centuries. The poor were left without the principal organized system of relief. Substitute provision for the burden of charity was overlooked, and while wars were waged for religious opinion, the care of the sick and the poor, a supreme trust of Christianity, was neglected. A general lack of interest in monastic life hindered successful introduction of reforms in those institutions which remained.

Another effect of the Reformation was to complete the withdrawal of medicine from monastery to university. Medicine thus found a refuge denied nursing. Medical advance was assured while the technics of nursing remained unchanged in the guardianship of the Beguines and other secular orders and those relatively few nuns who found it possible to continue their practice of them. Prominent among the latter were the Augustinians of the Hôtel Dieu and Heilige Geist hospitals. University learning in medicine, however, affected but faintly the activities of the general practitioner. His methods and his point of view remained medieval and typified Galenic ideals. While a few physicians realized the need of something better, apparently the average among them was satisfied with a low type of nursing service. Even when the ignorant midwife was not available to assist at labor, her place was seldom assumed by the doctor, but oftener a substitute officiated who was even more ignorant than she.

Only the women of the industrial class worked outside of the home unless compelled by dire necessity to become a teacher of children. Women who found places in hospitals as nurses were not acceptable even to industry. They were usually immoral, drunken, illiterate— the very lowest grade of human society. A decline in quality of public service for the sick, noticeable toward the end of the Middle Ages, became deeper and deeper.

A change was apparent now in the organization of hospital service. What had been for so many centuries gratuitous was changing over slowly and grudgingly to a paid service. The public would take painful centuries to adjust to the idea of paying money for care during illness, and to restore vocational desirability to nursing, inevitably a pivotal hospital function. The public must learn, too, to separate nursing from domestic service, for with this it had become entangled during an early development beside household occupations in groups of volunteer social workers and home-makers dwelling in convents. Meanwhile, this entanglement was being made worse by mismanagement, inadequate staffing, and even by deliberate exploitation. Women lost control of nursing, as men who were civil appointees undertook leadership and withheld authority from women called *matrons* whom they put in charge of a secular riffraff taken on as nurses. The fact that among the latter were some whose responsibility for ward management dignified them by the title "Sister" was a concession to policy. "Sister" was a word retained to please the public, for among rich and poor it had come to be associated with a sympathy and encouragement radiating characteristically from the nun in the monastery.

The latter half of the period between 1500 and 1860 A.D., saw nursing conditions at their worst. By that time new hospitals had been built, but something of the harshness of feeling aroused by religious controversy and persistent warring of human beings seemed to attach itself to them. Severe utility replaced the beauty which medieval builders had brought into institutions for the sick. Unsanitary conditions made them a source of outbreak for many of those epidemics which served to keep life expectancy down to an average of about eighteen years. The poor, or the paupers, as men called those for whom they provided the great, sinister, dirty buildings, associated them with extremity of wretchedness. Within those dreary, almost windowless walls were great wards holding as many as a hundred patients each. Women and men were not always segregated, diseases seldom. It was not uncommon for the sick to be thrown into beds already occupied by several bedfellows—the dead or the delirious, side by side, perhaps, with those who still lived and retained their reason. In a room leading off such a ward, a nurse who had been on duty all day slept at night so that she might be within hearing and call of her patients.

In wards like these, beds were so close together that even had there been people to do it, cleaning was almost impossible. All kinds of rubbish collected and remained under them. Only a few iron beds were yet in use, and the wooden bedstead, the straw mattress or the feather one, and the bedbug were better known. Nursing procedures, simple as they had been up to this time, became simpler. Feet or faces, that had once been washed before a stricken beggar entered a hospital bed from the dirty street, now went unwashed. Bed baths were not attempted. The usual treatments ordered for all conditions were bleeding and purging, a fact which at least spared harassed nurses the present-day rapid-fire adjustment necessitated by more individual consideration.

While respectable women were not expected to undertake nursing under such conditions, there was still criticism of drunkenness, heartlessness, and immorality in those who did. Such women received very small pay and very poor food. Much was expected of them in return. Housework, scrubbing, and laundry took up a great part of the time, and the hours of service fluctuated between twelve and forty-eight at a stretch. For night duty, old women were commonly engaged. For day duty, they were somewhat younger. No previous training was looked for, nor was character a consideration.

No change was to come until the middle of the nineteenth century. This was the influence that went with the Pilgrim emigrants to New England, and this was the background of their hospital and nursing development. Indeed, few discernible differences are to be met in descriptions of hospitals of this period, whether their location lie in Britain, in continental Europe, or in New England.

The person who suffered from mental illness was even worse off than he who was stricken by bodily disease. In spite of attempts to free him from restraining chains, he was far from being treated as a human being. His cell was apt to be small and damp, his food poor, the accepted remedies harsh. Fly blisters or mustard plasters might be applied to the head, strong purgatives or emetics given, or he might be ducked in cold water, or beaten. The family to which he belonged was made to feel itself disgraced.

Prisons   Among all unfortunates to be institutionalized, however, the worst off were those who became prisoners. Society felt a justifiable grudge against them, and dealt with them accordingly. The following descriptions of prisons, one continental, the other English, present what are conceded to be faithful pictures of its method:

"A prison taint was on everything there. The imprisoned air, the imprisoned light, the imprisoned damps, the imprisoned men, were all deteriorated by confinement. As the captive men were faded and haggard, so the iron was rusty, the stone was slimy, the wood was rotten, the air was faint, the light was dim. Like a well, like a vault, like a tomb, the prison had no knowledge of the brightness outside."[3]

[3] Charles Dickens.

"Brandon was taken to Newgate, the most loathsome prison in London at that time, it being used for felons, while Ludgate was for debtors. Here he was thrown into an underground dungeon foul with water that seeped through the old masonry from the moat, and alive with every noisome thing that creeps. There was no bed, no stool, no floor, not even a wisp of straw; simply the reeking stone walls covered with fungus, and the windowless arch overhead. One could hardly conceive a more horrible place in which to spend even a moment. I had a glimpse of it by the light of the keeper's lantern as they put him in, and it seemed to me a single night in that awful place would have killed me or driven me mad. I protested and begged and tried to bribe, but it was all of no avail; the keeper had been bribed before I arrived. Although it could do no possible good, I was glad to stand outside the prison walls in the drenching rain, all the rest of that wretched night, that I might be as near as possible to my friend and suffer a little with him."[4]

Augustinian Nuns   In the twilight and the darkness that enfold nursing in these centuries between 1500 and 1860 gleams a tiny light. It is borne by an order of nuns following the rule of St. Augustine. This first purely nursing order of the Church, established in 1155, bore a heavy share of difficulties arising in hospitals in times when religious and political strife kept disease-ridden countries in seemingly endless turmoil. Their nursing was carried on chiefly in the great city hospitals, which we have seen developed, and the freedom of action accorded the abbess and her nuns in former times was no longer theirs. Rather, they were under close direction of the clergy, sometimes working also under a lay hospital board. It is not surprising that they incurred criticism for disobeying orders given by doctors, and that it was found necessary to teach them that good nursing of patients involves loyal cooperation with physicians. It must be acknowledged, at the same time, that the asceticism which motivated stern devotion to their chosen work must have placed us in their debt for preserving nursing procedures as monasteries disappeared, and secular nursing was yet imperfectly developed.

The life of the Augustinian nun was strictly monastic. She renounced the world and home ties following a novitiate which lasted twelve years or longer. Her life, henceforth, was passed in a hospital, its monotony broken occasionally by service as a private nurse in homes. She wore a white robe and, when a full sister, donned a hood. In the notorious "Hôtel Dieu," as Paris strangely named the great hospital she now ran, these nuns became heroic figures, although the precedent for unremitting toil that they established has proved, in some ways, a bit unfortunate for nurses of a later day.

[4] Charles Major in "When Knighthood Was in Flower."

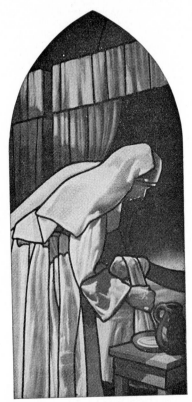

An Augustinian Nun
("They Caught the Torch." Courtesy of Will Ross, Inc.)

From one to the other the Augustinians passed on a routine of nursing; from year to year their duties of housekeeping and management increased. There were no lectures, no classes, little or no recreation. They nursed and scrubbed, cooked, sewed, and washed clothes, without benefit of any of our modern facilities. It is difficult, perhaps, to picture their method of performing the function of laundresses, but it is still a common one in France. It is also difficult to imagine the choice of white uniforms under prevailing conditions. Every day there was a "little wash" for their household of over six hundred patients; every six weeks there was what must have been

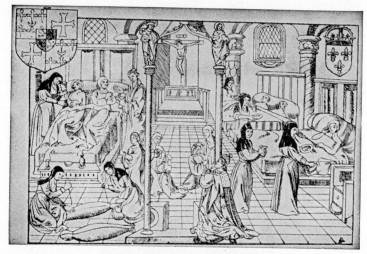

A SICK-ROOM IN THE HÔTEL DIEU, PARIS
(Castiglioni, Arturo, M.D.: A History of Medicine. Alfred A. Knopf, New York.)

named correctly, a "great wash." The work was done in the river Seine, regardless of season or water temperature. Knee deep in the stream the nuns dipped, soaped, slapped, and rinsed until all was done. Then they went back to confusion and the care of sick people lying, often, six in a bed. When they asked for assistants for the sake of these patients, the now classic reply came that they were "always trying to do nothing."

SUMMARY, 1500 to 1860

New inventions, religious beliefs, and social ideas challenged the minds of those who lived during the period extending from 1500 to 1860. As in our time, men were finding that changed conditions outmoded conventional methods. To those filled with the spirit of adventure that was leading to widening horizons, the confinement of monastery or feudal estate became intolerable. People were beginning to think as they had not done for many centuries. In the field of literature, too, a rebirth of interest, beginning in Italy, soon spread throughout Europe, while, in the field of art, painters, architects, and sculptors expressed themselves with a new spirit of freedom.

Whole countries soon revealed a popular will that was distinctively Protestant or Catholic. At the same time, advantages of commerce and expansion of power were always beckoning from beyond. America was discovered. Spain, France, and England each claimed a portion, and a New Spain, a New France, and a New England appeared across the ocean. In the field of science, great men like Copernicus, Kepler, and Galileo were changing the course of human thought.

In the practice of medicine came a rebirth of the science of a classical past with new viewpoints, new methods, and outstanding men to exploit them. Numerous names now became prominent where no name had equaled that of Hippocrates for two thousand years. Where time-worn traditions had flourished, a progressive spirit reinvigorated the practice of internal medicine. More understanding methods in relation to the treatment of the insane were introduced by William Tuke of England and Philippe Pinel of France. In the practice of obstetrics, also, improved methods were adopted. The science of bacteriology, the use of ether as a general anesthetic, and other discoveries caused an abrupt change in the practice of surgery. A new emphasis on provision for pure water supplies and proper disposal of sewage and garbage ushered in the era of sanitation and the beginnings of Boards of Health. With the general cleaning up, many bacteria were eliminated and health conditions improved to a noticeable extent.

The passive role that had been forced upon women began to change to a more active one as the privilege of learning was extended to them. They were beginning to expect from men the gentle manners and the devotion introduced in the age of chivalry. There was much writing of romantic poetry and drama. By the time of Florence Nightingale (1820–1910), women of the upper classes had become part of an aristocracy which disapproved of manual labor. Since the only accepted sphere of activity was that of a dutiful wife and mother, those among them who longed to use their intelligence more actively had to resist the forces of rigid convention. Brave demands were made in regard to the equality of women with men, and even in regard to equal educational opportunity. At the same time women of the lower class, who had none of these privileges, lost morale, coarsened, and grew hard.

The status of nursing, already affected by the Renaissance, the Reformation, and the position of women, lost ground still further through decline of interest in the monastic life. The suppression of monasteries by Martin Luther and Henry VIII brought on a period of rapid deterioration. As city hospitals came into existence, there was available no longer the unselfish devotion of religious orders, but the paid service of secular women. The rôle of the Augustinians nuns in these hospitals was an exception to the general rule. Control of nursing passed into the hands of men with civil appointments. Lower-class women who did the work were accused of drunkenness, heartlessness, and immorality.

TOPICS FOR DISCUSSION

1. Give a description of general social conditions as the year 1500 dawned on the western world.
2. (*a*) Make an outline of famous authors, sculptors, and painters of the Renaissance, adding several names to those mentioned in the text, giving the principal accomplishments of each. (*b*) Add the names of several scientists of the period, including Copernicus, Kepler, and Galileo.
3. Procure from an art store or from the Perry Pictures Company, Malden, Massachusetts, copies of famous paintings which will include the following:
   Spring—by Alessandro Botticelli
   Pinkie—by Sir Thomas Lawrence
   The Blue Boy—by Sir Thomas Gainsborough
   The Duchess of Devonshire—by Sir Thomas Gainsborough
   The Last Supper—by Leonardo da Vinci
   Mona Lisa—by Leonardo da Vinci
   The Sistine Madonna—by Raphael
4. (*a*) Compare the activities of Martin Luther of Germany and Ignatius Loyola of Spain during the Protestant Revolt. (*b*) What was the relationship of the Ursulines to the Jesuits?
5. Give an account of the colonization of America by Spanish, French, and English governments.
6. Tell what you know of the Industrial Revolution and its effect on the average citizen.

7. (*a*) Make an outline of famous physicians and their contributions during this period. (*b*) Show how superstition lingered in spite of progress in some directions.
8. (*a*) What do you know of the practice of medicine in colonial America? (*b*) Name several of the early medical schools of this country.
9. What general conditions in regard to sanitation prevailed?
10. Discuss the status of women of the Renaissance from the following standpoints:
    (*a*) Type of life expected of a good woman
    (*b*) Attitude toward work outside of the home
    (*c*) Circumstances under which she married
    (*d*) Attitude toward the feminist groups appearing
11. Discuss the Dark Period of Nursing from the following standpoints:
    (*a*) General causes
    (*b*) Type of women employed, and their preparation for the work
    (*c*) Title by which the nurse was known, and its significance
    (*d*) Type of person by whom nursing work was supervised
    (*e*) A purely nursing order of the Catholic Church that carried on courageously amid many difficulties
12. What was the contribution of the Augustinian nuns during this period?

REFERENCES

Dark, Sydney: The Story of the Renascence. Modern Readers' Bookshelf. New York, George H. Doran.

Dexter, Elizabeth Anthony: Colonial Women of Affairs. Boston and New York, Houghton Mifflin Co., 1924, Chap. 4.

Dickens, Charles: Martin Chuzzlewit. New York, Charles Scribner's Sons, 1911.

Dock and Nutting: A History of Nursing. New York, G. P. Putnam's Sons, 1907. Vol. 1, Chap. 14.

Fox, Ruth: Great Men of Medicine. New York, Random House, 1947.

Hayes, Moon, and Wayland: World History. New York, The Macmillan Co., 1941.

Kent, Rockwell (editor): World-Famous Paintings. New York, Wm. H. Wise and Co., 1939.

Quennell, Marjorie, and C. H. B.: A History of Everyday Things in England (4 volumes). New York, Charles Scribner's Sons, 1922–35.

Raynor, Edwin: Famous Cathedrals and Their Stories. New York, Grosset and Dunlap, 1935.

Raynor, Edwin: Famous Statues and Their Stories. New York, Grosset and Dunlap, 1936.

Robinson, James H.: The Story of Our Civilization. New York, Wm. H. Wise and Co., 1926. Vol. 1.

Schoolman and Slatkin: The Story of Art: The Lives and Times of the Great Masters. New York, Halcyon House, 1940.

Schubert, Marie. Famous Paintings and their Stories. New York, Grosset and Dunlap, 1934.

Wells, H. G.: The Outline of History. New York, Garden City Publishing Company, 1931.

Early Hospitals and
Nursing in America

NEW SPAIN

When Italian *Columbus* enlisted the aid of Spain's Queen Isabella in his scheme to open up western trade routes to the Orient, and ended the adventure by setting foot on an island near the edge of a strange new land, he brought opportunity within reach of many a dashing cavalier. Unwittingly also, the way had been opened to fellow-Europeans. Stories of fabulous wealth inflamed adventurous hearts. Stories of benighted Indians fired anew the Crusading spirit. Spain's bravest took ship for a new world as soon as they could. Immediately a close, continuous contact with the native population was set up. The American immigration problem started. The northern continent was the one to which findings enabled Columbus to give direction, and, naturally, the neighborhood of his landing was subjected first to foreign influence.

Hernando Cortez, efficient soldier of the King of Spain, and an organizer as well, conquered what we call Mexico. He met with cruelty the approach of the well-meaning Aztec ruler, *Montezuma*, whom legend had taught to believe in a white god, presumably now appearing in the form of Cortez. Spaniards soon profited from the wealth, not of the Aztecs alone, but also of those Toltecs, Mayas, and Incas whom we have found stretching Indian territory from Mexico into Peru. In Indian cities a civilization existed that included systematic provision for care of the sick, physicians, nurses, and hospitals. Indian culture had made some advance also into adjacent regions, north and west, inhabited by the Pueblo Indians. These had reached the agricultural stage, but elsewhere, on mountain and plain, were roaming tribes whose friendliness to the stranger varied, apparently, with the harshness or gentleness of the climate in which they lived.

Among these hunters were men still in the Stone Age of development. The Medicine Man of primitive peoples was their doctor; the squaw or herbwoman, his assistant and their nurse. Some lived in wigwams or in teepees, others in caves side by side with animals. Northern natives were energetic, fierce, and warlike. Those whose surroundings were semitropical were slothful and indolent, but frequently docile. The majority seem to have been dirty in habit, the Indian of northerly regions where cleanliness was most difficult, especially so. To women, Indians usually accorded the position of burden-bearer, cook, manager of the home, and helper in the fields. Among certain Indians, however, women were accorded the dignity of seats in the tribal councils, and often the tracing of descent to a common mother gave her prestige.

Need for additional provision for care of the sick was created when the first boatload of adventurers started out from Europe. Crude conditions of travel led to deadly outbreaks of scurvy, as well as of disease contracted before leaving the homeland. On his second trip, Columbus was careful to bring a physician. Explorers, conquerors, and conquered—all were exposed to infections for which they had no immunity. Unfortunately, it was almost simultaneous with this urgent need that the period of depression in European nursing was being induced by the Renaissance and the Reformation —a depression to be prolonged by revolutions to establish religious freedom and the civil rights of man. A great era of discovery opened up and facilitated the spread of disease, at a time when opportunities for its control were becoming fewer and less adequate than ever.

Spanish, French, and English colonizers met the problem of medical care and nursing in different ways. Spain, whose immediate financial rewards were greatest, was also best prepared for pioneering abroad. Protestantism had not weakened her church as it had in other countries. The three new missionary groups which Europe had brought into being—Dominicans, Franciscans, and Jesuits— stood ready, organized, and eager to help. Spain made use of them, and so did France. Protestant England had no corresponding sup-

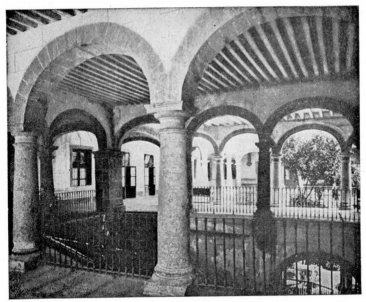

HOSPITAL OF JESUS OF NAZARETH, MEXICO CITY

The first real hospital known to have been built on the American continent. Founded by Cortez, about 1524, as the Hospital of Immaculate Conception. (Guillermo Kahlo.)

port, and medicine and nursing were left in the hands of individuals. Orders of the Catholic Church accompanied the Spaniards to America, pushing back frontiers by exploration, supplanting paganism by Christianity, protecting, as far as they could, the public health. As they penetrated wildernesses and lived among tribal peoples, they devoted themselves with a will to any necessary task, encouraging the weary pioneer, teaching his children if there was no one else to do it, and often, as nurses or doctors, caring for the sick and injured without distinction between friend and foe. The Jesuits kept especially systematic records. In diaries called "Relations" they transmitted minute details of everyday happenings to their home office. These have become a valued source of early American history.

Rise of Missions   The problem which faced all orders was very similar to that met by the monks who long before had dealt with

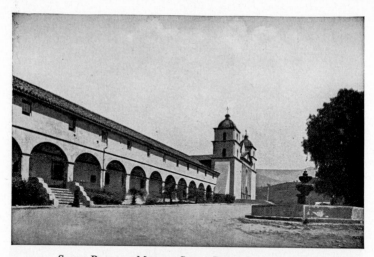

SANTA BARBARA MISSION, SANTA BARBARA, CALIFORNIA

Founded in 1786 and still occupied by Franciscan Fathers. (Published by Cardinell-Vincent Co., San Francisco.)

those barbarian ancestors of theirs who brought about the Fall of Rome in 476 A.D. The key to solution was the same, for the native American had to be brought to a state where he and the white man could live side by side. In the absence of established monasteries, a monastic type of institution known as the "Mission" sprang up in the path of the missionary from Spain or France. Friendly advances were made to the Indians, a place of worship set up, and barbarians gathered about it in self-supporting communities that might reach the number of several thousand. Agriculture and the trades were taught as well as religion.

Well-organized care of the sick in these earliest missions could hardly be expected. There were overwhelming epidemics of measles or smallpox, times of stress in which the well had to help the few friars with the nursing.

The first real hospital in America, the Hospital of Immaculate Conception, was built by Hernando Cortez in 1524, on the spot where he had met Montezuma and the men whose land and gold he had come to take from them. As the Hospital of Jesus of Nazareth it stands today in Mexico City, reflecting all the beauty and spacious-

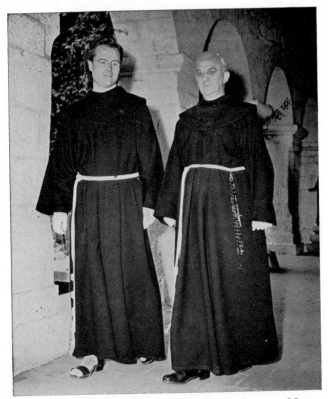

Two Friars of the Franciscan Order of Santa Barbara Mission
Santa Barbara, California, 1950.

ness of Spanish hospital architecture under Moslem influence. To Cortez, it represented thanksgiving for victory and the expiation of sins that he might have overlooked as he made his peace with Heaven. He intended it to shed its mercy on white and Indian alike, and put their care into the keeping of a nursing Brotherhood.

Seven years after the founding of the Hospital of the Immaculate Conception in Mexico City, the hospital of Santa Fé (Holy Faith) was built in what is now New Mexico. This was the undertaking of padres (fathers) whose ambition led them to expand one mission to the scope of an ancient monastery.

Missions gradually extended from Mexico City in a direction north and west through New Mexico and Arizona into the peninsula of lower California. They became part of the Spanish scheme of colonization, with control centered in the homeland. Military protection was afforded them in a line of presidios or forts. In little more than two hundred years the line of missions and forts was extended about six hundred miles along the coast of what is now the state of California. *Junípero Serra*, a Franciscan friar, was made responsible for this great project, and, by 1776, when England's colonists were declaring their independence, his arduous zeal had placed his paternally governed missions with their schools and manual training centers as far north as the Mission San Francisco, so named in honor of St. Francis of Assisi.

With a determined little group of brown-robed followers of St. Francis, Father Serra had brought Christianity to the California Indian. Through the brush and over the hills of California on foot he had made his way, laying out as far as possible the route that would be the El Camino Real, or King's Highway, and so made communication between the missions a possibility.

The California missions ultimately gathered together thousands of Indian children of the Christian faith, followers of the cross that Father Serra planted on the hills. He had opened a new land to the white man. His work was hampered continually by outbreaks of white men's diseases, of which mission cemeteries tell the story. Only occasionally was a doctor's help available, and the burden of medicine and nursing fell, in the main, on him and his friars.

NEW FRANCE

Not long after Cortez began the colonization of Spanish America, *France* hastened to claim the lands adjacent to two great waterways—the St. Lawrence River with its source in the Great Lakes, and the Mississippi flowing south almost from that point into the Gulf of Mexico.

CANADA

In 1535 *Jacques Cartier* erected a cross and set up the flag of France at Cape Gaspé near the mouth of the St. Lawrence. Explorers, Franciscan friars, Jesuits, and settlers followed him. By 1607 there were settlements in Nova Scotia and Quebec, and Frenchmen had reconciled themselves to the work of getting their share of gold out of the fur trade instead of from mines or ready hoards of native treasure. Theirs was a difficult task, made worse by Indian hostility.

As far as sickness was concerned, the same complications arose as in New Spain. Measles, smallpox, and tuberculosis played havoc among the natives to whom Europeans transferred these diseases. The native rightly blamed the white man for the blight that fell upon his race. Dirt and cold, both of a degree beyond their experience, made it almost impossible for the friars to combat disease that swept like forest fire, let alone to advance religion in roving groups that lived during long winters in smoke-filled wigwams, crowded with men, women, children, all infested with lice, and surrounded by many flea-ridden dogs. In his zeal for saving souls the poor priest even tried living in these surroundings, but found that he must content himself with a contact less close. His days were more than filled as he moved about baptizing the dying, doing what he could for the sick.

The letters that went home to France from Franciscan, and later from Jesuit missionaries, carried a touching picture of bravery in face of overwhelming odds. They arrived at a time when certain public spirited groups were busy erasing the worst ugliness from another picture of misery that had been disclosed at home. Canada (Huron Indian for "settlement") profited by the new social-mindedness of France which was, through the ancient art of nursing and the companion art of teaching, reaching souls that needed saving. The same means seemed applicable to the strengthening of her position among these disturbing Indians.

Founding of Hôtel Dieu and Ursuline Convent of Quebec in 1639

The idea of establishing in Canada a permanent hospital came from one of the Jesuits, and it caught the attention of a socially minded woman, the wealthy *Duchesse d'Aiguillon*. Niece of *Cardinal Richelieu*, one of the most influential political men in France as well as in the Catholic Church, she made it her business to obtain a grant of land with permission to start this hospital in the city of Quebec, then a community of about two hundred and fifty people, principally Indians. Three nuns of the Augustinian Order, then supply-

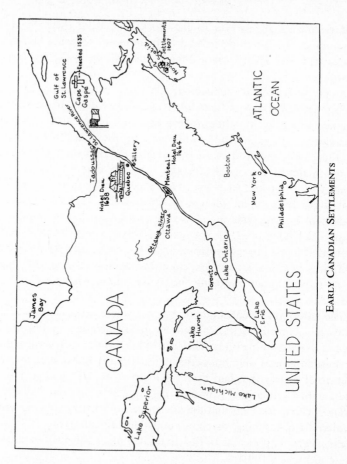

EARLY CANADIAN SETTLEMENTS

ing so many of the great city hospitals of Europe, were selected as nurses.

Meantime, the value of an orphanage and a school for the education of the little Indian and French children was suggested, and another member of the nobility pledged herself to this scheme. *Mme de la Peltrie's* enthusiasm carried her farther than that of Duchesse d'Aiguillon. She determined to go in person to Canada to start the work. The order of St. Ursula answered her appeal by supplying nuns who were trained teachers. In May 1639 Mme de la Peltrie and the little company of Augustinian and Ursuline nuns sailed from Dieppe. It took them two and a half months to reach the trading post of Tadoussac at the mouth of the St. Lawrence River. The tiny ship in which they had been buffeted about on the great and little known Atlantic left them there. The seasickness, the shortage of drinking water, the threatening sea, and the floating iceberg faded quickly in memory as they traveled wearily up the great river in a little boat, subsisting for two other long weeks on a diet of uncooked salt cod.

It was August first when they reached Quebec where they were given such a welcome as made up for all. The guns of the fort saluted, the village went on holiday. As they landed, Mme de la Peltrie and the nuns kneeled down to kiss the soil of that dreamed-of land they had dedicated themselves to save and keep for God and France. After mass, they were taken to Sillery, four miles beyond, to view the pride of the Jesuit priests, the nucleus of a mission. Within a palisade built for protection against attack by hostile Iroquois bands, stood a church, a mission-house, an infirmary, and the log-cabin dwellings of converted Indians. As no buildings of their own had been provided for the new missionaries, the infirmary at Sillery was given to the Augustinian nuns for their temporary use as a hospital.

Before the Augustinian sisters unpacked their few belongings, the sick were gathered about, besieging them for help. The bed linen brought from France was insufficient even when they attempted to eke it out by cutting it into pieces. The beds overflowed so that log-cabins had to be built and the church used for extra patients. August heat can be almost unbearable around Quebec, and the nurses had no time to recover from a long, hard trip. They felt it keenly, and as their work became even more emergent in character following an outbreak of smallpox, they were sorely tried. The effort to carry out accustomed nursing procedures for relief of dirty Indians crowded into inadequate quarters, unfamiliar customs, difficulties of providing suitable and sufficient food, lack of sleep, all told on them.

Their companions, the Ursulines, were no better off. They had been housed in an empty wooden warehouse on the bank of the St. Lawrence River just below the heights on which stood the fortifications of Quebec. Indian children overran the school-to-be just as their relatives had overrun the hospital. Smallpox broke out here also, and the Ursulines must be nurses before they could be teachers. The beginning of pioneer life for them, too, was marked by hardship. Fear of the epidemic drove the Indians from all about into Quebec. The Ursuline shack, as it really was, had to have berths put up along its interior walls for rows of patients, and mattresses laid close together on the floor for others. The nuns did their best and, fortunately, were not infected. "In those days of peril and catastrophe nobody had time to catch a disease. So it was with the Ursulines. Like Hotspur, they lacked the leisure to be sick."[1] In both of these emergency hospitals many Indians died—so many, in fact, that others stopped coming. Some months later the disease ran itself out, and enough peace descended upon all the harassed first nurses of Canada to allow them to make progress at last.

The Augustinians applied themselves enthusiastically to development of the work at Sillery. They called their hospital the "Hôtel Dieu," and here they were free, as they had not been sometimes in Europe, to make the spirit emanating from it that of a true House of God. Its goodness penetrated the palisade and touched the entire community. The Indian, sick or well, could rely upon friendship; and kindness to him helped to protect the colony. Old Indian women and children, to whom fortune and the winter weather alike showed harshness, found a home. An out-patient service in which the nuns dispensed quantities of medicine drew many others to their door, and sent them away cheered by the helpful words dispensed with it.

Never did there seem to be enough room or enough time for all good works that the generous nuns found to do, and every arriving ship brought more patients, to say nothing of complicating infections. The year 1658 saw them moved into a new Hôtel Dieu of Quebec built near the fort where they would have protection in case of attack by their savage and uncertain neighbors. Here they built up an institution that endured many hazards, and remains to the present time, a mainstay for the city that grew up about it, and a monument to three capable nurses who a long time ago were called upon to make a great adjustment, and accomplished it.

Meanwhile, in the hospital which they had been called upon to organize so suddenly, the Ursulines were especially successful in

1 Repplier, Agnes: Mère Marie of the Ursulines. Copyright, 1931, reprinted by permission of Doubleday, Doran & Company, Inc., New York.

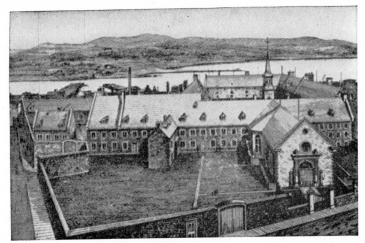

Hôtel Dieu of Quebec in 1825 Showing Stockades as Protection Against Indian Attack

(From Hospital Management, September, 1939.)

utilizing the help of Indian women, as both orders did. Their teacher training, doubtless, set its own stamp of quality on this *earliest instruction and supervision of nurses in America.* As soon as it was possible, they returned to the work that they had set out to do. Little Indian girls in health sorely needed teachers if they were to grow up in the ways of civilization and Christianity, and make good wives for French and Indian men. They had to learn how to keep their small bodies clean, how to wear and take care of the queer French clothing, how to behave in a mannerly fashion while eating at table, at the same time that they learned how to cook, sing, and read, and how to pray and give the right attention to chapel service. They must be led to practice kindness instead of cruelty. This was a stumbling block over which all missionaries had tripped when trying to change their savage elders. The mothers of these very girls could accept with joy their time-honored privilege of helping to torture captives. Their daughters must be taught to find joy in other ways.

The staunch little group of Ursuline nuns had a long struggle with poverty before one of their dreams was realized and a beautiful stone convent replaced inadequate quarters. In 1660 such a school was theirs, set high on the cliff of Quebec, in seven acres of ground, and proclaiming itself the finest building in New France. Quebec had given them the land, and friends had sent from the homeland the workmen who fashioned it out of native rock. The great convent of the Ursulines stands on the same site today. Here the young women who braved the Atlantic storms because they were willing to become colonial wives for France found protection. This was the locus of the marriage mart where they chose husbands from applicants presenting themselves.

The Relations of the Jesuits and the letters from nuns in Quebec spread the tidings of adventure over an ever-broadening field in France. The life that held so many hardships was suffused in the distance by the golden glamour of romance. Its inspiration, the religious zeal of the Catholic, was ever more being urged by the advance of Protestantism toward expression in missionary activity. Trading companies and political leaders learned to rely upon the establishment of missions as fundamental to control of the savage. In France and in Spain, Christianization of the Indian, acquisition of wealth and the satisfaction of nationalism were dominant motives behind colonization.

Settlement of Montreal   The next phase in development of Canada, after Quebec had been set going, was the foundation of a second settlement about two hundred miles farther up the St. Lawrence, on what already had been named the "Island of Montreal" (Mount Royal rises behind it). Promoters of the new colony profited by Quebec's experiences. They included in their original plans a hospital and a school, and decided that the hospital was the immediate necessity if choice had to be made. In 1641 the first ship sailed carrying forty colonists, a governor and four women. One among these visioned herself merged in whatever pious work might come to hand in a land where the Christian could find so many opportunities to practice his religion. Since her childhood, *Jeanne Mance* had shown herself to be of unusual religious bent. She had not become a nun, however, and the inspiration that drew her now to far-off Canada she owed to her reading of the popular *Relations*, and the example of Mme de la Peltrie. Her own fortune had not been sufficient to supply funds necessary for her venture, but the generous donations of *Madame de Bullion*, who became interested in her, had made it financially secure, for the present.

The colonization party was forced to land at Quebec because August was too late in the year for clearing land, for sowing, and for building cabins of logs made from great trees that must be felled. The winter would close down upon them, and, perhaps, destroy them before all was finished. A settler made room for them at his farm near Sillery and the Augustinian nuns. Mlle Mance saw, at close range, the life of a pioneer, in health and in sickness. She learned, intimately, the problem of dealing with the savage Indian. Mme de la Peltrie at the Ursuline school became her friend and extended her kindness to the little group of enthusiasts who were busied with boat-making in preparation for their trip up river in the spring. When that happy time arrived, Mme de la Peltrie went with them. In May, 1642, they reached the island on which they were to develop the tiny settlement that grew into the great city of Montreal.

Hôtel Dieu of Montreal Founded. By October, 1644, Mlle Mance was established in a building sixty by twenty-four feet, divided into a hospital of two wards, servants' quarters and kitchen, and a room for herself. A palisade surrounded all, for the fierce tribes of the Iroquois were ever-threatening neighbors who prowled about and shot arrows from forest hiding-places, and shared with other savages the delights of torturing captives. From France came hospital supplies, household and chapel furnishings, and animals wherewith to stock a small farm. Provision for medical aid was overlooked, and the colony depended on the common sense of Mlle Mance and the knowledge of medicine possessed by missionary priests. Fortunately, pioneer life made men rugged, and they seldom needed care unless beset by epidemic disease, or were victims of accident or war.

For the next fifteen years, in the little mission hospital, Mlle Mance nursed the sick and stretched resources to interpret Christian hospitality to all who came her way. In 1659 the difficulties surrounding colonial organization and its support impelled her to visit France to see what could be done to improve them through a closer contact. While there she secured the services of three hospital nuns from the Society of St. Joseph de la Flêche, one of whom was made the first superior of the hospital. Mlle Mance did not withdraw completely from management of the institution, and was the actual administrator of its affairs until her death in 1673. Many vicissitudes beset it in the intervening years, and even greater ones followed them. Within the next century, all French developments at Montreal, and at Quebec also, passed into English control as a result of the Seven Years' War, and French support of its Canadian missions was suspended.

The change in political administration naturally created economic disturbances that shook the lives of all who had tried to make a place for themselves in this section of the New World. The nuns of Quebec were close to the hazards of war, for its decisive battle was fought at their very door. In the Ursuline convent and the Hôtel Dieu wounded French and English soldiers found nurses to care for them, and it was to the Ursuline chapel that France's hero, *Montcalm*, was carried for burial.

The nuns at the Hôtel Dieu of Montreal were at a loss to know how to keep their hospital going at all, until one of them, resourcefully, devised the idea of selling bread. Their ovens immediately became a source of income and, before long, produced hundreds of loaves daily. In time, also, the great kettles began to turn out quantities of soap, and two household industries had been developed on a major scale. With sewing, candle-making, and other lesser activities, they went far toward maintaining an institution which the general poverty made more and more essential to community health.

The story of pioneer life for women in America, in the church and out of it, appears unutterably hard, until we remember that in pioneer living at any time and place will be found compensations. In the pioneer environment, conventions slacken and social distinctions disappear. Dullness is unknown, for something is always happening. There is a freedom of action and of thought that has been lost by older societies. A helpful spirit rules those who live in isolation. The one who has lends to him who has not. Good things and evil things that befall individuals are shared, and much joy is to be got from trifles. There is a deep sense of comradeship, and always there is somebody who can see the funny side of things. The sense of humor is as oil to machinery in difficult situations. Among Quebec's early settlers, one of the best loved was a happy Ursuline nun whom people learned to call the "laughing nun." There were priests who could share the amusement of those who watched them learning to

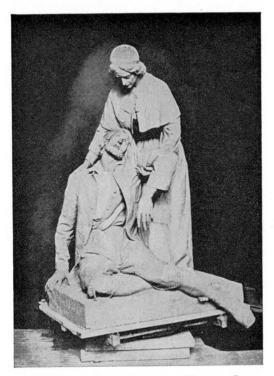

STATUE OF JEANNE MANCE TENDING A WOUNDED SOLDIER

The sculptor was Philippe Herbert. Photograph from the clay model in the artist's studio, from which the bronze statue now standing in the courtyard of the present Hôtel Dieu of Montreal was cast in the year 1909. (From "History of Medicine in the Province of Quebec" by Maude E. Abbott, McGill University Montreal, Canada, 1931.)

use snowshoes. There were many nuns among them who could smile with friends or patients whose interest was caught by the many and varied patches that were spread over worn habits and made it hard to pick out the original cloth.

Perhaps beyond all other compensations in point of reward are those of being able to adjust more and more quickly to changing circumstance, of inventing, and of seeing the fruits of labor and thinking ripen. In pioneer America Europeans had to make many concessions to social exigency and physical environment. They had to learn his languages if they were to gain headway with the Indian. There were necessary modifications in farming and building. Cherished class distinctions tended to disappear even in spite of French royal efforts to establish feudalism and a system of nobility. Clothing had to be adapted to new types of weather, food became necessarily coarse and extremely simple. There were times when money was all but gone and, as pinching failed, new ways of providing sustenance must be found. White habits of nuns became brown when the former proved themselves unsuited to conditions; coarse but beautiful weaves in cloth replaced the fine ones of the old land. Indian moccasins were substituted often for shoes. Indian squaws taught herbal medical lore. Slowly, surely, progress was made. Tents and wooden buildings were replaced by stone ones, farms supplanted forests. Schools, churches, towns began to grow, and social gaiety was more frequent.

Two colonial ambitions met early fulfillment. Wealth flowed homeward to France through the trading companies, and missions were established among the Indians. So far, however, there had been only slow growth of population. The country must, in some way, be permanently settled. Men emigrated to follow the fur trade as it developed in New France, "coureurs de bois," she called them, but they became used to a half-wild, carefree life in the woods. Their occasional visits to the settlements were full of irresponsible gaiety. They did not promise to develop into the substantial type of citizen upon which a country could depend. The question of a growing population in her colony became a serious one to France. It was obvious that if it was to develop there must be more men who would farm the land, and women who would help them to build permanent homes and rear children. Indian girls educated by the Ursuline nuns sometimes fulfilled expectation by marrying a French settler, but oftener reverted to native life. The idea of one husband who could not be divorced was foreign to them, and not pleasing.

Marriage Mart. The year 1654 saw the first of a series of importation from France of young girls who had agreed to become the wives of French colonists. Some of these girls had been brought up in orphan asylums, some were convent bred. All were carefully selected on the basis of character. Experience proved the most satisfactory group to be derived from the farm homes of France. On the voyage

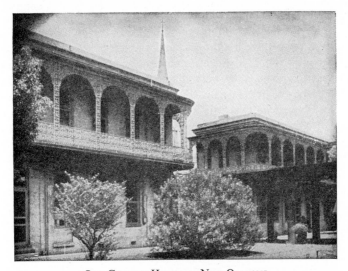

OLD CHARITY HOSPITAL, NEW ORLEANS
Established in 1727. (Sister Henrietta, American Journal of Nursing, March, 1939.)

across the Atlantic they were accompanied by a nun or a paid matron. Upon landing in Canada they were under the protection of the Ursulines. To the convent came prospective husbands with whom the girls were free to converse and interchange questions. Some girls were slow in making the great decision, some were difficult to please. They might turn down suitors but, until safely married, they stayed with the nuns. At the end of twenty years nearly one thousand new homes had been created through their cooperation. Royal dowries often went with them, and bounties might be offered for children. France seldom numbered less than ten in her colonial families.

LOUISIANA

Within the next hundred years France was busy acquiring land, building up her fur trade, and establishing outposts on settlements along the St. Lawrence and Mississippi waterways. Another French colony had developed about the mouth of the Mississippi and needed teachers and nurses. New Orleans was the front door to territory bordering the great river to its source, and called "Louisiana" in honor of France's king, whose "home town" also had been remembered in naming the infant capital. Six or seven Ursuline nuns answered the call from a far-off land, and left France in 1727. Their passage was an adventurous one, dragged out for five months. Storms beset them, they were chased by pirates, and finally landed in the harbor of Belize on the coast of Honduras. Another hazardous week was spent on two little freight boats that took them across the Gulf of Mexico to New Orleans. Here they fared somewhat better than the nuns of Quebec. Their new home was ready, and slavery provided helpers. Colonial life was less primitive, and the site of their future labor was a fruitful land in contrast to rocky Quebec, but the mosquito produced a new enemy in yellow fever. Many epidemics of this disease, of cholera, and of smallpox had to be met in another port of immigration and trade. Political disturbances brought war dangers. It was under stress of many difficulties that the little house developed slowly into the present great Charity Hospital of New Orleans. The convent school, which probably had first place in the Ursuline objective, was established too.

NEW ENGLAND

The Spanish were well established in Mexico, and the French called the region about the mouth of the St. Lawrence theirs, before English seamen joined this new "Gold Rush." These subjects of Queen Elizabeth followed along as pirates who stole the treasure that ships of Spain were busy carrying home. Some of them became explorers, and one sailed around the world. Another country contributed its quota to the group of advance agents who prepared the way for civilization to supplant barbarism once more. Another people was being stirred by that restlessness which has kept the human race ever on the move, adding to its experience, seeking new knowledge, and steadily spreading over the earth better ways of living. In 1584 England laid claim to a portion of the Atlantic coast lying between the claims already staked by Spain and France, and the area was named "Virginia" in honor of her virgin queen, Elizabeth.

Europe, meanwhile, in her zeal to take advantage of what was proving to be an outlet for expansion, found new occasion for national enmities, and extended her wearisome struggles to the seas. By 1588 Spain had developed a marine power that was her national pride. A great fleet of ships, known as the "Invincible Armada," arrived off the coast of England, bent on doing away with their greatest rival. Its destruction gave Englishmen supremacy in naval power, a position of utmost advantage for protecting foreign possessions.

In 1607 English colonization really got its start. A colony called "Jamestown," for Elizabeth's royal successor, was planted at the mouth of a river called the "James." Its growth was impeded by the disappointment of men who came to carry away gold and found none. They could not believe that life in Jamestown was worthwhile, saw no way of making a living, and completely failed to adjust. Many of them starved to death. The colony's spirit was changed and its destiny saved by constructive *Captain John Smith* who declared against unwillingness to work, brought out men of proved stability of character and manual skill, built cabins for permanent settlers, and set up trade with the Indians. A few years later the industry of raising tobacco was introduced, the privilege of individual ownership of land was granted colonists, and real progress began. An era of great estates and fortune-making followed. Tobacco ultimately proved to be a substitute for gold, lucrative as the furs which had been the solace of France.

Before any of this came about, however, the colony had a miserable history of hardship and Indian massacre, sickness and heavy mortality. Its members were adventurers, frequently dashing young cavaliers belonging to noble families. The lure was sudden wealth and they meant to take it home. No one understood sanitation necessary in camp life. Medical care was lacking, for doctors appointed by the colonizaton company would not stay. There was little that could be called nursing, and homesickness was depressing. Women do not appear in the picture until 1619 when a shipload arrived at Jamestown to be auctioned off as wives. In the same year the first slaves were brought from Africa. The problems of instability and labor and income having been removed, the settlement improved like an infant victim of malnutrition for whom the proper food at last has been found. Immigrants flocked to it.

Meantime, various things had been happening in the homeland which made emigration more and more desirable. There was bitter struggle for religious freedom, and political justice was threatened by a king who claimed to rule by divine right and imposed ever heavier taxes. When feudalism had broken over a century before, it left a trail of unemployment behind it. However, now that no bond tied men to the soil as serfs, restlessness in the laboring group could be satisfied by moving, and, particularly, by having land of their own. Another colony was planted farther north, and, to some extent, it profited by the experiences of Jamestown.

Northern colonization had difficulties peculiarly its own, and the little group of about one hundred men and women who undertook it in 1620 experienced hardship too. The little ship, "Mayflower," in which they chose to make their pilgrimage to America, acquainted them with danger, seasickness, and scurvy. It landed them on a rocky wooded coast in the middle of winter. The pitiful little huts they were able to build were wholly inadequate as homes, and even when, later, the frost disappeared and they were able to clear the land, it made stony, unfruitful farms. In the meantime, half of the colonists had died.

The survivors succeeded ultimately in their determination to make permanent homes, develop orderly government, and worship in their chosen way. The Indians proved friendly and, although missionary effort among them was limited, there was an attempt to be kind and just with them. Other settlers followed, and other colonies were developed. While Spain and France had sought to transplant both feudalism and Catholicism, England's policies were formed at a time when her laborers wanted land of their own. She could see the advantage of toleration afar off, if not at home. America was roomy enough to afford separate homes for all of those groups into which Christians were dividing themselves as they broke away from the one Church in which, for fifteen hundred years, they had worshiped together one God.

Provision for medical care of settlers remained inadequate, as it had been in Jamestown. *Samuel Fuller,* a deacon of the church who arrived on the Mayflower, acted as physician to fellow colonists in New England for thirteen years, and his was the precedent followed for long years after. Prayer was a large part of treatment, for patients expected it, and men like Fuller considered it a part of their duty to the sick. No degree was required, and the educated man among the colonists—clergyman, governor, or school-teacher—was held equipped to essay the role of doctor. The ignorant quack throve. Ideals of health protection and care during illness in these early days could only be reflected from countries where the general outlook was of the Middle Ages. Indian folk-lore soon clouded this outlook further.

"Obviously this clerical and lay medicine would have to be very primitive. It was a peculiar mixture of religious medicine, folk-medicine, and scientific principle. One invoked the word of God, let blood, or prescribed drugs, to the best of one's understanding. We must not forget that at this period European medicine, even when practiced by physicians, was effective only in exceptional cases."[2]

English pioneers lacked the organized service of the mission or the convent, and the institutional experience of nun and priest. Women were scarce, although the wives of Englishmen accompanied their husbands more frequently than did those of the Spaniards or the French. The wife of Samuel Fuller was brave enough to assume the busy function of colonial midwife, and there were always some who followed this occupation, or helped in families during illness. When strangers fell ill, or if it was not feasible, for some reason, to keep the patient in his own home, the custom was to depend on the generosity of neighbors. When the doctor, in the midst of his long round of widely separated visits, found someone whose recovery depended on close supervision, he took him to his own home. Out of these repetitions of primitive hospitality, the hospital would take shape, but, unlike the Spanish or the French, these early English builders of America took considerable time to get around to introducing it.

The missionary spirit of New England colonists demonstrated itself in the preparation of religious tracts for the Indian, and in establishment in 1638 of Harvard College and in 1750 of Dartmouth College, where he might be prepared, with their own sons, for the ministry. Their conception of care in illness unfolds itself in two groups of selected quotations, the first the work of a biographer of *Cotton Mather* (1663–1728), the second taken from the diary of *Samuel Sewall* (1652–1730). Both were Puritan ministers of Massachusetts, men of public spirit, graduates of Harvard, and both shared the belief of their time in witchcraft. Cotton Mather was interested in medicine and, to some extent, used his knowledge. It

[2] Sigerist, Dr. Henry E.: American Medicine. New York, W. W. Norton & Co., Inc., 1934, p. 37.

did not prevent him, however, from prosecuting witchcraft trials, in which his friend Mr. Sewall, in the capacity of Chief Justice, was forced to take the responsibility of endorsing a legal decision. That the latter's faith in witches wavered as a result of weighing popular testimony against them, is evidenced by the fact that later he arose in his pew at the old South Meeting House, in Boston, to acknowledge publicly that he deplored his part in a judgment of human beings which gave their fellow creatures authority to hang them.

"At this time medicine had far to go. Men were credulous in this as in all scientific fields. Mermaids and mermen were accredited facts. A sailor on the boat that in 1686 brought the bookseller Dutton to Boston had seen both on voyages to the East Indies."

"Deformities were ascribed to witchcraft. Cotton Mather's own first son, born in 1693, lacked an anus, and in spite of efforts to relieve him, died in three days. Mather more than suspected witchcraft, his wife having been frightened some few weeks before by a *Spectre*."

"He was sure that he could confer one benefit upon Boston—he had never forgotten his medical interest—by spreading the news of inoculation, a treatment he had learned from a publication of the Royal Society lent him by Dr. William Douglas, the only physician in Boston with a medical degree and the one most inhospitable to the new idea. This was not vaccination in the modern method, but inoculation which induced a mild form of the disease. Though it had never been tried in America, Mather felt sure that many lives could be saved by it. Therefore he prepared a statement for the Boston physicians embodying a summary of the Royal Society publications."[3]

"N. B. Tuesday, Dec. 22, 1675, about the time of the Eclips Sister Sewall was delivered in my chamber of a daughter, Goodwife Brown being Midwife."
"This night Eliza Damon, servant to Nash the Currier, dyes about midnight of the small pocks, to our great startling, lest it should spread as in 1678. Had hop'd the Town was clear of it. But one that I know of dyed on't before, and that a great while since."
"About one at night, Jane comes up with an unusual Gate, and gives us an account of Mothers Illness, not being able to speak of a considerable time. I went to Capt. Daviss and fetched some Trecle Water and Syrup of Saffron; Dame Ellis made a Cake of Herbs to try to strengthen Mothers Stomach. In the morn Roger Judd is sent to Cambridge for Dr. Oliver, mother chusing to speak with him and no other. When he comes he advises to a Plaister for the Stomach, which is aplied; and a Potion made of Bexar (Bezoar) to be taken in Syrup of Saffron and Treacle water; of which took once or twice. About 8. or 9. I call'd Mr. Willard at her desire, who prays with her."[4]

[3] Boas and Boas: Cotton Mather, 1928, pp. 40, 42, 170, 226. By permission of Harper and Brothers, New York and London, publishers.
[4] Samuel Sewall's Diary, edited by Mark Van Doren, Macy-Macius, New York, 1927, pp. 8, 42, 123.

Growth of Hospitals   The growth of hospitals was slow. In over one hundred and fifty years elapsing before the War of American Revolution (1775–1783), only five hospitals appear to have been founded in the English colonies outside of Canada. In only two of these did the quality of nursing improve beyond that which we have seen to be characteristic of city hospitals in the homeland. Two were located in what is now New York City, two others in Philadelphia, and a special hospital for the insane found its location at Williamsburg, in Virginia.

When Dutch New Amsterdam on Manhattan island was taken over by England, it boasted already more in the way of institutionalized charity than existed in English colonies. There was a home for the poor financed by the Church, and a small hospital built in 1658 was maintained by the Dutch West India Company. This hospital, about which information is limited, was probably nothing more than an emergency shelter for homeless sick people such as sailors, or the slaves coming into port as cargo on company ships. A nurse is said to have been appointed to care for the patients, and it has been suggested that he or she, too, may have belonged to this slave group.

New Amsterdam became New York, and there arose as adjunct to its hospital a *Publick Workhouse and House of Correction*, an institution lately devised in England where hard work was being used as a cure for crime and indigency, and to reduce the cost of maintaining the petty criminal and the homeless unemployed. Criminal and pauper from now on staffed the hospital. Buildings changed according to need, the city assumed a share of the expense of charity, and, in time, these small beginnings of the present great *Bellevue Hospital* of modern New York were concentrated on the bank of the East River.

The *Philadelphia General Hospital*, or, as it was then called, "Blockley Hospital," originated in 1731, also with an almshouse as its background. Both Bellevue and Blockley, like St. Thomas' and St. Bartholomew's of London, were in their early days comparable to the xenodochia of ancient times. They cared for the destitute, the insane, the vagrant, or the homeless. Both, however, looked not to the Church but among their inmates for workers, and for nurses too. Their management was complicated by frequent epidemics and conditions of increasing poverty due, in part, to individual difficulties of immigrant adjustment, in part to the influence of the Industrial Revolution. The penniless of Britain were moving to America. Under this new pressure, and lacking, as they undoubtedly did, the public interest, these institutions became neither better nor worse than institutions of their type and time abroad.

Treatment of the insane was modeled on that of Newgate and places like it. Men and women victims of smallpox might lie in the same ward, the dead might be left on the floor, undisciplined attendants devoid of training might allow filth to accumulate, and run away from yellow fever or typhus. When nurses were sought by hire, only the roughest element among women and men could be secured. Drunkenness among them was common. Nurses like Betsy Prig and Sairey Gamp of Dicken's novel, had come to the new land, and were accepted as necessary evils. Even those nurses who might be of more motherly quality lacked education, and worked under disadvantages which are difficult for us to understand. There were no thermometers, no conscious application of hygienic principles, no knowledge of asepsis or antisepsis. Surgery was done without anesthesia by surgeons whose frock coats gained distinction as they accumulated dirt and bloodstains, who used unboiled instruments and unsterilized sea sponges for mopping blood, and were content to stick needles and thread into velvet pin cushions.

It was all of a piece with conditions of the Old World during that period of decline in nursing which, unfortunately, coincided with growth of foreign colonies. Bellevue and Blockley only followed the current model in city hospitals. The public responsible for New World institutions were in the position of the nurse who knows the ways of one hospital. What they had to give was limited by a narrow experience. They could transfer only what this had taught them, and already they were finding that ways must be investigated for making knowledge grow to adequacy in a new sphere. Doctors were protesting, and the fame of the well trained Sisters of Charity, who heralded nursing reform in France, was so great as to cause reforming spirits to seek to introduce some corresponding group of nurses to America.

The *Pennsylvania Hospital* founded in 1751 and the *New York Hospital* founded in 1771 were the next two hospitals to be developed. They both departed from the xenodochial type, in limiting admission to the sick only, and from the city hospital tradition by depending for support on privately donated funds. Both were unique in the care given to selection of the women who were to nurse their patients, and both initiated methods of training them for their work. Physicians of the Pennsylvania Hospital taught simple procedures in nursing, and *Dr. Valentine Seaman of the New York Hospital* augmented similar teaching by lectures on anatomy, physiology, maternal nursing, and care of children. *He is the first doctor known to have lectured to nurses in America.* In 1776, war intervened to complicate nursing difficulties and suspend any other possible progress.

AMERICAN REVOLUTION (1775–1783)

The war of the American Revolution involved all the young English colonies scattered along the Atlantic Coast. Some of them wanted to be free to develop in their own way; others wished to remain with England. England's colonial children, however, found themselves badly prepared to assume burdens of expense and organization necessary to wage a conflict on their own account. Their hastily mobilized army had no medical corps, no Red Cross, no trained nurses. The only organized units of nurses in the country were the nuns of the Catholic Church. They nursed wounded soldiers in their hospitals, as well as those who fell victims to epidemic disease, for there was scarlet fever and dysentery, and smallpox broke out in spite of the fact that the new variolation was used on fighting men.

Enthusiasm and loyalty to a cause, to some degree, made up for the lack of system and experience, but, in the light of modern methods of warfare, much makeshift appears. Soldiers were apt to get poor or meager rations. There were times when shoes and clothing wore out, and they marched barefoot in tatters. There were women who followed their husbands even to the battlefield, and, under the greatest difficulties, nursed them through serious illnesses. Other women made clothing and bandages, and parted with precious pewter that went to be made into bullets. Homes were turned into hospitals, and so were barns. One farm-woman, at least, baked huge batches of bread, day after day, and served it by the roadside to hungry soldiers, and many tales are told of such resourcefulness. In heroism, woman did not fall behind her male relatives.

The war descended on the colonies just as they were getting a financial start. It left the usual poverty behind, with invalids who needed care, cripples for whom there were no rehabilitation centers, and none of the modern highly organized social service. Among these poor and sick people were many who never in their lives had asked for public help and now were unable to get along without it.

PHILADELPHIA DISPENSARY

Out of a deep social distress came a new type of social institution which has proved itself the forerunner of today's clinic or out-patient department of the hospital. This institution, like the Pennsylvania Hospital, owed its origin to the social spirit of Quakers in a Quaker City. In 1786 the *Philadelphia Dispensary* was established. Independent of any hospital, the dispensary finances were met by appealing to public sympathy through a new plan of public service, the advantages of which were set forth by its sponsors somewhat as follows: Large numbers of persons needing treatment were not sick enough to be hospitalized, and the expense of their care in the hospital was unnecessary. People who had enjoyed better circumstances could be assured that publicity would not be given to their post-war status as it was, unavoidably, when they accepted care in a charity hospital. A staff of volunteer physicians would treat both groups without charge, and make visits in patients' homes when necessary.

The Philadelphia Dispensary was a success, and the idea spread to other cities. Boards of Health were rare. Pending establishment of city or state health departments, a dispensary came to be looked to as a means of controlling disease. Vaccination against smallpox was one of the earliest preventive treatments which it made widely possible. Dispensary physicians knew those streets from which epidemics commonly derived, and, one having appeared, the hospital would supply the physicians with addresses of patients. After verification of the suspected source, newspaper publicity then informed the citizens of the hidden menace to their health, and roused sentiment in favor of abolishing it. The next thing was a health law.

Later history shows the dispensary, which began with so much promise, sinking into neglect and obscurity as an institution when public and professional interest becomes focused on hospitals. The dispensary dwindles then until its main functions are a badly managed first-aid service, and the issuance of medicine free, or at cost. Frequently, it loses its identity in the hospital. Only recently has it been revitalized and recovered its dignity as the portal of entry to the hospital, an indispensable factor in modern preventive medicine, and a radiating center for much of our community, health, and social work.

NURSE SOCIETY OF PHILADELPHIA

One of the physicians who gave their time to the Philadelphia Dispensary was keenly impressed by conditions surrounding the confinement of poverty-stricken young mothers. He hoped to get a hospital for them and a school in which to prepare nurses, but was forced to content himself with the *Nurse Society of Philadelphia*, established in 1839. This was an organization of women who undertook to supply a maternity service in homes.

The Nurse Society of Philadelphia chose its nurses from applicants who had stability of character and experience as heads of families. These were given instruction in obstetrics in common with medical apprentices, and in the form of lectures and practice on a manikin. *Dr. Joseph Warrington* taught these classes, and lady visitors from the society supervised practice in allotted districts. In 1850 a combined Home and School was opened. Further systematized instruction was arranged that included lessons in cooking, and experience in homes for two weeks at a time. The Society paid the salary of the nurse. In time, this service was extended to include medical and surgical patients, but no additional instruction was provided. Certificates were awarded, and the English system of renting rooms in the mother school and providing through it calls for private duty was adopted. Another brave attempt had been made toward instructing and supervising nurses under secular auspices, and so helping to fill a need that grew always more urgent.

After 1800, one evidence of returning growth was to be seen in a great development of hospitals and, as they were called, "asylums for the insane," the latter usually under the control of states or provinces. The tendency to specialize institutions seen in Williamsburg's asylum was seen again in the establishment of a Lying-in Hospital in New York in 1798. The same tendency, following woman's entrance to the field of medicine and her more frequent presence on hospital boards, became apparent later in the development of separate hospitals for women and children, or of hospitals combining these two groups. The following are a few out of many well-known institutions established up to 1860, and chosen to emphasize variety and spread rather than priority:

> Massachusetts General Hospital, Boston, Massachusetts—1811
> McLean Asylum, Somerville, Massachusetts (now in Waverly)—1818
> Montreal General Hospital, Montreal, Canada—1819
> Cincinnati General Hospital, Cincinnati, Ohio—1821
> Knight Hospital (later New Haven Hospital), New Haven, Connecticut—1826
> St. Louis Mullanphy Hospital, St. Louis, Missouri—1828
> St. Vincent's Infirmary, Louisville, Kentucky—1832
> Mt. Sinai Hospital, New York, New York—1852
> Buffalo General Hospital, Buffalo, New York—1853
> Nursery and Childs' Hospital, New York, New York—1854
> Woman's Hospital, New York, New York—1855
> Children's Hospital, Philadelphia, Pennsylvania—1855
> General and Marine Hospital, St. Catherine's, Canada—1855
> San Joaquin General Hospital, French Camp, California—1857
> Halifax Hospital (now Victoria General), Halifax, Canada—1859

Quite a number of institutions that still carry on public service originated during this period, and a steady increase in immigration made the hospital or the dispensary more and more necessary. Medical schools needed them for training ground. As the tide of settlement flowed westward, they went with it. From east to middle west, and thence to the west, hospitals accompanied immigrant public until they stretched from coast to coast, the dispensary, in the course of passing years, losing individuality as it becomes a hospital adjunct.

At the same time, some further improvement was made in nursing by introducing to America European sisterhoods, Protestant as well as Catholic. These nursed in homes, founded hospitals, and, in time, organized schools for nurses. In 1809 *Mother Elizabeth Seton* founded, at Emmitsburg, Maryland, the Catholic Sisters of Charity. In 1843, the Catholic Sisters of Mercy came from Ireland to Pittsburgh, and four years later founded the hospital which bears their name. In 1845 the Protestant Nursing Sisters were organized in New Jersey through the efforts of *Reverend Muhlenberg*. In 1848 *Reverend William Passavant* established a hospital in Pittsburgh, which he staffed with deaconess nurses imported from a Protestant mission house at Kaiserswerth on the Rhine in Germany. Of this mission and its system of training deaconesses for nursing we shall hear again, for it was here, only a few years later, that Florence Nightingale was to glean some of the ideas that enabled her to set in motion a scheme for world-wide reform in methods of caring for the sick.

SUMMARY

Settlement of the New World followed schemes of colonization developed largely by Spain, France, and England. These mother countries regarded their colonies as existing primarily for advantage of the homeland, and organized trade with them from that viewpoint. Christopher Columbus and Hernando Cortez, at different times and with different objectives, promoted the interests of Spain. Their explorations and conquests brought into Spanish possession the great wealth of the Aztecs, Toltecs, Mayas, and Incas. In contrast to the culture that had been developed by these Indian peoples was that of other roaming tribes of hunters whose Medicine Men were acting as doctors and whose herbwomen were assuming the functions of nurses. Oddly enough, however, in some instances women of these tribes were accorded much respect.

For care of the sick and other forms of social work, the Spanish were well prepared, for did they not represent a Catholic country whose Dominican, Franciscan, and Jesuit Orders stood ready to offer help when needed? As after the Fall of Rome there arose the necessity for civilizing and Christianizing great numbers of barbarians, also with colonization of America there came similar need for training and educating American Indians. As the monastery developed to fill the needs of the first instance, so a similar institution, the mission, appeared in the second. Founder of the great chain of missions reaching along the Pacific coast was *Junípero Serra*, a Franciscan padre. Mission Dolores, the last one established, was erected in San Francisco about the time the Liberty Bell was ringing in Philadelphia. This mission and several other of these links with an heroic and colorful past are today in a good state of preservation and may be visited by interested persons.

Mexico has the distinction of possessing the first hospital to be erected in the Western Hemisphere. In 1524 it was built in her capital city by Hernando Cortez, and was intended to offset, within his own conscience, many acts of cruelty perpetrated against defenseless natives. A nursing Brotherhood originally provided care for the sick. As the "Hospital of Jesus of Nazareth," it operates today with all the facilities of a modern surgical institution.

While Spain was developing what is now Mexico and the western coast of the United States, the French were as busily taking possession of the rich valleys of the St. Lawrence and Mississippi Rivers. Like the Spanish, the French had the benefit of Catholic orders in all of their social undertakings. Their first hospital was opened in Quebec in 1639, and three Augustinian nuns were imported from France to do the nursing. The *Duchesse d'Aiguillon*, niece of influential Cardinal Richelieu, had obtained a grant of land for the hospital, and she sponsored the undertaking which grew into the great Hôtel Dieu of Quebec.

At the same time, an orphanage and school for Indian and French children, with Ursuline nuns as teachers, was the special project of *Madame de la Peltrie*, another Frenchwoman who came with the nuns to supervise it. Upon their arrival, an epidemic of smallpox forced Ursulines, as well as Augustinians, to act as nurses. The Ursulines made use of their skill as teachers by instructing Indian women in care of the sick. This is believed to be the *first instruction and supervision of nurses on the American continent*. The Ursuline convent ultimately erected, like the Hôtel Dieu of Quebec, is still in existence. It was to the protection of this convent that French country girls were brought when imported as available wives for French trappers.

When plans were devised for building Montreal on an island in the St. Lawrence River, *Jeanne Mance* came from France to found a hospital. Though religiously inclined, Jeanne Mance was not a nun. Funds with which a hospital building was erected in 1644 were provided by *Madame de Bullion* of the mother country. Around it were placed palisades to afford protection from fierce tribes of Iroquois Indians. Here, for fifteen years, Jeanne Mance did all the nursing, until hospital nuns of the Society of St. Joseph de la Flêche came from France to assist her. She earned for herself the reputation of being the *first lay nurse of Canada*, and of North America as well.

During the Seven Years' War (or French and Indian War) both the Ursuline Convent and the Hôtel Dieu of Quebec functioned as military hospitals, caring for French and English soldiers alike. At its close, governmental control passed from the French to the English, and it was to be some time before provision could be made for upkeep of hospitals and convent. At the Hôtel Dieu of Montreal, ingenious nuns saved the day by earning money through sewing, baking bread, making soap and candles.

What proved to be the beginnings of another large hospital and another convent developed in 1727 at the mouth of the Mississippi River in what is now New Orleans. Ursuline nuns took an active part in the founding of both. Over one hundred years later, in 1834, the order of Sisters of Charity assumed management of the hospital, now known as the "Charity Hospital" of New Orleans, and one of the largest in the United States.

In founding English colonies, the names of Queen Elizabeth, Sir Walter Raleigh, Captain John Smith, and the ship *Mayflower* stand out as significant. The determination of colonists to work out religious beliefs in their own way, and the desire to escape heavy taxes imposed at home were largely influential in causing emigration from the mother country. These English seekers for freedom were Protestants and, therefore, lacking in certain social benefits to be derived from Catholic religious orders. Any who were educated were expected to have some knowledge of medicine, and were called upon during illness. On the voyage of the Mayflower, *Samuel Fuller*, a deacon of the church, acted as ship physician, while his wife assumed the duties of midwife.

English colonists had no organized plan for converting Indians to Christianity or to a more civilized way of living. Save for a few individuals such as John Eliot, Richard Bourne, and Jonathan Edwards, they had few ministers who would assume a responsibility commonly borne by French and Spanish Catholic priests. However, with establishment of Harvard College in 1638, and with the later founding of Dartmouth in New Hampshire, they provided not only for the preparation of Englishmen for the ministry, but of Indians as well.

The growth of hospitals in New England was slow. Early treatment consisted largely of prayer which was intermingled with much superstitious medical practice. Of the first hospitals to finally appear, two were in New York and two in Philadelphia. Bellevue Hospital, founded in New York in 1658, and Blockley Hospital, founded in Philadelphia in 1731, were of the xenodochial type, caring for many types of needy persons as well as the sick. Inmates acted as nurses. The next two hospitals, Pennsylvania Hospital founded in 1751, and New York Hospital in 1771, were for the sick only, and they used care in the selection of nurses. While the Pennsylvania Hospital has the distinction of being the *first real hospital in the United States*, the New York Hospital is known for providing the *first lectures for nurses on the American continent*. It was here that *Dr. Valentine Seaman* taught anatomy and physiology, obstetrics, and pediatrics. Honoring him today is a plaque showing his profile in the entrance hall of the institution.

At the beginning of the Revolutionary War in 1776 there was no medical corps, no Red Cross Society, no trained nurses. Catholic Orders were the only organized groups with some knowledge of nursing. They and their hospitals were placed at the disposal of the military authorities. Colonial women followed their men to the battlefields, doing what they could to alleviate suffering. After the close of the war, the Philadelphia Dispensary was established for the benefit of discharged soldiers and other ambulatory patients, many of whom were entirely without funds. In some cases, home visits also were provided. The plan proved so successful that the idea spread to other cities.

To provide maternity service in the home, the Nurse Society of Philadelphia came into being in 1839. With this, another American physician achieved renown for early instruction of nurses. *Dr. Joseph Warrington* lectured on obstetrics, while district practice was supervised by Quaker ladies who sponsored the Society. After this time, development in hospitals was rapid, and many of them specialized in particular branches of medicine. The tendency toward more careful selection of nurses gained impetus through introduction of European Sisterhoods, Protestant as well as Catholic. Among these groups were Catholic Sisters of Charity, Protestant Nursing Sisters, Catholic Sisters of Mercy, and Protestant Deaconesses from Kaiserswerth, Germany.

TOPICS FOR DISCUSSION

1. By what three European countries, and in what general locations, were colonies developed in the Western Hemisphere?
2. Show how differences in religion affected early provision for medical and nursing care.
3. How did Spain go about the task of developing her new possessions, and making sure that they would show allegiance to her?
4. (*a*) What do you know of the first hospital to be erected on this side of the Atlantic? (*b*) The first one in Canada? (*c*) The first one in the United States? (*d*) By whom was each sponsored? (*e*) How was nursing care provided in each?
5. Where, and under what circumstances, was instruction first given to those who would do nursing on the American continent?
6. Deriving information from several sources, write a short article on the life work of the first nurse of Canada.
7. (*a*) What political upheaval greatly changed conditions surrounding the management of the Hôtel Dieu of Quebec and the Hôtel Dieu of Montreal? (*b*) What novel adjustment was made in one instance?
8. What is the story of the founding of the Charity Hospital of New Orleans?
9. (*a*) How did English colonists make provision for care of the sick? (*b*) How soon did their first hospitals appear? (*c*) What was their attitude toward the Indians?
10. (*a*) Name the first four hospitals to be established by English colonists. (*b*) Which two were comparable to xenodochia? (*c*) What type of nurse was to be found in each?
11. (*a*) In what hospital, by what physician, and on what subjects were lectures first given to nurses? (*b*) With what undertaking was Dr. Joseph Warrington associated, and for what is he remembered?
12. How far had nursing developed in the United States at the time of the Revolutionary War?
13. To what groups could appeal be made for supplying nursing care to soldiers?

14. Compare activities of the Philadelphia Dispensary and the Nurse Society of Philadelphia.
15. (*a*) When did rapid growth of New England hospitals get under way? (*b*) Give names and locations of several of these early institutions.
16. Improvement in nursing service was made by the importation of what European nursing sisterhoods?
17. Tell something of the origin and history of the modern hospital clinic.
18. Collect data in regard to the founding of the hospital with which your school of nursing is associated.

REFERENCES

Abbott, Maude E.: History of Medicine in the Province of Quebec. Montreal, Canada, McGill University, 1931.

Andrews, Charles: The Fathers of New England. New Haven, Yale University Press.

Atherton, William Henry: The Saintly Life of Jeanne Mance: First Lay Nurse in North America. St. Louis, Catholic Hospital Association of the United States and Canada, 1945.

Beard and Beard: The Rise of American Civilization. New York, The Macmillan Co., 1927.

Boas and Boas: Cotton Mather. New York and London, Harper & Brothers, 1928.

Crawford, Mary Caroline: In Days of the Pilgrim Fathers. Boston, Little, Brown and Co., 1920.

Denis, Alberta Johnston: Spanish Alta California. New York, The Macmillan Co., 1927.

Dexter, Elizabeth Anthony: Colonial Women of Affairs. Boston and New York, Houghton Mifflin Co., 1924, Chap. 4.

Foran, J. K.: Jeanne Mance or "The Angel of the Colony," Montreal, P. Q., The Herald Press, Ltd., 1931.

Groves, Ernest R.: The American Woman. New York, Greenberg, 1937.

Lyman, George D.: John Marsh: Pioneer (first doctor in California). New York, Charles Scribner's Sons, 1930.

Macmichael, William: The Gold Headed Cane. New York, The Macmillan Co., 1927.

Repplier, Agnes: Mère Marie of the Ursulines. New York, Doubleday, Doran, 1937.

Sigerist, Dr. Henry E.: American Medicine. New York, W. W. Norton & Co., Inc., 1934.

Starkey, Marion L.: The Devil in Massachusetts. New York, Alfred Knopf, Inc., 1949. (Historical novel about Salem witchcraft.)

Van Doren, Mark (Editor): Samuel Sewall's Diary. New York, Macy-Masius, 1927.

Sporadic Efforts
At Social Reform

Social conditions in Europe, such as have been described, undoubt-edly were direct results of religious, industrial, and political revolu-tions which threatened to destroy any social recovery accomplished up to this time. Antagonism and ambition had replaced human sympathy as dominant in the emotions of upper and middle classes. The intellectual revolution gave them an attitude of cold skepticism, and the distraction of new interests. While they strove for wealth, leisure, and power, the masses huddled into slums where they sank deep into the mire of poverty, immorality, and brutality. War, fam-ine, industrial abuses, and pestilence made the inadequacy of nursing strike home as those who had destroyed its main source realized what had been done.

CATHOLIC SOCIAL REFORM
SOCIAL SERVICE ESTABLISHED

The need of reform could never be completely lost sight of, and here or there, in the darkness of social desolation, shone the beck-oning light of a constructive idea. The first to forward substantially the new adjustment was *St. Vincent de Paul* (1576–1660), an unas-suming French Catholic priest whose experience of life included parish work, missionary work among galley slaves, and travel and captivity in a foreign land where he picked up some knowledge of medicine before he reached Paris, the scene of his real achievement. Here, he lived close to a hospital where many rich and influential citizens were giving volunteer service as nurses to help out the overworked Brothers of St. John of God. St. Vincent joined them, and proved his usefulness by doing surgical dressings and otherwise assisting with care of patients. Soon, however, his interests reached out into provincial communities, and an accidental occurrence gave him the idea which set the trend of his future labors.

In response to a request from a parishioner, the priest at once appealed in church for help for a family overcome by burdens of poverty and sickness. The little home found itself inundated by well-meaning visitors, and St. Vincent learned the lesson of charity's waste through lack of control. In order to make it a regular community function, and to spread more equably the bounty of the charitable, he suggested forming a working group among the women who would divide among themselves community tasks of service to the poor. From this small beginning, associations of women came into existence in numerous towns and villages. These carried on home visiting, and bore the expense of buying food which they cooked and served to the sick. They paid also for burial of the dead, and frequently assisted at funerals.

By this time St. Vincent had come to believe that prevention was possible for some of those evils in poverty which arise from broken human spirit. Everywhere the social virus of professional begging was present. Observation disclosed to him three groups among the poor: those unable to earn a living, those able to earn a partial living, and those who could earn a complete living were they given opportunity. The time seemed to have arrived when the old system of almsgiving would no longer work. The young, the healthy, and the strong were dependent as well as the old, the sick, and the weak. Five years of work resulted in many changes. Much was done toward stopping indiscriminate alms. Many tramps were taken off the highways and given some supervision by the establishment of public night refuges, trade workshops were organized for teaching manual arts to idle youth, and jobs were hunted up for able-bodied adults. He had organized a system of *Social Service* or a method of *helping people to help themselves.*

Order of Sisters of Charity Founded   St. Vincent de Paul had still another famous piece of work to do. While he was in Paris, a friend sent to see him a widow of noble family and great piety who wished to be guided into a life of good works, and had already had

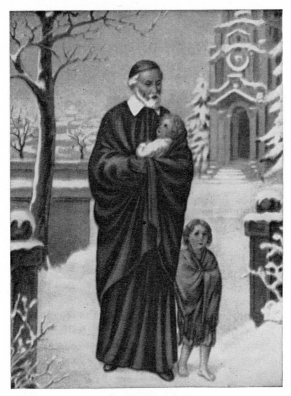

ST. VINCENT DE PAUL

(From "Miniature Stories of the Saints," Book One, by Rev. Daniel A. Lord, S. J. [Catholic publications].)

experience in visiting nursing with a group of volunteer women working near her own home. *Saint Louise de Marillac* as she is now known, had longed as a young girl to become a nun. On account of delicate health, friends dissuaded her, and she married into the Court circle. Early environment had fitted her well for the social sphere. Louise de Marillac, however, avoided society, devoting all her leisure time to that work among the poor which now, after her husband's death, she urged St. Vincent to help her to continue.

Several years of training followed in which Saint Louise de Marillac gained the reformer's viewpoint of a new and flexible type of human service. St. Vincent de Paul then sent her on a tour of the provinces to visit his various associations of women and observe their activities. Living in simplicity equal to that of the poor themselves, she made long journeys in springless carts or on horseback. Her enthusiasm was contagious as she set out to make herself a co-worker in reform. She found that she could teach improved procedures in nursing to association members, and she carried religious instruction among children and adults, as the need appeared.

On her return to Paris two years later, Louise de Marillac hit upon the plan of making her own house a home and a training school for peasant pupils. In 1633, the Community of the *Sisters of Charity* was established, its object the service of the poor in different parts of Paris, its guiding motto "Caritas Christi urget nos" ("The Charity of Christ Presseth Us"). They are words that give out the intensity that drove its two founders and their followers on and on to ever greater service, down to the present time.

A little over a year after the Community was formed, on March 25, 1634, Saint Louise set the example by formally taking a vow and becoming the first Sister of Charity of St. Vincent de Paul. The date later became the annual one on which the sisters rededicate themselves to their work. If they do not wish to renew the vow, they are free to marry or to choose some other form of occupation outside the Community. A few rules on which to base selection for enrollment of these peasant girls began. They must be of good family and good character. They were not allowed to enter without the consent of a male relative.

Uniform Dress. The first members brought with them the peasant costume which they had worn at home, and which now became the dress which they wore as they went about their duties. It was not long before the gray-blue gown of rough woolen cloth, with blue apron and spreading white headdress became the conspicuous reminder of humility and kindly human service which we still recognize in it. Their period of training lasted five years and instruction included a basic education enabling them to read, write, and make use of some arithmetic. At the same time, they were taught by Saint Louise all that she herself knew. The unavoidable limitation of this knowledge is dramatically apparent when we learn that one of the earliest of her graduates was a sacrifice to ignorance of any means of preventing infection. Coming across a patient sick with plague on the highway, she took her to her lodgings and put her in her own bed. Patient and Sister of Charity both died.

St. Vincent was always aware of the danger of losing his new order to the monastery. The young girls and their friends were accustomed to associate religion and good works with monastic life in which care of the personal soul was of prime importance. It was necessary to build up in their minds, as he had in the mind of Louise de Marillac, the idea of a Sister of Charity doing her work where she found it. Often far removed from institutional protection, Sisters must learn how to protect themselves, and their relatives sometimes were fearful. St. Vincent de Paul explained, advised, and combated influences which arose to interfere with his ideal of their carrying religion and help to the people as St. Francis of Assisi had done before them.

No rule was made for the Community for nine years, but this ideal of a new kind of community life was kept constantly before the members in words like these:

"Nuns must needs have a cloister, but the Sister of Charity must go everywhere."

"You have no grating to shut you off from the dangers of the world; you must erect one in your inner self."

The vision before him, St. Vincent de Paul painted in beautiful language for the whole world to understand:

"Their convent must be the houses of the sick; their cell the chamber of suffering; their chapel the parish church; their cloister the streets of the city or the wards of hospitals; in place of the rule which binds nuns to the one enclosure, there must be the general vow of obedience; the grating through which they speak to others must be the fear of God; the veil which shuts out the world must be holy modesty."[1]

In their nursing, St. Vincent made it plain that the patient's needs came before religious offices. He emphasized strict obedience to the orders of the physician as essential to the welfare of the sick, urged them to observe all procedures so that they might be more efficient as medical assistants. At the same time he made it possible for them to harmonize these aims with a thoroughly religious life and spirit.

[1] Quoted in Dock and Nutting: A History of Nursing. New York and London, G. P. Putnam's Sons, 1907. Vol. I, p. 436.

The motto so happily chosen has been the inspiration of a long line of servants of the poor reaching down to our own time, and into far places, as St. Vincent prophesied in his address to the first small group:

"The little snowball will one day become an avalanche; in the future you will be called to Africa, Asia, and farther still."[2]

The Sisters of Charity, at the time they were founded, were a product of Catholic reform. Their first service outside of France was naturally done in countries adhering to the Catholic Church. Increasing religious tolerance and their own high reputation gradually extended these limits. In 1809 *Mother Elizabeth Seton* introduced Sisters of Charity into America. The rule of the Motherhouse in France was obtained and a Community established at Emmitsburg, Maryland. In spite of its proximity to France and its dominant Catholicism, Ireland lacked the benefit of the Sisters' work until 1815 when *Mother Mary Aikenhead* organized a Community in Dublin. In this twentieth century, they may be found all over the world, nursing, teaching, doing social work, guarding the orphaned and the foundling, the aged, the leper, any who need their friendship anywhere.

Only sixteen years after the foundation of their Order, the Sisters of Charity were called to nurse soldiers on a battlefield in France. Not long after they saw war service in Poland. In the Crimean war it was their efficient service to the soldiers of France that inflamed neglected British soldiers to a discontent that aroused England to action, and sent Florence Nightingale to Scutari.

Seen in summary, the accomplishment of Saint Vincent de Paul and Saint Louise de Marillac attains deserved importance as a reform in nursing. Their organization was based on study and knowledge of existing conditions. The order eventually performed two needed types of nursing service. It reached the poor in their homes, and provided partial or complete nursing service for hospitals. In arranging the latter service the legal contract was used to prevent exploitation and preserve identity of the order. The scheme of organization of the Sisters of Charity called for the following:

2 Quoted in a pamphlet, "Saint Louise de Marillac," translated from the French, and published in Emmitsburg, Maryland.

(*a*) A selected group, with set regulations restricting acceptance

(*b*) A common home with experienced supervision

(*c*) A system of instruction

(*d*) A probation of two months followed by a training period of five years

(*e*) Protection by the use of uniform dress of a type which would distinguish them from the people about them, and at the same time be secular

(*f*) Annual renewal of vows, or freedom to leave for marriage or change of occupation

PROTESTANT SOCIAL REFORM

While the Catholic Church was thus busy adjusting its social service to accord with new conditions, Protestants in Germany, England, and the Netherlands were making an effort to replace the lost nun with the deaconess. Unfortunately, she was selected from the ranks of the married woman who had other work to do, and no provision was made for care after her working days were over. With organization and instruction both lacking, leadership proved too weak for the status of a movement to be realized. Although scattered bands of Sisters of Charity had alleviated some phases of social mismanagement, many institutions, including hospitals for the insane, lazarettos, prisons, workhouses, orphanages, factories and their slums, remained to grow into magnets for the reformer.

The general condition of hospitals has already been described. The English model was being copied with unfortunate faithfulness in New England, while the continental European model influenced New Spain and New France. Bethlehem Hospital or "Bedlam" in London and the "Lunatics' Tower" in Vienna were typical of mental asylums to which the sane bought admission tickets and repaired with their friends when they wanted amusement. In the prisons were to be found everywhere great numbers of citizens, put there often for minor offenses, and once in, it was often difficult to get out. Gaolers could demand fees, prisoners often could not pay, and then the great gates did not open even if the law had granted acquittal. Two hundred and fifty different crimes were considered of a degree to merit death. The fact that the close of this period saw these reduced to three illustrates the injustice that had crept into old Roman and Anglo-Saxon law.

A young American girl, victim of an envy which impelled her to strip another girl of hat, shoes, and bright buckles, was hanged in Massachusetts. Tortures were still in use. People who failed to pay back borrowed money or who could not meet their bills might be thrown into debtors' prisons. In this way, swindlers tricked clients and often disposed of them. Respectable merchants, poets, gangsters, thieves—all languished together in places so unsanitary as to be breeding places for disease. Wives and children, suddenly made indigent, sometimes lived with the prisoners. Idleness favored coarse brutalities and gambling, and often upset mental balance. The tremendous public expense was met by parsimony in care. Prison mortality was very high.

A new type of institution was developed in England which found itself burdened with the support of increasing numbers of beggars after the monasteries closed. This country organized a system of "workhouses" in which paupers and minor offenders against the law were detained, and given work to do that brought no personal profit. Hard work gradually became synonymous with correction and the cure of vagabondage. Institutional upkeep was purposely made cheap, and harsh treatment was countenanced. The workhouse became the dread of the poor, while it protected the rest of society from offending sights that might have brought about earlier changes. Hardly less humane than the workhouse were the numerous orphanages built to house the abandoned children and orphans whose numbers increased with war, immorality, and epidemics of disease.

Other social problems were arising to disturb England. It was here that the capitalist first replaced the feudal lord in control of the worker. None of the old paternal attitude went over into the new system which, in fact, was at first unconscious of any responsibility beyond profit making. After 1750 huge factories were built in centers that grew from industry, by builders who knew nothing of sanitary requirements. They were surrounded by equally unsanitary and carelessly erected homes for the workers. Houses were set as close together as possible, and as little land as possible was used for streets. Depreciation of property was rapid, and slums developed. The public health in these neighborhoods was doomed. Epidemic disease was rife and uncontrolled. The factory machinery was put into the hands of operatives without adequate instruction. Accidents were many, and industrial insurance or any form of industrial compensation was as yet undeveloped. The lowest possible wages were paid. The problem of overproduction was solved by shut-down, and great numbers of men, women, and children would be thrown out of employment.

Little children had to work with their parents to make enough to support the family, although this was not new, for they had always done so. Now the conditions were more difficult and their treatment more evident when they were gathered together in public view. All the evils of a lost family life became apparent, but the first Factory Act to legally control industry did not come until 1819. Hours for adults had arisen by that time to as high as eighteen a day, and children often began at three in the morning and worked until nine in the evening. Hours of women and children were now set at twelve a day, and children under nine years of age were not allowed to work.

Fortunately, time had permitted the new group of Christians to settle differences of opinion and arrange themselves in various sects—Baptists, Quakers, Methodists, Presbyterians, Unitarians, and others. Protestantism had reached a point where it was ready to give its own expression to the real work of Christianity, the practice of Christian love. The missionary spirit was apparent in its ranks, and the plight of victims of society's disruption, with the persistence of plague epidemics, was an increasing source of anxiety to the thoughtful or humane.

PRISON REFORM

John Howard   One of the early exponents of this changing attitude was *John Howard* (1727–1789), an English grocer's apprentice, to whom a legacy gave opportunity for travel abroad. A twist of fate made him a prisoner of war in France, and that unlooked-for experience gave him a life work far removed from the grocery business. After regaining his freedom, Howard began to look around through other prisons to see if they were all as bad as this one. He made seven continental tours, and managed to find his way into places about which many people had never heard.

Allowing himself no more than six hours of sleep, he spent the time when he was not investigating filthy jails and foul, dark dungeons in writing up his observations. These he had the courage to publish, or to present directly to rulers responsible for the conditions in different nations. The whole story of the degradation of often forgotten human beings was laid before them, and many changes rewarded his courage and initiative. To Howard, whose primary interest was in prisons, there was some connection between the care of patients, as he had seen it there, and those institutions designed for disease segregation. He visited many hospitals incidentally, and wrote a book on "Hospitals and Lazarettos." His comments were to the point, his observation critical and not biased by his faith as a Calvinist. The work of the nuns in Catholic countries impressed him, and he spoke favorably of the Beguines and the Sisters of Charity.

Elizabeth Fry   Howard died in 1789 and about twenty-five years passed before the next chapter in the history of prison reform began to be written. Its author was an Englishwoman, *Elizabeth Gurney Fry* (1780–1845), a member of the Society of Friends, or Quakers. About 1811 *Stephen Grellet*, a young French-American among her friends, had begun a round of English prisons, his primary interest being military prisoners from France. Finally he came to London's Newgate, most celebrated of all. It had been destroyed by rioters a few years before, and rebuilt. The new exterior was beautiful, but also windowless. Conditions within the walls may be gathered from a description which the visitor wrote after seeing the women's quarters to which interest and curiosity had led him:

"They occupied two long rooms, where they slept in three tiers, some on the floor and two tiers of hammocks over one another. . . . When I first entered, the foulness of the air was almost insupportable; and everything that is base and depraved was so strongly depicted on the faces of the women who stood crowded before me with looks of effrontery, boldness and wantonness of expression that for a while my soul was greatly dismayed."[4]

When the same visitor saw the infirmary, he was moved to write:

"On going up, I was astonished beyond description at the mass of woe and misery I beheld. I found many very sick, lying on the bare floor or on some old straw, having very scanty covering over them, though it was quite cold; and there were several children born in the prison among them, almost naked."[5]

[4] Whitney, Janet: Elizabeth Fry. Boston, Little, Brown & Co., 1936, p. 193.

[5] *Ibid.*, p. 184.

It was to help the babies that he hastened to seek out his friend, Elizabeth Fry, a woman on whom he could rely for action. She bought flannel immediately, gathered together a group of women to help with the sewing, and next day took a bundle of clothing to the prison. The sights which met her were strange and harrowing to one who never before had entered this type of institution. She saw sick prisoners lying on filthy straw that could not be changed because no funds had been provided for this necessity, and they had no money of their own with which to buy it from their gaolers. Adults as well as children were in obvious need of clothing, and all were ill-nourished. All were in need of occupation and diversion.

The upshot was that a school for children was started in Newgate Prison. After that, Mrs. Fry contrived to organize instruction and find books and materials for the women themselves who wanted to read and to sew. Already interested in the monitor system which lately had been introduced into English schools, she tried the experiment. Dividing the women into groups, she allowed them to choose their own monitors, and the system worked. The amusing fact that prison authorities, when approached for a large room to be used for a workshop, offered the laundry, is in itself an explanation of prison hygiene in the early nineteenth century. What laundry was there to be done where people slept on the bare floor or on dirty straw, and wore their own clothes until they fell to pieces?

The laundry it was that Newgate cleaned and made ready for Elizabeth Fry's workroom. She started the women prisoners on the making of gay patchwork and layettes, wisely bringing both color and a ready interest into drab lives. Her next idea was that of producing goods which could be sold outside the prison. Income from sales would go to the worker. By 1840 there was a prison shop where the latter could purchase simple food and the tea dear to all England. By that time also, the financial depression had lifted, and returning family demands made inroads upon her time. Elizabeth Fry and her reform of one of the worst prisons in the world already had a fame that spread far beyond England, and influenced the steady, slow upward trend of circumstances bearing on the life of the prisoner. As opportunity permitted, she continued to be active in various types of social work until illness compelled her to stop.

Mrs. Fry was adding her share of stimulus to the movement

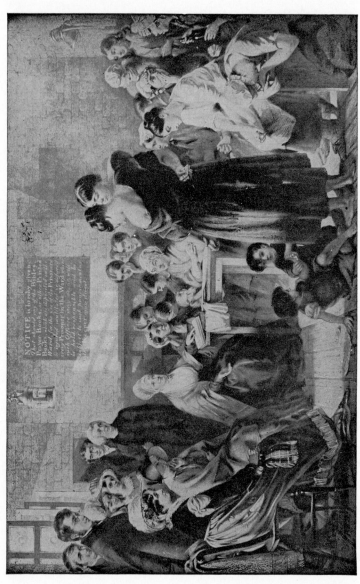

ELIZABETH FRY READING TO THE PRISONERS AT NEWGATE PRISON

(From "Elizabeth Fry, Quaker Heroine" by Janet Whitney. Little, Brown and Company, publishers.)

toward development of social consciousness. Her work, in reality, was but one side of a greater movement progressing throughout England. Distraction of war prevented a corresponding advance on the continent, but since Philippe Pinel and William Tuke had demonstrated the possibility of freeing insane persons from restraint, this idea had begun to filter through English "asylums," as mental hospitals were then called. Already, political influence was being invoked to hasten segregation of the mentally ill from the criminal.

REFORM IN CARE OF THE MENTALLY ILL

Dorothea Lynde Dix   The next great figure on the stage of social reform came on the scene in America. *Dorothea Lynde Dix* (1802–1887) had been born into the New World just in time to focus her much-needed activities on these two inescapable problems, care of the criminal and the mentally ill—problems which her country was then meeting with outworn Old World measures. Miss Dix was thirty-nine years of age when she began the work that earned for her the title, "The John Howard of America." For years before, she had run a private school in Massachusetts for children of the well-to-do, a responsibility to which her social spirit prompted her to add separate classes for the instruction of children of the poor. Overwork and the invasion of the popular public school finished this career and brought on a physical breakdown. Fortunately, she was able to arrange a sea trip which took her to Liverpool, England. The returning ship left behind an invalid who found refuge in a hotel. An influential American friend, however, had paved the way for her social reception by an influential resident of Liverpool, and *William Rathbone* sought her out.

We shall meet Mr. Rathbone later, as a philanthropist pioneering public health nursing, but now, for more than a year, he and his family undertook the care of Miss Dix. At their beautiful suburban home, she not only regained health but experienced keen pleasure in contact with friends of people whose interests spread over the field of social betterment. Industrial revolution had but lately embroiled Liverpool in its usual complications of crowding, poor housing, poverty, spells of unemployment, and disease. Miss Dix could lend both sympathy and interest to reformers, for she had seen much the same sort of thing in the mill towns of New England. She could give some help, too, for she was not unfamiliar with the Sunday schools and the missions organized to combat some of industry's evils. With broadening social outlook she listened to the experiences and the plans of humanitarians, among whom were those who pushed improvement in prisons and asylums.

Returning to America after a year and a half, Miss Dix found adjustment difficult. In her former busy life, her circle of friendships had been small in comparison with that which she had enjoyed in England. Health and circumstances forbade her to resume teaching as a vocation. An inheritance had relieved her of the necessity of earning a livelihood but, though new interests drew her toward social work, opportunity eluded her. She had small personal acquaintance with that considerable group of Americans who were unsatisfied with some of those social institutions established by their ancestors on a foundation of foreign tradition and pioneer necessity. People in New England especially, where industry and new facilities for travel were bringing wealth, leisure, and culture, were reading and writing and publicly declaiming as they planned and tried social experiments, or set balls rolling toward abolition of slavery, temperate drinking, better educational methods, better care of mothers.

The interest of Miss Dorothea Dix eventually attached itself to care of the mentally ill, and led to her determination to study the problem from a state-wide point of view. Beginning in Massachusetts, she was able, through systematic investigation and careful recording of observations, to prepare such a story as could be presented to a legislature and influence its action. On the whole, conditions had been found to be little better than those observed by Elizabeth Fry in England. Until 1839, when the Boston Lunatic Asylum was opened, the city kept its mentally ill in the almshouse, the jails, the House of Industry, and in the state hospital. Enlargement of the state hospital crowned this earliest work of Miss Dix with success. Thereupon she extended her work to other states, south, and as far west as the Mississippi, then into Canada.

The whole present system of mental hospitals under government control has gradually come into being as a result of twenty years of effort on the part of Miss Dix. Their foundation principles of expertness of supervision, legal commitment based on medical diagnosis, and abolition of restraint, were advocated by one who knew from observation and experience the value of such a basis. Success enabled her to carry this experience effectively into Britain and the countries of Europe. The title of "The John Howard of America" was a title hardly won, for travel conditions of the time were extremely uncomfortable.

PREVAILING NURSING METHODS EXPOSED

Charles Dickens   The social awakening which Vincent de Paul had stimulated two hundred years before, by changing beggars into skilled workers, interesting women in better nursing service, and calling attention to the need of the foundling, John Howard and Elizabeth Fry had hastened through their efforts to reform prisons, and Dorothea Dix by influencing legislatures to improve care for the mentally ill. *Charles Dickens* (1812–1870) added his weight to the movement by writing humorous, pointed descriptions of evils that he saw. Success enabled him to extend his public by offering cheap editions of his works, and his influence spread over two continents. A lecture tour of America brought the further opportunity of observing and depicting evils there.

Of the middle class himself, Dickens found in middle class manners and doings material for his satire. Always in touch with the very poor, industrialist group whose condition in his time kept them apart as a definitely lower class, his sympathy with their misery was deepened by an intimate, forced association with them in childhood. Dickens' father had been locked up in a debtors' prison, and there the entire family had resided until freed by a fortunate legacy. Few who read his descriptions in "David Copperfield" realize that they are the story of experience. England's indifference to housing and unsanitary conditions under which her slum dwellers were forced to live are never lost sight of by Dickens. The institutions which society kept up for them also are subject to analysis. In "Oliver Twist" he is occupied with the workhouse and its education of children in the ways of crime. The harm wrought by cheap schoolmasters and poor educational method he makes known through "Nicholas Nickleby"; the sad lot of the foundling finds its way to the reader's heart in "Cricket on the Hearth."

"Martin Chuzzlewit" is a study of selfishness, the outstanding vice of a period when social consciousness lay half dormant. In his study appear two characters of especial interest in our story of trends in nursing. *Betsy Prig* exemplifies the type of institutional nurse employed by the important London Hospital of St. Bartholomew. Her friend, *Sairey Gamp*, is the prevailing type to be found in private work. Both are tricking their employers, and trying to eke out a better living by accepting double responsibility. Mrs. Prig is a night "watcher" at the hospital. Mrs. Gamp accepts a day case while on night duty with the delirious patient whose care she shares with Mrs. Prig as day nurse. Before us is laid a picture of mismanagement in institutions otherwise displaying considerable efficiency, the helplessness of the sick public, the lack of education, good manners, and habits in nurses of the time. A conversation passing between the nurses as they change places in the evening is only one of many disclosures:

" 'I began to think you warn't a coming!' Mrs. Prig observed, in some displeasure.

" 'It shall be made good to-morrow night,' said Mrs. Gamp, 'honorable. I had to go and fetch my things.' She had begun to make signs of inquiry in reference to the position of the patient and his overhearing them—for there was a screen before the door—when Mrs. Prig settled that point easily.

" 'Oh!' she said aloud, 'he's quiet, but his wits is gone. It an't no matter wot you say.'

" 'Anythin' to tell afore you goes, my dear?' asked Mrs. Gamp, setting her bundle down inside the door, and looking affectionately at her partner.

" 'The pickled salmon,' Mrs. Prig replied, 'is quite delicious. I can partick'ler recommend it. Don't have nothink to say to the cold meat, for it tastes of the stable. The drinks is all good.'

"Mrs. Gamp expressed herself much gratified.

" 'The physic and them things is on the drawers and mankleshelf,' said Mrs. Prig, cursorily. 'He took his last slime draught at seven. The easy-chair an't soft enough. You'll want his piller.' "

And yet Dickens, assigning his ideal of a good nurse to a poor one so that the ridiculous may emphasize the contrast, makes this same Sairey Gamp exclaim:

"What a blessed thing it is to make sick people happy in their bed, and never mind one's self as long as one can do a service! I don't believe a finer cowcumber was ever growed. I am sure I never see one!"[6]

One of the author's contemporaries, *Leigh Hunt*, has given us his own version of the midwife specialist, which Sairey also professed

[6] Dickens, Charles: Martin Chuzzlewit. New York, Charles Scribner's Sons, 1911.

to be—a frequently recurring feature of the household in those days of large families. For variety it is quoted, but for the fact, too, that his final sentence betrays, as Dickens has already done, a public opinion itself turning in the direction of better nursing and appreciative of intelligence, education, and good breeding in nurses.

"Her greatest pleasure in life is, when lady and baby are both gone to sleep, the fire bright, the kettle boiling, and her corns quiescent. She then first takes a pinch of snuff, by way of pungent anticipation of bliss, or as a sort of concentrated essence of satisfaction; then a glass of spirits—then puts the water in the teapot—takes another glass of spirits (the last having been a small one, and the coming tea affording a 'counteraction')—then smoothes down her apron, adjusts herself in her arm-chair, pours out the first cup of tea, and sits for a minute or two staring at the fire, with the solid complacency of an owl—perhaps not without something of his snore, between sneeze and snuffbox."[7]

Hunt softens the whole picture, and gives hint also, of dawning public appreciation of what nursing might be, by adding:

"The Monthly Nurse as you ascend in society, is not seldom a highly respectable woman, who is nearly all that she should be—mild, firm, and well-meaning; and we have known instances—or rather we should say, as far as our personal knowledge is concerned, one rare instance—in which the requisite qualifications were completed, and the precious individual (for when can a mother's luck be greater?) was an intelligent gentlewoman! This is what the assistant-moulder of the first month of the existence of a human being ought always to be, and what she always would be, if the world itself were older, and the humblest and earliest form of education regarded as the important and sacred thing which it is."[8]

Leigh Hunt's was a dream already on the way to realization, for a Protestant pastor in a tiny German village on the Rhine was busy blazing the trail that would help the nursing situation in Protestant countries, as St. Vincent de Paul's Sisters of Charity had been changing it in Catholic countries.

ORDER OF MODERN DEACONESSES FOUNDED

In the early days of the nineteenth century, in Kaiserswerth, a little town near Düsseldorf, on the Rhine River in Germany, Theodor Fliedner, pastor of the local Lutheran church, and Friederike Fliedner, his bride, embarked on a project that gave to Protestants a model social substitute for the lost monastery, and incidentally

[7] Hunt, Leigh: Essays—The Monthly Nurse. London and New York, Frederick Warne & Co., 1889.

[8] *Ibid.*

changed the concept of nursing far beyond the borders of Germany. Behind the success that attended the Kaiserswerth Institution lay a long trail of attempts at organized nursing through Protestant sisterhoods, or through the restoration of the old church order of deaconesses. Much loyal service was given, as it always had been, by individual women.

Luther's plea for provision of means for education, charity, and nursing among his immediate followers had not been met satisfactorily, but some seeds of enterprise along these lines that had been sown through the past three centuries were pushing above ground. Professional men and laity were alive to the need for better and more widely distributed nursing. Manuals of nursing procedures were being written. The women of Germany had developed only recently a system of war relief and nursing of compelling adequacy. Hamburg had its *Amalie Sieveking* whose home-visiting association, "The Friends of the Poor" was attracting attention, and other cities were making attempts to give to attendants improved methods of hospital nursing.

Pastor Fliedner arrived at Kaiserswerth in 1821 to find himself head of a congregation that was learning the meaning of financial depression. The silk mills, which gave its members their daily bread, closed down a few weeks later. There was no chance of paying the new ministers salary. An offer of another church tempted him, but the young preacher, in his earnestness, wanted to be "a true shepherd, not an hireling." Faithful to an ideal in faithfulness to his flock, he set out to solicit abroad the funds which could not be found at home. These unfortunate sheep of his must not suffer for loss of Christian service that they needed now more than ever. He journeyed through Holland and England and got the money. More than this, he met a great many people of influence, among them Elizabeth Fry whose work in Newgate prison made a deep impression on him. He inspected public institutions, schools, almshouses, hospitals, and prisons, and in Holland he observed the work of deaconesses. As he re-entered little Kaiserswerth it was with great eagerness to bring prison reform into Germany, and deaconesses who would take hold of its problems of education, poor relief, and nursing. He and Friederike, both able organizers, entered upon a difficult path that led them to fame.

Pastor Fliedner looked after the church and parish duties, but every now and then had to fare forth on journeys that brought the necessary income. He succeeded in getting a German Prison Association started, but found responsibility for leadership in helping the prisoner left to himself. When he tried to interest women in prison work he met discouragement, for popular sentiment condemned the association of good women with degraded wrong-doers, and decreed that all decent women stay at home. One day a homeless girl, who was an ex-convict, came to beg shelter of the Fliedners. Gladly, but with some misgiving, they installed her in a little one-room house that stood in their garden. The attic above was her bedroom which she must reach by an outside ladder. *Minna* became a loyal friend, and the little house became a prisoner's refuge which grew and grew with its success in bringing about the better adjustment of criminals to society. This asylum, as it was called, was the first of numerous units that eventually went to form the institution thus informally introduced to Kaiserswerth and the world.

The next unit was a hospital, a responsibility assumed with two purposes in mind. One was the care of the sick, and the other was to provide a field for the instruction of deaconesses. By this time, his observations and friendships at home and abroad had acquainted Pastor Fliedner with the general lack of good nurses. The deaconess seemed to him and his wife to offer a solution for a widespread problem. Friederike's own experience as Kaiserswerth's first deaconess led her to believe that it was useless to try to revive the old-time order without due consideration of changed times and an altered outlook in young women. Both realized that it was an idea that cost money to put into effect. They realized, too, the limitations of a tiny town when it came to keeping a hospital filled with patients from whom deaconesses were to derive nursing experience.

Faith in a divine goodness that had given them means to carry on their work up to this time, supported this pious pair as they dared a promise to pay for the best house in town, which stood empty, inviting them to be its owners and make it a hospital. It was a faith that the outcome justified, for when the time to pay arrived, they were able to do it. Even before then, there was enough furniture in the house to begin work, and the first patient was admitted on October 16, 1836. The first probationer arrived shortly afterwards.

She was *Gertrud Reichardt*, a doctor's daughter who had helped her father with his patients. Notwithstanding her old friendship with the Fliedners and her resolve to become a deaconess, Gertrud found staying difficult. The hospital looked very bare after her comfortable home, and there seemed so little to work with that she was moved to doubt God's favor toward the whole undertaking. " 'No I cannot work here,' she said, 'God cannot be with you, or He would at least provide you with necessaries.' She was about to put on her cloak when the rumbling of a heavily laden wagon was heard, and a gruff voice called out: 'Does Pastor Fliedner live here?' As the driver unloaded the precious freight of hospital necessaries, Gertrud Reichardt was convinced that God was indeed with Theodor Fliedner."[9] Under the leadership of Friederike Fliedner, Gertrud Reichardt served ultimately for seventeen years. The first year of her training saw the advent of six other young women who aspired to become deaconesses, too.

The burden of organizing the work of the hospital, of selecting the right women to become deaconesses, of instructing them and assigning their work, all fell upon Mrs. Fliedner. How well fitted she was for the responsibility is clear from the systematic way in which she arranged things from the beginning. There were wards for men, women, and children, with a deaconess in each, and an orderly nursed the men under her direction. Housecleaning, cooking, washing, and the care of linen fell in turn on the deaconesses. The garden which supplied vegetable foods and fruits was theirs to care for, and one of them regularly spent her summer there.

An interested physician, with the help of a manual in use at the Charity Hospital in Berlin, gave clinical and theoretical instruction in the art of nursing. Students had opportunity, too, to study pharmacy, and took the state examination for pharmacists. All of this looks simple, perhaps, to us who live in a highly organized age, from childhood accustomed to routinized procedure, but to Friederike Fliedner it was pioneer work that grew so rapidly that it was hard to keep up with it, and that had to be accomplished with minimum funds. There were inescapable family duties besides. Nine babies of her own came to her so that her personal household was large in

[9] Gallison, Marie: The Ministry of Women: One Hundred Years of Women's Work at Kaiserswerth, 1836–1936 (a pamphlet). The Lutterworth Press, London.

spite of the fact that four of them died at birth. Nevertheless, her beloved hospital and school for deaconesses soon came to be known beyond Kaiserswerth and Germany, and Elizabeth Fry journeyed from England to see them. Her story brought Florence Nightingale, and there were many others interested in humanitarian and health problems who made similar pilgrimage. The policy of Kaiserswerth was one of generosity in sharing experience and achievement, and visitors were made welcome.

The work of the Kaiserswerth Deaconess Institution had features in common with the ancient xenodochium, the monastery, and the New World missions. It profited, no doubt, by the example of St. Vincent de Paul, whose Sisters of Charity had proved the superiority of their preparation for nursing during two hundred years in which they had earned a world's affection. Its prime purpose was to instruct women of such religious bent that they wished to be admitted to the ancient church office of deaconess and participate in its social service. The training of the deaconess was designed to fit her for *teaching or nursing*, but with these specialized vocations it combined the study of relief work among the poor, prison work, and rescue work. A simple vow was taken to work for the love of Christ and to follow Him in caring for the poor, the sick, or those in need of any help.

One of the most amazing things about Kaiserswerth in its early stages of growth is the amount of work accomplished under conditions close to poverty. Donations are never a reliable source of income, and times were hard, but "Father Fliedner's" faith was great, and sometimes its reward savored of the miraculous. A framework of organization was developed with passing years which proved worthy to become a model for deaconess institutions wherever they were established. About the original home of the pastor and his garden house there eventually clustered the following units offering facilities for the instruction of his deaconesses:

A hospital of one hundred and twenty beds
A "Lunatic Asylum" for female patients
An Infant School for forty children of all creeds
An Orphan Asylum for Protestant girls
A Day School for girls which was also attended by the orphans

A Normal School containing infant, elementary, and higher
grades for practice teaching in preparation of deaconesses for
school and governess work
An asylum for released female prisoners and "Magdalenes"

All deaconesses were assigned, in turn, to definite stations, and
teaching deaconesses were given a term of service in the care of sick
children. The field available for the practice of those deaconesses
who would devote themselves particularly to nursing is outlined in
an undated prospectus of the institution published, probably, in
1866, just two years after Pastor Fliedner's death. Condensing a
little, the list of stations shows them serving in separate wards for
men, women, and children, as well as in units for communicable disease, for convalescents, and for sick deaconesses. Additional stations
appear as follows:

Apothecary's Room
Office of Porteress
Office of Chapel Sister, "who has to keep the church and
churchyard in order, to prepare the corpses of women and
children for interment" and perform other duties.
Kitchen
Laundry
Sewing room, "where linen is sewn and mended and the gowns
and bonnets of the deaconesses are made"
Writing room, "where some sisters assist the superintendent in
her correspondence"
Garden, where vegetables and fruits are produced for the
household[10]

A further, momentary glance at the system regulating school organization and acceptance of students will make more obvious the
relationship existing between Kaiserswerth methods and those of the
specialized, secular school of nursing which later owed some inspiration to this source:

[10] Fliedner, Theodor: Some Account of the Deaconess Work. Property of
Public Library, Boston, Mass.

Three years' course

Eighteen years as minimum age for admission

Letters from clergyman and physician in certification of good character and health

Probationary period of three months to a year, for as time went on a preparatory school was organized to make up educational or other deficiencies

Allowance of pocket money (about twenty-five dollars a year)

Instruction by class and lecture

Rotation of practice in departments of hospital and institution

Division of students into junior, senior, and head sister groups

Uniform dress

Student deaconesses at Kaiserswerth came from no one group in society, and their days were passed under most democratic conditions. Princesses and peasants alike got up at five o'clock in the morning, and worked and studied side by side until nine o'clock at night. Night duty was covered by day nurses in turn. About once a week, instead of going off duty at nine o'clock, a day nurse would stay on until midnight. The night nurse who relieved her was one who had retired on leaving the wards at nine o'clock, and arose at midnight to begin a day that would end twenty-one hours later. The uniform dress is described as of dark blue material for work days, with plain black for Sundays. A bibbed apron, said to have been a blue one after the manner of the Sisters of Charity, but appearing to be white in pictures, was worn with the blue dress, while a white hood-like cap with ruffle about the face had broad ties for strings becomingly set in a perky bow under young chins, a picture further enhanced by a becoming white collar. A black bonnet in the fashion of the day, and likewise held fast by white strings, covered the head for street wear.

Both Pastor Fliedner and his wife instilled ethics into their pupils, and developed for them to follow, a semimilitary code of etiquette that facilitated harmonious relations in their growing group. Students were taught the necessity of loyal cooperation with the physician for the benefit of his patient. While thus avoiding one of the stumbling blocks that beset the Augustinian nuns of the Hôtel Dieu

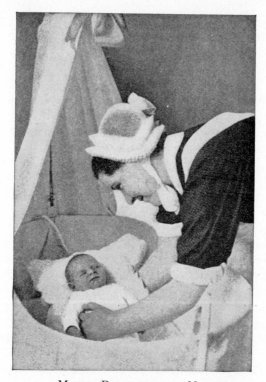

MODERN DEACONESS IN THE NURSERY

Kaiserswerth Deaconess Institution, Kaiserswerth, Germany. (From British Journal of Nursing, October, 1936.)

in Paris and other ecclesiastical nurses who found adjustment to new loyalties difficult in the confusion of church, civil, and professional authority, the Fliedners were not without mistakes. The placing of education in institutions dependent on voluntary subscription made the economics of its position hazardous. Necessity often induced the temptation to keep deaconess nurses on private cases in the home and thereby increase the institutional income. Long hours of work, and a rest period depending on conscience, were dangerous advantages to set before more commercial souls than those possessed by Theodor and Friederike Fliedner. The arrangement by which deaconesses must perform household duties, not only of their home but of the institution at large, could be only temporarily blessed. Sooner or later, the tradition of no paid help would become as firm as it was elsewhere in nursing institutions, and the loophole made for non-educational duties would show itself to be very elastic. Instruction and, often, health would become unfortunate sacrifices.

The *Motherhouse System*, however, did make up in some measure for abuses that were sure to come. It offered deaconesses a certain amount of security in providing for them a permanent home. They were children of Kaiserswerth, and from this home they were sent to district, hospital, and private duty assignment, and often to distant mission fields, but always they were under the direction, supervision, and protection of the Institution. Always, they knew that in Kaiserswerth there was a place for them when their work was over. Obviously, the motherhouse system was an offspring of the old monastic system. In Europe it is in use to this day, but the self-reliant American girl has been inclined to discount its values.

So honorable a reputation did the deaconess earn in society that Pastor Fliedner finally had to give up his pastorate, and give exclusive attention to establishing branch Deaconess Houses, to assignment of graduates to teaching, prison, or relief positions, and to the introduction of nursing staffs in hospitals. His work took on the proportions of a movement, and other pastors followed his lead by establishing schools, not all of which were as good as Kaiserswerth, Kaiserswerth deaconesses soon found themselves established at Jerusalem, Smyrna, Beyrouth, Constantinople, Alexandria, Cairo, Bucharest, and Budapest. In 1850 Father Fliedner took several of them to Pittsburgh in America, where, at the request of Pastor Passavant, they staffed his hospital, to be known as the "Passavant Hospital." About the same time a Deaconess Home and Hospital was founded at Milwaukee, young city in a great Middle West that straightway took the deaconess idea to its heart. When Father Fliedner passed away in 1864 there were nearly five hundred deaconesses scattered in small groups over four continents.

Friederike Fliedner, ambitious and energetic cofounder of Kaiserswerth, had died over twenty years before. To her the movement owed a primary stimulus, unmeasurable, perhaps, but unforgettable. She was one of those first women who insisted on emerging from the retirement into which medieval conditions forced women, and who dared to combine family with public duty. Her capacity in both fields is acknowledged. On her shoulders rested the main burden of devising those details of general management, of curriculum, and of student practice which were the basis of the Deaconess Institution's success.

After the death of Friederike, Pastor Fliedner had been blessed further in finding a worthy successor to sustain his family life and his deaconess project. *Caroline Bertheau*, former pupil of Amalie Sieveking, was in charge of the nursing at the Hamburg Hospital when Fliedner met her. She brought both experience and devotion to the Kaiserswerth institution. She was a good mother to Friederike's children, bore eight children of her own, and directed Kaiserswerth for twenty years after Pastor Fliedner died.

The deaconess movement came at a welcome time for women, many of whom were beginning to chafe at the dullness of home life, and a few of whom had been given, through education, a vision of activities in which custom as yet permitted them little opportunity to take part. A long series of wars had diminished the number of eligible husbands, while it increased the needs of poor people. The nunnery remained an outlet for religious zeal in a restricted group. The diaconate offered a corresponding opening for others. It was another great body inspired by religion and giving free service to God's poor. Its visiting nurse service, and its service in epidemic or disaster, took their place beside those of the Sisters of Charity. Its traditions were those established by Phoebe, first deaconess of the Christian church, and by those others who sustained these traditions, unnoticed, through the confusion of medieval times.

The diaconate helped to popularize women as executives in charge of nurses at a time when great hospitals were discovering their mistake in allowing this authority to pass into the hands of their new lay directors. It brought up the standard of nursing performance. Unfortunately, perhaps, it did not manage to avoid the pitfall of exploitation. Burdens of expensive domestic detail again fell on the willing shoulders of youthful zealots of the early nineteenth century. Deaconesses probably had a great deal to do with passing on the ever-recurring myth of floor scrubbing as an accepted feature in nurse education. Their Motherhouse was built around the family ideal, their times accepted domestic labor as woman's sphere, economy necessitated it in the deaconess establishment. No work done in the service of God and humanity lacked dignity.

While Protestantism took more than three hundred years after Luther's revolt to get around to accomplishing anything in connection with nursing, things happened rather quickly after that. One immediate result of the experiment at Kaiserswerth was the establishment in England of an Institute of Nursing Sisters. Here, in 1840, Elizabeth Fry undertook to interpret her appreciation of Pastor Fliedner's work by gathering together in this home a selected group of women. They were known as "*Protestant Nursing Sisters*," wore an attractive uniform, and did district and private nursing among the poor. The only training was a short term of experience in Guy's Hospital, London, but this, with their superior character, unexpectedly led to Sisters being carried off into the private duty field.

The strongest church influence in England at this time was the national, or established church, which deviated in considerably less degree from the old church than did the numerous sects grouped as "non-conformists." What followed was natural. A series of Sisterhoods under this English Church made their appearance, beginning with the Protestant *Order of Sisters of Mercy* in 1845. In 1848 there came into being the first Protestant Sisterhood with nursing as its major interest, and with an organized system of preparation for this vocation. It was the *Sisterhood of St. John's House*, the name being derived from its location in the district of St. John the Evangelist in London. *Sisters of St. John, first Protestant religious order devoting itself wholly to nursing, took a place beside the Augustinians, oldest nursing order of the Catholic Church.* Just as the latter had entered the hospital field through the Hôtel Dieu of Paris, so the nurses of St. John went into King's College Hospital in London. Before long they had supplied improved nursing staffs for a number of other English institutions. Wherever they took over a hospital service, however, the Sisters of St. John's House established the new precedent of reserving to the Sisterhood the right to control its nursing activities.

In 1851 the *Sisterhood of All Saints* was established and, in 1854, that of *St. Margaret*. Other communities followed these, and there was a nursing fraternity known as the *Cowley Brothers*. The main accomplishment during these years of English experiment which cast its reflections on America was the introduction of a minor group of more or less poorly prepared better-class women into district and private nursing.

Although they gave abundantly, and some of them still function, the new orders were not adequate to fill the public needs, and the public mind was divided on the question of religious motive as a requisite for good nursing. In the main, the orders themselves held nursing a secondary interest to spiritual self-development and missionary work. Ancient tradition set nursing aside as a service inspired by religion, and free. Acceptance of material coin in payment for the service changed its value, and lowered the public estimate of the nurse. Nursing must be both free and accompanied by self-sacrifice. In their district work, the Sisters of St. Margaret submerged self in all sorts of menial duties, and carried the scrubbing of floors into patients' homes. People like Mrs. Fry, who felt that good women might do good nursing in secular groups, and for remuneration, were "moderns."

Various proposals were forthcoming, and there were hints of plans for more substantial nurse training, but up to 1860 no great change was seen. Rich private patients and a limited group of the very poor reaped the advantage of any improvement made. England was not ready to use the principles of nurse preparation being demonstrated at Kaiserswerth. America made limited use of them, too, but continental Europe profited most, for here the deaconess throve side by side with the Beguines and the Sisters of Charity. Some of the filth of hospitals of this dark period was cleaned up. Some patients received better care but, in spite of all, the majority of institutions remained unchanged. At the same time, more and more influential people were learning to appreciate the personal advantage of culture in women who took care of them and their families during illness. The urgency of vocational education for these women was admitted slowly. In hospitals and outside of them, however, the ground was being broken and cultivated by women who used as tools whatever training they could get, and made ready for rich harvest when the seed of new ideas could be sown.

FLORENCE NIGHTINGALE: REFORMER OF HOSPITALS AND NURSING

EARLY LIFE

Florence Nightingale belonged to the layer of English society in which dwelt those business men who had grown well-to-do through development of the natural resources of their country, or through trade. Lead mining, marble works, groceries, in the capable hands of relatives had bestowed upon her parents, by inheritance, financial freedom and the privilege of collecting rents. In youth, both parents had been sheltered and subject to the best influences of their time. Their lives were set in a milieu of people who shared with them the pleasures of what is known as "good society," and who, like them, enjoyed the privilege of social excursions and friendships among the aristocracy. Politicians, literary men, artists, and some who merely played, were in their "set." Their religious affiliation, somewhat unique among many daring sectarian choices of the time, was Unitarian. Florence's mother, described as beautiful, appears to have been a woman of conservative tastes, thoroughly Victorian in her outlook, the daughter of a member of Parliament whose hobby had been collecting pictures. Her father had more elasticity in his nature, and took gentle pleasure in literature and art. He was a college graduate, knew mathematics, was a master of foreign languages, and read in the classics, natural science, history and philosophy.

Travel at that time was difficult in comparison with travel today, but Mr. Nightingale was interested enough in it to overlook difficulties, and took advantage of his opportunity to make use of any comforts available. It was in Italy that his two daughters were born, Parthenope in Naples, and Florence, on May 12, 1820, in the city from which she received her name. It was a name which the fame of this distinguished owner made popular for girl babies of generations who followed this little Florence of the Nightingales. When the family returned to England, a comfortable new home was built at Embley Park, not far from Romsey. Here "Parthe" and "Flo" spent happy months of every year amid the trees and flowers and birds of a southern English garden.

The monotony of country life was varied by an annual carriage drive to London, and another to a northern home called "Lea

Hurst," situated in Derbyshire, near the Derwent River and the lead mines of a chill area, the barrenness of which industry had made more forbidding. Long visits were made in both places, and governesses became part of the household that Parthenope and Florence might not go unschooled. Mr. Nightingale himself took particular pleasure in teaching Latin and Greek to Florence, with mathematics, science and languages, and in educating her to enjoyment of his books. Good friends that they became, these two read and talked, and, when separated in after years, carried on lengthy correspondence. Mrs. Nightingale leaned toward the older and less original sister, content to have a beautiful voice and a grace of walk and manner her chief gifts, in preference to Florence whom she found it somewhat hard to understand.

At seventeen, Miss Nightingale, the young lady, was given another stay in continental Europe, a finish to her education. This time the family traveled for a year and a half in France, Italy, and Switzerland, enjoying scenery, art, and society. It was on this trip that Florence was introduced to one of the great salons where she met some of the most distinguished men of France and, incidentally, learned some of the social methods of distinguished Frenchwomen. It was a time when the talk of liberty and war for liberty was stirring Italy as it had shortly before stirred France. She was interested in politics and people, but charitable institutions strangely intrigued her, and everywhere she tried to acquaint herself with social conditions, for the conviction had come to her that some day God would appoint her to fulfill a mission of mercy for Him. She must be ready when the time came. Years after she explained this as she wrote:

"Thoughts and feelings that I have now I can remember since I was six years old. It was not I that made them. A profession, a trade, a necessary occupation, something to fill and employ all my faculties, I have always felt essential to me, I have always longed for, consciously or not. . . . The first thought I can remember and the last, was nursing work; and in the absence of this, education work, but more the education of the bad than of the young. But for this I had had no education myself."[11]

Meantime, Miss Nightingale went on doing what she could toward self-education, and she was always especially happy when helping someone. At home, she found opportunity in the industrial village

[11] Cooke, Sir Edward: A Short Life of Florence Nightingale, 1925, p. 40. By permission of The Macmillan Company, publishers.

beyond the trees of Lea Hurst for observing at close range the life of the poor, and doing something toward relief of the sick.

"One sees in every cottage some trouble that defies sympathy."

"All that poets sing of the glories of this world appears to me untrue; all the people I see are eaten up with care or poverty or disease."

"To find out what we can do, one's individual place, as well as the general end, is Man's task."[12]

For this end of discovering her vocation, if for no other, the experience had value for Florence Nightingale.

Diary writing, a current fashion in which men as well as women indulged, was not an altogether satisfactory outlet for this young dreamer, but it helped her to come to a decision as to the kind of work she would choose to do if choice were before her. As she wrote up her daily doings, she was reminded of unsatisfactory nursing conditions in hospitals and of a need for Sisters in England like the Sisters of Charity of St. Vincent de Paul. Nursing would be just the work she would like best to do. She would be a nurse. To her orthodox mother, useful occupation was not an impossible thing for a daughter of hers, but the acquisition of a husband was of first importance. A married woman, under protection of a husband and his name, could do things that Victorian ideas of propriety did not permit an unmarried woman to do. An Elizabeth Gurney Fry might visit those terrible people in Newgate, but an Elizabeth Gurney! No, certainly not! Mrs. Nightingale could not picture her daughter in company with drunken immoral nurses, tending the unwholesome bodies of sick people in a great prison-like, smelly hospital. She, too, had heard people talk about hospitals and nurses. She would try to make Florence forget a foolish, youthful notion.

In her own home, however, Florence was meeting people whose interests lay in many kinds of social work and reform—women and men who were free to carry on prison work, educational reform and workhouse reform. Among them was a leading physician of the town of Salisbury in the neighboring shire. She thought it would be nice to go to the hospital in that town to learn nursing by doing it, and pick up what knowledge she might by observing what those women did who earned a living by this means. The big drawing

[12] *Ibid.*, pp. 12, 14, 15. By permission of The Macmillan Company, publishers.

room at home, she said, made her wonder how it could be made over into a hospital ward. She knew friends who were doing things away off in America, too. When Julia Ward Howe and Dr. Howe visited her home, she asked him if it would be a very terrible thing to devote her life to nursing. Indeed, it was not long before all sympathetic listeners came to know that young Florence Nightingale wanted to be a nurse, and that she was restrained from this thoroughly useful occupation only by parental unwillingness.

Accepting the parental dictum as best she could, Miss Nightingale turned to the study of the new sanitation that her friend, *Sir Edwin Chadwick*, was succeeding in bringing before the public. Friends abroad sent her what they could in the way of information regarding the Fliedner undertaking of which she had heard from Mrs. Fry. She continued to cherish her dream of becoming a nurse, and, perhaps, of forming some day a Sisterhood of educated women who also would be proficient nurses. In 1847 came an opportunity to visit the continent again, and in Rome she turned from the study of art to the study of a community of nuns. The sister Superior found kinship in the attractive stranger, and permitted her to stay in the convent during ten days of retreat. Miss Nightingale was privileged to listen to the addresses that she gave to nuns and novices, and to study their mode of life. Systematic person that she was, she wrote notes of her observations for use when the longed-for opportunity to improve the nurses and the nursing of England should be hers. In Rome, too, she had the pleasure of running across Mrs. Herbert and Sir Sidney Herbert, the man in whose hands fate, unknown to all of them, was preparing to place the key to this opportunity. Just now she and the Herberts could share particular interests, for they told her of their intention to start a hospital when they got home to England. The plans for it were discussed, and she was invited to visit it.

Other opportunities for gaining social understanding came to this girl who wanted to study nursing, and could find no way of going to a school for nurses, but inevitably she ran into the ever-recurring question of marriage. Indeed, one among the admirers proved so attractive that Florence found it hard to refuse him, and only after considerable deliberation made a decision disappointing to him, and equally so to a mother who wanted to see her daughter "settled."

The old desire to work with such a soul-filling motive as inspired some about her stood in the way. Florence Nightingale was one of those "new" women of the nineteenth century, and she wanted a career.

"I could be satisfied to spend a life with him combining our different powers in some great object. . . . Voluntarily to put it out of my power ever to be able to seize the chance of forming for myself a true and rich life would seem to me like suicide."[13]

Marriage without full community of interest looked impossible. She had only sorrow for the social-minded woman whom marriage thrusts into a little routine, and compels to live apart from the larger life of the husband to whom her affairs were trivial.

"Such a woman," she writes later when she had seen more of life, "longs for a profession . . . struggles to open to woman the paths of the school, the hospital, the penitentiary, the care of the young sick, the bad,—not as an amusement, to fill up odd times, to fancy they have done something when they have done nothing, to make a sham of visiting—but systematically, as a reality, an occupation, a 'profession.' . . . Without the right cultivation and employment of all the powers . . . there can be no repose, and with it repose may be found in a hell, in a hospital of wounds and pain and operations and death and remorse and tears and despair."[14]

Two years after the visit to Rome, Miss Nightingale accompanied friends to Egypt. On the way home, she was to have a long-promised visit to Theodor Fliedner and Friederike, his wife, the two persons who seemed to have realized an ideal that eluded her. Meantime, the city of Alexandria gave opportunity to learn intimately the work of the Sisters of Charity of St. Vincent de Paul. In Greece she met American missionaries and studied the school and orphanage which they were running. In Berlin she made the rounds of hospitals, and finally Kaiserswerth, her Mecca, was reached. For a happy two weeks in August, 1850, she observed what had been done, and heard of the Fliedner plans and hopes. Then, more than ever impressed with the need of systematic training for that life-work toward which she groped, she returned home.

[13] Cooke, Sir Edward: A Short Life of Florence Nightingale, 1925, p. 34. By permission of The Macmillan Company, publishers.
[14] *Ibid.*

Not long afterwards, opportunity came. In 1851, her sister was advised to go to Carlsbad Mineral Springs for her health. The resort was in Germany, and while her mother and Parthenope remained there, it was decided that the time was opportune for Florence to go into residence at Kaiserswerth. The visit was to be kept from the knowledge of friends, but the Sidney Herberts knew of it, and came to see her and the institution. Three months spent at this time with the founders of the Deaconess Institution made a lasting impression, and gave Miss Nightingale valued material to use in the foundation of a profession that seemed always so remote.

After that, Miss Nightingale of Embley Park and Lea Hurst again sought satisfaction for the emptiness of life, in writing. She was thirty-three before her mother, at last convinced of her determination to follow a "career," sent her abroad once more, this time to study the work of the Sisters of Charity in Paris. At the last moment the opportunity almost slipped away from her. Her father tried to keep her at home by offering her a little house to convert into an institution. Her mother could not refrain from objecting. A sick relative needed her. In the end, however, she found herself installed in Paris with a public permit authorizing her to look over its hospitals, infirmaries, and religious houses.

FIRST POSITION

Every possible bit of printed information about methods of hospital management and nursing were meticulously written up. There were interruptions. Miss Nightingale got the measles while with the Sisters of Charity. She had to go home for a while to nurse her grandmother in a fatal illness. Undaunted, she returned to the task to which she had set herself. Persistence and ambition, at last, were rewarded by news of a vacancy in the position of superintendent of a small institution at 1 Upper Harley Street in London, which offered shelter to homeless ladies, and nursing care to sick governesses.

It is interesting to follow Miss Nightingale through the now everyday excitements of making formal application for a position, and appearing before the Board of Managers for personal interview. She knew her own mind, and succeeded in arranging for her share of authority without interference, as well as for conveniences like bells, hot water, and such an innovation as an elevator. The Board, in turn, would not act without assurance that her parents did not object. Finally all was settled, and Florence at the age of thirty-four entered upon the professional career for which she had been preparing herself since she was seventeen. Everything went satisfactorily and her ability was acknowledged. Her desire to organize a training school for nurses had to be curbed in deference to the ruling of a Board that could not understand it. Energy and imagination, however, led her to incorporate a degree of social work into her duties. Besides nursing her governesses, she characteristically undertook to find convalescent homes or jobs for them when they left her, or through her friend, Sir Sidney Herbert, to locate them in America through a placement society of his sponsoring.

CRIMEAN WAR SERVICE

Friends thought the position at Harley Street not quite worthy of her talents, and one of them tried to have her appointed superintendent of nursing at King's College Hospital. A vacation at home was interrupted by a cholera scare in London, and a hurried return to the city was followed by some emergency nursing work in Middlesex Hospital. She was soon back with the governesses, but not for long. Little more than a month later, newspapers were full of complaints of neglect of English soldiers wounded in a war on the Crimean peninsula in the Black Sea where England and France were assisting Turkey in a war against Russia. Sisters of Charity were there nursing France's soldiers, and Sisters of Mercy were nursing those of Russia. "Why have we no Sisters of Charity?" somebody asked in the London Times. On the same day, Mr. and Mrs. Nightingale once more found themselves called upon to give parental sanction, and their daughter was writing to her friend Mrs. Herbert to tell her that she thought of accepting the charge of a privately financed expedition of four nurses as an immediate answer to a public need. This plan was changed on receipt of a letter from Sir Sidney Herbert who was on vacation, and, strangely enough, had written Miss Nightingale to ask if she would consider going to the Crimea under appointment by the government. The young woman who one day was to write, "The Lord helps those who keep moving," was learning this truth. She had never stopped even when it seemed that her life must be passed in still places. Always learning, always going ahead, she was ready for a great opportunity.

In his position of Secretary at War, Sir Sidney knew the situation thoroughly, and understood the reluctance of army officials to introduce women to the service. He knew, too, that personality, knowledge, administrative capacity, and social prestige combined to make Miss Nightingale the "one person that I know of in England who would be capable of organizing and superintending such a scheme."[15] Five days later, official orders were put through, and Florence Nightingale began the work of preparation "as calm and composed in this furious haste as if she were going for a walk."[16]

It was with great difficulty that suitable nurses were found, but at last there was a unit numbering thirty-eight in all, ten Roman Catholic Sisters with eight Sisters of Mercy and six Sisters of St. John's House, both orders of the English church, and fourteen practical nurses from hospital staffs. The government put them under her control, as Superintendent of the Nursing Staff, or, as she came to be called, "Lady-in-Chief." On October 21, 1854, one week after she had written her letter to Mrs. Herbert, Miss Nightingale and the nurse corps were on their way. From London, they traveled to the coast, crossed the English Channel to Boulogne, thence to Paris, and on to Marseilles on the Mediterranean. There they boarded ship for Scutari, suburb of Constantinople and site of a hospital base opposite that city on the Straits of Bosphorus. From the Crimean Peninsula on the other side of the Black Sea were coming the wounded, crowded into unsanitary ships, and without anything that could be called nursing care. Back in England, Florence Nightingale, still a stranger to them, was already famous as the leader of a brave rescue. Public opinion was behind her, and soon the government as well.

On November 4, 1854, England's new nurses landed at Scutari, and found, not one, but two hospitals filled and awaiting them. Ten members of the unit were assigned to the General Hospital, and the remainder quartered at the Barrack Hospital, a half-hour's walk distant. This had been a soldiers' barracks, and still was only partially adapted to housing of wounded men. A three-story building in the

---

[15] Cooke, Sir Edward: A Short Life of Florence Nightingale, 1925, p. 74. By permission of The Macmillan Company, New York, publishers.
[16] Ibid., p. 79.

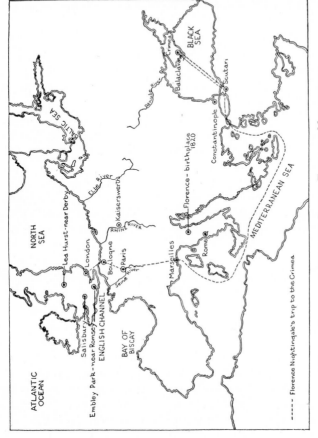

PLACES ASSOCIATED WITH THE LIFE OF FLORENCE NIGHTINGALE

form of a square, it had wards opening off corridors, the total length of which was four miles. A tower arose from each corner, and the rooms in one of these towers became the nurses' quarters. In the cold hospital wards were nearly eighteen hundred patients, bed-bug-ridden and lice-infested. Sanitary arrangements had proved themselves inadequate. Ventilation was poor. Rats and mice ran free. Candles in bottles supplied illumination. Overflow patients lay on the floors, and all lacked adequate covering. Dysentery from a poor water supply and fever added their complications. Food was so poor that the men could not eat it, and, besides, there were neither knives nor forks. "Not a basin, nor a towel, not a bit of soap nor a broom could be found."[17]

No time was to be lost, for more wounded were even then being landed. What could be done toward feeding the sick in the wards and replacing dirty clothing was the first move. Miss Nightingale secured brushes and cloths, and her group went to work at cleaning up. When they had done what they could, she realized that a healthful hospital was still an impossibility unless water supply and sewer system were changed. These were things that must be reported to the government. An inadequate laundry service which broke down completely, she remedied herself by renting a house in Scutari, having boilers installed, and paying soldiers' wives to do the washing. In the already crowded quarters of the nurses, in a central room on the first floor off which their bedrooms opened, space was made for a combined diet kitchen and storeroom, and a smaller room was used for an office.

In the three diet kitchens eventually opened, the nurses cooked tempting, nourishing foods for the very sick. From the same storeroom which provided stoves and some of the food came other supplies which Miss Nightingale had had the foresight to bring with her, and which were issued on requisition signed by a medical officer. These supplemented army deficiencies, or offset unbreakable "red tape." In a letter to Mrs. Herbert, Miss Nightingale described herself as a "kind of general dealer in socks, shirts, knives and forks, wooden spoons, tin baths, tables and forms, cabbages and carrots, operating tables, towels, soap, fine tooth combs, precipitate for destroying lice, scissors, bedpans and stump pillows."[18] In the first three months, ten thousand shirts alone were given out. In order to provide necessary beds for eight hundred new patients, she even found it necessary to remodel unused wards at her own expense, so as to have them ready in time for their occupants. The money thus spent was later refunded by Parliament.

The office became the seat of business and conference, and, often

[17] Cooke, Sir Edward: A Short Life of Florence Nightingale, 1925, p. 96. By permission of The Macmillan Company, New York, publishers.

[18] Official History of American Red Cross Nursing, 1922, p. 3. By permission of The Macmillan Company, New York, publishers.

long after midnight, of a huge and personal correspondence that must be done all by hand. Social prestige made possible a direct confidential relationship between Miss Nightingale and people of political power. In other words, she had that useful possession now known as "pull." Comprehensive reports of sanitary conditions written here aroused such concern among authorities in England that experts were sent to investigate. Changes made according to her suggestion, together with nursing care and dietary treatment, brought dramatic proof of the authenticity of Miss Nightingale's observation and knowledge through a drop in death rate from about 40 to 2 per cent. Graphic descriptions of surroundings and nursing brought large sums of money from individuals and groups who were eager to help. After the war was over her expenditures were systematically embodied in a published report to subscribers. The following description of her personality was written while she was thus earning the gratitude of a people and the approbation of a Queen:

"In appearance, Miss Nightingale is just what you would expect in any other well-bred woman, who may have seen perhaps rather more than thirty years of life; her manner and countenance are prepossessing, and this without the possession of positive beauty; it is a face not easily forgotten, pleasing in its smile, with an eye betokening great self-possession, and giving, when she wishes, a quiet look of firm determination to every feature. Her general demeanour is quiet and rather reserved; still I am much mistaken if she is not gifted with a very lively sense of the ridiculous. In conversation, she speaks on matters of business with a grave earnestness one would not expect from her appearance. She has evidently a mind disciplined to restrain under the principles of the action of the moment every feeling which would interfere with it. She has trained herself to command, and learned the value of conciliation towards others and constraint over herself. I can conceive her to be a strict disciplinarian; she throws herself into a work as its head. As such she knows well how much success must depend upon literal obedience to her every order. . . . Miss Nightingale . . . in my opinion, is the one individual who in this whole unhappy war has shown more than any other what real energy guided by good sense can do to meet the calls of sudden emergency."[19]

Power, admiration, and respect gradually came to the young nurse who had longed for opportunity, but they were not won without opposition. There were medical officers and others who, mistaking her eager aggressiveness, looked upon her as a nuisance. There were those who went so far as to work against her, and there were patients who never knew the benefits of the care which her sister nurses

[19] Cooke, Sir Edward: A Short Life of Florence Nightingale, 1925, p. 134. By permission of The Macmillan Company, New York, publishers.

offered but could give only when the doctor did not object. The hard-earned prestige was also threatened by bungling at home. Miss Nightingale had asked for more nurses, stipulating that they be given preliminary training in London hospitals. A group of forty-six women arrived, but they were under a new and untrained head, and knew almost nothing about nursing themselves. Their orders, more-over, assigned them, not to Miss Nightingale, but to the military officer in command. The complications resulting almost ended in her resignation, but ultimately were straightened out and the young women distributed.

Other groups of nurses followed, and lady volunteers with neither training nor experience beyond home nursing. The number of women working under Florence Nightingale's direction gradually came to be one hundred and twenty-five. Some returned home of their own accord, or were sent back for misdemeanor or incompetence. Some became too ill to continue in the service, and nine died.

Two hospitals located at the front in the Crimea were staffed with nurses and equipped with diet kitchens like the three already men-tioned in Scutari. Miss Nightingale crossed the Black Sea to take charge of the nursing in these hospitals at Balaclava. On horseback or in a carriage given her by the army, she covered the distances between them, ignoring darkness and loneliness, danger, storm, cold, and weariness. By special permission she went on the battlefield itself. It was in the midst of this strenuous work that she contracted Crimean fever. Always indifferent to contagion, it had caught up with her finally, and now it brought her very close to death. After her recovery, part of her time was spent at Scutari and part at Balaclava.

Army nursing under Florence Nightingale gradually expanded into a health service, working hand in hand with the new sanitary science. How she made up for poor functioning of the army stores department has been told. Drunkenness among the soldiery was lessened by setting up reading rooms, providing amusements and lectures, and establishing a canteen. She eased minds of sick men by writing letters for them, starting the allotment of their pay to needy families at home, and providing employment and care for those wives who accompanied their husbands to the scene of war. Always, it was her custom to make rounds in the wards at night, stopping to

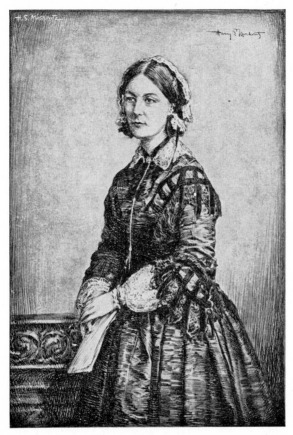

FLORENCE NIGHTINGALE

observe the condition of the sickest patients. She was lighted along her way by a lantern or the oil lamp famous in the army before Henry Wadsworth Longfellow endowed with immortality "Santa Filomena," the Lady of the Lamp.

While the soldiers of England were thus benefiting under the supervision and care of Florence Nightingale and her nurses, in the hospitals of their enemy, sick and wounded men were finding corresponding help and encouragement through the efforts of one of their countrywomen. The *Grand Duchess Pavlova*, having secured the enlistment of three hundred ladies of Moscow and St. Petersburg who were willing to give assistance, used them to staff Russian army hospitals of the Crimea. So much did she accomplish and so great was the appreciation of her group, known as "Sisters of Mercy," that it was said of them, "She provided them with everything necessary and these saintly women were blessed by thousands of soldiers."[20]

Professionally, some of the English nursing group proved to be excellent nurses, some were very poor, and some gave a lot of trouble. As the army had not heretofore made the acquaintance of women nurses, they had no defined position in its organization, and a defined position is a sacred thing to military men. With little help from tradition, in any given situation, a method of discipline suitable to the circumstances of army life had to be worked out and established. Even under the advantage of accepted power of control, this was not easy among women of varying social status, varying education, varying religion, in times when people were highly conscious of class and sectarian barriers, and anxious to maintain them.

It was Florence Nightingale's first real job of nursing supervision, for the Harley Street institution had been small, and visiting hospitals to see how others interpreted nursing was different from personally shouldering responsibility for every act of individuals in a large, mixed group. Her own broad views prevented discrimination between sect or church. She asked only that they work together in "a common brotherhood of love to God and man."[21] No one knew better than she came to know what she owed to those women who stood by her loyally, adapting themselves to new and difficult circumstances, and giving the best that was in them to their patients and hers. She learned to have an intense pride in their accomplishment, and understood how much she gained from them of expertness in distinguishing good from bad in nurses and nursing. Any shortcomings they might have betrayed had served only to make her more alive to the need of education for all nurses.

[20] From The Origin of the Red Cross ("Un Souvenir de Solferino") by Henri Dunant, translated from the French by Mrs. David H. Wright. The John C. Winston Co., 1911, pp. 80–81.

[21] Cooke, Sir Edward: A Short Life of Florence Nightingale, 1925, p. 80. By permission of The Macmillan Company, New York, publishers.

INSCRIPTION . . . *"Of the vast throng passing from the mystery of birth to the mystery of death, certain ones so live that their deeds become impressed upon the memory of the race. Among these we name Florence Nightingale, whose life has been, is today and will ever continue to be, a mighty influence against man's cruelty to man. To her memory, this statue, symbolizing the protection of the flame of life is dedicated, and to all those following in her footsteps in the care of the sick."*

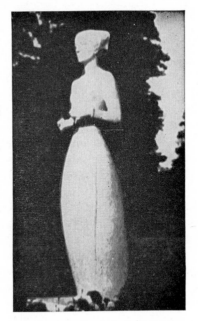

STATUE OF FLORENCE NIGHTINGALE IN LINCOLN PARK, LOS ANGELES

(David Edstrom, sculptor, Pacific Coast Journal of Nursing, July, 1940.)

Army Dress In her dress while in army service, Miss Nightingale favored practical but sombre shades. It was customarily of gray or black, with the then fashionable simple white cap over her dark hair. A black handkerchief was sometimes tied over the cap. Often she added a rough apron which, perhaps, may be taken as symbolic of her intensely practical outlook, for this leader in nursing was a doer who knew nursing and who let slip no detail in the care of the sick. A heavy cloak and bonnet were worn outdoors in this country where the winters brought storms of snow. The dress of her nurses was of corresponding sobriety. They wore dresses of gray tweed, wool jackets, and caps so unbecoming that at least one nurse declared she would never have come had she known about the head gear. A brownish linen scarf embroidered in red with the same "Scutari Hospital" was worn as a protection in going about an eastern port town. Short woolen capes completed the outfit.

The time finally drew near for the group to break up, to discard those conventions of army life so hardly learned, and readjust to civil life. They were tired out, just as was Miss Nightingale, and this readjustment would be hard. Some among them would be fortunate in having a convent enfold them in its sheltering peace, others would go back to luxurious homes, but there were those also who must go back to work. While they were still in service, London too was thinking of the nurses, and considering the matter of employment for the professional among them. Miss Nightingale gave her assistance by sending careful and detailed reports of all.

In March, 1856, the war was over. The nurses, gradually detached from service, sailed off on different transports. It was August before the hospitals were evacuated and Santa Filomena herself could take ship for England. Before leaving Scutari, she visited the cemetery where lay so many who might have been saved had men known more about what army medical service, army hygiene and sanitation, and army nursing might be. "While I live, I fight their cause," she pledged herself. It was a dedication ultimately to fill the days of her life, but just then she was so exhausted with excitement and responsibility, with work and illness that she must reach the quiet of home as speedily as possible.

POST-WAR ACTIVITIES

All England was waiting to do her honor when the ship that would bring her back should reach port, but the people's heroine slipped in unknown to them. Avoiding their band play and all the other well-meant publicity, her first thought was to see about sending off to Lea Hurst a collection of those mascots dear to all soldiers for what they have meant in making possible affection where hate abounds, familiar, gentle contact amid the harshness of the army mechanism, and humaneness amid the strange, overwhelming inhumanities of war. The Nightingale family was called upon to make room for a one-legged sailor boy named "William," a little Russian orphan picked up on a battlefield, and a black pup called "Rousch" given her by the soldiers. Alone, the beloved Florence followed after, and no one met her at the little country railway station because, again, no one knew when she would come. She walked home, seeking peace now behind those tall trees that had once seemed a barrier between her and the longed-for work of a busy, unhappy world that she had wanted to help.

Miss Nightingale, however, soon found that she could not rest by doing nothing. She had never been content in idleness, and in spite of periods of exhaustion, physical and mental, knew that she must get back to work while public interest was warm. People would forget this war as they had forgotten others. Ideas had come to her that must be carried out if there was to be any permanent improvement in army medical service. The mail in far-off Scutari had borne two letters that seemed keys to opportunity. One of these was from Queen Victoria who had expressed a desire to meet her on her return. With it had come the badge of honor that she had worn at Christmas dinner in the British Embassy at Scutari. This decoration carried the Cross of St. George, England's royal emblem, done in red enamel, with the name "Crimea" and the Royal monogram surmounted by a crown of diamonds. Surrounding all stood out the words "Blessed are the merciful," and on the back was inscribed: "To Miss Florence Nightingale, as a mark of esteem and gratitude for her devotion to the Queen's brave soldiers. From Victoria R. 1855." She must make haste to have that royal audience brought about, for royal cooperation, if it could be won, would help to push the reform of army hospitals.

Nightingale Fund   The other letter had come from her old friend, Sir Sidney Herbert, thrilled to tell her of a great public meeting held in London on November 20, 1855. The purpose of this meeting had been to find some way of expressing the gratitude of the British people for the unselfish service that she had given. Important men and women had taken part, and, unanimously, a resolution had been passed to raise a "Nightingale Fund" that she could use to make that old dream of hers come true by establishing a school in which a superior group of women might be taught the art of nursing and go thence to teach it to all the world. This answer to her years of longing meant a great deal to Miss Nightingale, but she knew that fulfillment must wait until she had done what she could toward improving the health protection of the army. What had been accomplished in the Crimea was only a passing good unless governmental measures ensured permanent changes in the medical service.

Army Sanitation   Florence Nightingale must keep that vow given in the soldiers' cemetery at Scutari, and to do this she would have to fight to bring influential men and conservative military officials to see why things should be different.

"No one can feel for the Army as I do. These people who talk to us have all fed their children on the fat of the land and dressed them in velvet and silk while we have been away. I have had to see my children dressed in a dirty blanket, and an old pair of regimental trousers, and to see them fed on raw salt meat; and nine thousand of my children are lying, from causes which might have been prevented, in their forgotten graves. But I can never forget. People must have seen that long, dreadful winter to know what it was."

"In the Sebastopol trenches, these men would refuse to report themselves sick lest they should throw more labour on their comrades. They would draw their blankets over their heads and die without a word. . . . But surely the blood of such men is calling to us from the ground, not to avenge them, but to have mercy upon their survivors. . . . It remains for us to strive that their sufferings may not have been endured in vain—to endeavour so to learn from experience as to lessen such sufferings in future by forethought and wise management."[22]

It was, therefore, to the work of improving health conditions in the army that Miss Nightingale now gave herself. She rooted out statistics that showed the death rate among England's soldiers *in times of peace* to be double that among her civilians. This, as she pointed out, was obviously unnecessary in face of advances made in sanitation. In the light of such knowledge, it was criminal. No other group of men was "so dependent upon their employers for health, life, and morality as the army." Sympathizers gathered about her, a meeting was held at the home of the Royal Physician, and it was made possible for her to present her views to the Queen. She was requested to write her experiences and her suggestions for reform that they might be brought before the government; for direct parliamentary contact, like the suffrage, was not permitted to women of her day.

Political obstacles began to turn up in Miss Nightingale's path, but in six months she was ready with "Notes on the British Army." In 1857 the notes were printed at her expense, and privately circulated. Their appearance marked a turning point in the history of military medicine. From this time curative measures became second-

[22] From Cooke, Sir Edward: A Short Life of Florence Nightingale, 1925, pp. 171–172. By permission of The Macmillan Company, New York, publishers.

ary in importance to preventive measures. Reforms were outlined to make health possible, and such innovations suggested as sanitary officers, reorganization of medical and supply services, a Department of Statistics, and a Social Service through education, recreation, allotment of pay, and trade training in organized workshops. Even her enemies recognized the clarity of her thinking and the value of her contribution. She was requested to supplement this report with another on what she considered feasible in the way of army nursing by women. "Subsidiary Notes as to the Introduction of Female Nursing into Military Hospitals in Peace and War" was her answer.

A considerable portion of the next sixteen years was spent in behalf of the army. Miss Nightingale moved to London, found time and strength to extend her acquaintance with experts, and, for a time, resumed her habit of hospital visiting. Many of her suggestions went into the building of a model military hospital, and other military hospitals and barracks were remodeled to provide what they had not had—good water, ventilation, light, and heat. Their dietary and sanitary facilities were revolutionized. All of the practical experience and the knowledge that she had been collecting through the years was put to use, for constant search, a good memory and careful recording had helped to turn them into wisdom.

Hospital and Nursing Reform   In spite of ill health resulting from army experiences, Miss Nightingale also extended her exertions to include reform in civil as well as military hospitals. She began what proved to be a long series of articles and books for publication. In every odd moment, her pen went hurrying across the pages In 1859, "Notes on Hospitals" was published to spread the message of better care for the sick through better construction, better sanitation, and better management, with more careful statistics, a new viewpoint on housekeeping, and changed ideas of nursing. That this book filled a great need was proved by its widespread circulation. In a time when such information was scant and hard to obtain, it became an authority for persons in many countries who joined with her in bringing about an era of hospital reform. In the same year appeared, "Notes on Nursing." This book immediately became a "best-seller." Not only was it popularly read in England for its novel approach to one of the great home problems, but it became a textbook for nurses in the school she founded later. America put out an edition, and it was translated into foreign languages. Even today reprints are available.

On hospital and nursing reform such as Miss Nightingale advocated was to depend the success of the concurrent development of medical science. Her personal friendship for health reformers, such as the great public sanitarian Sir Edwin Chadwick and the military hygienist Sir Sidney Herbert, brought an unusual understanding of problems of health in their relation to the broader field of hospital environment, and the still broader one of national health. As a group they formed with her an advance guard, unknowingly clearing the way for *Louis Pasteur* who already was working along lines that would open up another and a great era in which bacteriological science would enable sanitarians to recognize and destroy the germs which he discovered to be the specific agents destroying health. After that, his later discoveries would uncover still another goal, that of assured individual protection against these germs through the science of Immunology.

Sanitation in India   It was also in 1859 that Florence Nightingale began to work for the health of the English Army in India. Here was repeated the dramatic success in reduced death rate obtained in the Crimea, and, later, at home. Again she turned from purely army problems to public health problems. This was a subject that held her interest for over twenty years, during which time she did much to arouse official and civilian England to improve living conditions for the native population of India. Her plan for India's health reform was discussed with important Indian officials who visited London and with powerful English friends, and through their influence it was initiated. When progress seemed slow, she wrote what she had to say, had it translated, and saw that it reached those educated leaders of rural India who could influence their backward brethren toward new ways of thinking. It was her dream that trained nurses, some day, might be sent to assist with their home care and teaching, and hold what we call "health clinics."

Two others papers were written, one on "How People May Live and Not Die in India," and the other on "How Some People Have Lived and Not Died in India." Sanitary regulations gradually controlled health conditions arising from the stress of great travel movements, such as India's fairs and pilgrimages. Hospitals, prisons, and other institutions were improved. Great cities put in drainage systems, sewage disposal systems, and other means of sanitation that kept down the common epidemic diseases. India was helped to begin a huge task of cleaning up, and was helping to earn for Miss Nightingale new titles among her friends, one of whom humorously addressed her as "Florence the First, Empress of Scavengers, Queen of Nurses, Reverend Mother Superior of the British Army, Governess of the Governor of India."[24]

In a few years, the heroine of the Crimea had arrived at the position of world-consultant on matters pertaining to health measures for armies, institutions, and towns. Plans for hospitals poured in for her criticism and advice. She drew about her experts on different phases of her many-sided work, but never again did she appear in public. The greatest accomplishment of a great woman's life now radiated from a simply furnished little apartment at 10 South Street, in London. Progressive, systematic, creative, wise, Florence Nightingale won the right to a place among the pioneers of those movements that have shown the early nineteenth century to be a period of exceeding growth in the humanitarian spirit. In all that she attempted, up to the time of his death in August, 1861, Sir Sidney Herbert was ever a mainstay. Personally, he gave her a wholehearted sympathy. His influence as Secretary at War, and later as Secretary of State, gave her political access. To both of them work was life, and life was work, and mankind owes much to an unusual friendship.

SUMMARY

Sporadic efforts at reform were numerous. The *first great reform movement* of international importance originated in Catholic France in 1633, when St. Vincent de Paul instituted a system of *Social Service*, and with the assistance of St. Louise de Marillac founded the nursing order of *Sisters of Charity* with a five year course of planned instruction. Assisting in hospitals, in homes, on battlefields, or wherever needed, the Sisters established interest in a type of nursing that was less restricted than that of the monastery and one which spread rapidly into other Catholic countries.

John Howard and Elizabeth Fry of England influenced prison re-

[24] From Cooke, Sir Edward: The Life of Florence Nightingale, 1913, Vol. II, p. 179. By permission of The Macmillan Company, New York, publishers.

form far beyond the boundaries of their own country. Dorothea Lynde Dix of America devoted her energies to reform of institutions for the mentally ill, and gave us our system of mental hospitals under government control. Far-reaching social results followed upon the satirical writings of Charles Dickens, whose descriptions of middle-class conditions revealed a shocking lack of social conscience. In "Martin Chuzzlewit," Betsy Prig is the typical nurse employed by the Hospital of St. Bartholomew, and Sairey Gamp is her sister in the field of private-duty.

The *second great reform movement*, originating in Protestant Germany, came with a revival of the ancient order of Deaconesses by Pastor Fliedner and his wife, Friederike. In 1836 they instituted a course covering three years of bedside and classroom experience for those deaconesses who would devote the greater part of their lives to nursing. From the famous Deaconess Motherhouse at Kaiserswerth on the Rhine, large numbers of deaconesses eventually went forth to found similar institutions in various parts of the Protestant world.

The *third and greatest reform, a nonsectarian movement*, was due to the work of Florence Nightingale, an English girl born in Florence, Italy, on May 12, 1820. Her youthful interest in social conditions led to a study of charitable institutions, and a conviction grew that she would some day fulfill a God-given mission of mercy. In 1850 she was able to spend two weeks observing methods and listening to the hopes and plans of the Fliedners at Kaiserswerth. One year later, she gathered still more valuable information during another visit of three months. In 1853 she studied the work of the Sisters of Charity in Paris, and later secured permission to investigate all hospitals, infirmaries, and religious houses of the city. Finally she was ready to apply her knowledge as superintendent of a small institution on Harley Street which offered shelter to homeless ladies and nursing care to sick governesses.

Miss Nightingale had been in this hospital but a short while when a remote situation, the Crimean War, brought to public light the inefficiency of English nursing. While soldiers of France were being cared for by the Sisters of Charity and those of Russia by the Sisters of Mercy, those of Protestant England, according to newspaper accounts, were suffering from neglect. Aided by the Secretary at War,

Sir Sidney Herbert, Miss Nightingale gained permission to sail for the Crimean hospitals with a carefully-selected group of thirty-eight English women, which eventually grew to a corps of one hundred and twenty-five. Under her supervision, army nursing joined forces with the new sanitary science to become an efficient health service.

An expression of gratitude from the British public for Miss Nightingale's war service was the "Nightingale Fund" to establish a school for nurses that would train a superior type of young women. Great as was her interest in planning the new school, Miss Nightingale felt that her first concern must be that of improving health conditions in the army. In carrying out her plans for reform of military hospitals, she produced statistics proving the death rate among England's soldiers in time of peace to be twice that among her civilians. In spite of the damage done to her own health during the war, she was soon attacking the problem of inefficiency in civil hospitals. On hospital and nursing reform such as advocated by Miss Nightingale was to depend the success of the concurrent development of medical science. Her exertions in behalf of the British Army in India resulted once more in a greatly reduced death rate. Her work was then extended to problems of public health, and the improvement of living conditions for all India.

In a few years the heroine of the Crimea had become an acknowledged authority on health measures for armies, institutions, and cities, as well as for training schools for nurses. Plans for hospitals poured in for her criticism and advice. She drew about her experts on different phases of her many-sided work, but never again did she appear in public.

TOPICS FOR DISCUSSION

1. Compare the training provided for Sisters of Charity with that of deaconesses of Kaiserswerth.
2. (*a*) What points of resemblance do you find between the organization of the Catholic Sisters of Charity and that of schools of nursing of today? (*b*) Between the Protestant Order of Deaconesses and modern nursing schools?
3. Describe the effect of development of factories on family life in England.

4. Discuss the contribution toward social reform of each of the following:

   St. Vincent de Paul

   St. Louise de Marillac

   John Howard

   Elizabeth Fry

   Dorothea Lynde Dix

   Charles Dickens

5. Compare the spirit of the ethical principle stated by Sairey Gamp with that put into practice by Betsy Prig and herself.

6. Give an account of the early life of Florence Nightingale as follows:

   (*a*) Her family life

   (*b*) Influences that led her to become interested in nursing

   (*c*) Opportunities of her time for studying nursing

   (*d*) Her means of becoming familiar with hospital methods

   (*e*) Her first position

   (*f*) Events that led to organization of a group of women for service in army hospitals of the Crimean War

   (*g*) Her demonstration of the therapeutic power of nursing to save human lives

   (*h*) Her post-war activities

7. What changes in ward management, introduced by Miss Nightingale at the Crimea, resulted in a greatly reduced death rate?

8. (*a*) Procure a copy of "Santa Filomena" for your notebook. (*b*) Who is its author?

9. Add new names to your map, and show the route of Miss Nightingale's trip to the Crimea.

REFERENCES

Andrews, Mary R. S.: A Lost Commander: Florence Nightingale. Garden City, New York, Doubleday, Doran & Co., Inc., 1933.

Cooke, Sir Edward: A Short Life of Florence Nightingale. New York, The Macmillan Co., 1925.

———: The Life of Florence Nightingale. New York, The Macmillan Co., 1913.

De Barberey, Helene R. B.: Elizabeth Seton. New York, The Macmillan Co., 1931.

Gallison, Marie: The Ministry of Women: One Hundred Years of Women's Work at Kaiserswerth, 1836–1936. The Lutterworth Press, 4 Bouverie Street, E.C. 4, London. (A pamphlet, price 6 d net.)

Marshall, Helen E.: Dorothea Dix. Univ. of North Carolina Press, 1937.

O'Malley: Florence Nightingale. Butterworth Publishing Co., England.

Quennell, Marjorie and C. H. B.: A History of Everyday Things in England (4 volumes). New York, Charles Scribner's Sons.

Richards, Laura E.: Florence Nightingale: The Angel of the Crimea. New York and London, D. Appleton & Co., 1927.

Stowe, Lyman Beecher: Saints, Sinners, and Beechers. Indianapolis, Bobbs-Merrill Co., 1934.

Strachey, Lytton: Eminent Victorians. New York, G. P. Putnam's Sons.

Whitney, Janet: Elizabeth Fry. Boston, Little, Brown & Co., 1936.

Willis, Irene Cooper: Florence Nightingale. New York, A. L. Burt Co., 1931.

Woodham-Smith, Cecil: Florence Nightingale. New York, McGraw-Hill Book Co., 1951.

Modern Development
of Social Agencies

1860-1893

NONSECTARIAN REFORM IN NURSING

In 1860, Miss Nightingale began the reform of nursing through establishment of a model school in which the art of nursing might be taught. The Nightingale Fund, raised in her honor for this purpose by subscription of the grateful people of her country, now amounted to approximately fifty thousand English pounds. This represented a much greater sum at that time than it would today. St. Thomas' Hospital in London, with medical school connection, rich and influential, charitable and long-established, had been chosen as desirable for making what was a radical experiment. The first need was to find some one to take charge of the school, for Miss Nightingale, although she had wished to do this herself, was not now in sufficiently good health. She would provide a plan, but another must carry it out under her direction. In those days when she had been trying to find nurses to accompany her to the Crimea, she had run across one matron apparently so able, and of so superior a personality, that she always remembered her. This Mrs. Wardroper would seem to be just the one to undertake supervision of the Nightingale School. Her position of matron in St. Thomas' Hospital, where she had improved the nursing considerably, made her a particularly advantageous choice.

Mrs. Wardroper was willing to accept the additional responsibility, and the Nightingale Fund Committee appointed her to the posi-

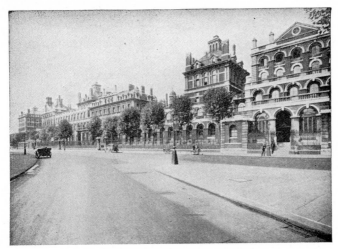

MAIN ENTRANCE TO ST. THOMAS' HOSPITAL
(From bulletin of The Nightingale Training School for Nurses, St. Thomas'
Hospital, London, England.)

tion. Miss Nightingale unfolded her plan. Well-bred young women, not less than twenty-five years of age, and not over thirty-five, were to have a course of class instruction and practical training in the hospital to prepare them to earn a living as efficient nurses. This first modern school of nursing was to be an endowed school. The Fund would pay the matron, ward sisters or head nurses, and medical lecturers for the time devoted to the school. Basic principles underlying the general plan, in addition to selection of a general hospital offering broad experience, were that the pupils must live in a comfortable, well-kept home, under supervision and discipline such as would ensure character safe-guarding and development, and learn nursing under the direction and instruction of a cultured Matron, assisted by a selected group of teaching Sisters, for a period of three or four years. This long training under nurses was an innovation, for, up to this time, nurses had been taught a few simple procedures by doctors or their assistants who themselves took temperatures, gave hypodermic injections, and sometimes changed the sheets under those patients who were critically ill or whom they did not want moved. The upper floor of a new wing at St. Thomas' was set aside for the school and fitted up for residence. Separate bedrooms were arranged for students, with a sitting-room to be used by them in common, and a suite for the Sister deputed to take charge of this, their home.

The regulation of life in this home was necessarily outlined in accordance with times which had necessitated Miss Nightingale's being accompanied to the shores of the Mediterranean by an uncle, and chaperoned throughout her whole Crimean experience by trusted friends of her parents. Its rules, unavoidably, belonged to the Victorian Age when women were just beginning to venture forth from the shelter of family life, and were formulated, besides, under the influence of Kaiserswerth and the convent. A student, for instance, might not go out alone, but must have with her another student as companion. A chaplain must give two sermons a week. Every act was to be watched that no criticism might be brought on the school by unguarded use of unaccustomed freedom, however much curtailed. Its founder knew well that it was under trial. The prejudices of "nice" families had to be overcome by promising protection to their gently reared daughters. The prejudices of those doctors and laymen who thought the old kind of nurse, with all her faults, good enough, had to be overcome by providing a better nurse. Even slight errors of judgment in conduct or practice must incur discipline by the matron.

There would be two social grades represented among the women in the school, as there had been in the nursing group at the Crimean War. Educated probationers from the upper class would pay about thirty pounds a year for tuition. A nonpaying group would represent a less distinguished stratum of society, but yet selected for fitness and character. Probationers would enter on a trial period of one month, and a primary course of study for all was to cover one year.

During the year of training, these probationers would serve as assistant-nurses, and were to be taught nursing procedures by the Sisters in charge of wards. They were to be kept free from subsidiary work and provided with all conveniences possible to make nursing efficient. Instruction was to be given also by the Resident Medical Officer of the hospital whom Miss Nightingale requested to prepare a form for what we would call a "Nursing Care Study"—written notes of observations of patients which students were to keep with the greatest care, and hand in for examination. The hospital staff was asked to supplement this teaching by a systematic course of lectures and bedside clinics. Matron, Ward Sisters, and Medical Instructors, all were to receive remuneration for services to the school from the Nightingale Fund. Students were to receive board, lodging, laundry, and uniforms, with about ten pounds for incidental expenses. A time-schedule to cover activities by day and by night was formulated as follows:

Day Nurses				*Night Nurses*		
Rise	6	A.M.		Rise	9	P.M.
Breakfast	6½	A.M.		Tea	9½	P.M.
Wards	7	A.M.		Wards	10	P.M.
Dinner	1	P.M.		Dormitory	6	A.M.
Wards	2	P.M.		Breakfast	6½	A.M.
Exercise	11½	A.M. to 1 P.M. or		Wards	7	A.M.
	3½	to 5 P.M.				
Tea	5	P.M.		Dormitory	10	A.M.
Wards	6	P.M.		Exercise	11	A.M. to 1 P.M.
Dormitory	8½	P.M.		Dinner	1	P.M.
Supper	9	P.M.		Bed	2	P.M.
Bed	10	P.M.				

When the members of both student groups had finished the studies of the first year, an examination was to be given and those who passed it were to be known as *Certified Nurses*, although it was decided to issue no printed certificates. Their classwork was finished, but there was to be a further course of training. This second part of their course would require three years for the nonpaying pupil, two for the one who paid, and would be devoted wholly to ward practice, on salary, at St. Thomas' or a hospital chosen by the Nightingale Fund Committee. A record of their service was to be kept and sent to the Committee which, after the two or three additional years of hospital service, would find them suitable hospital positions on salary.

The latter arrangement helped to fix in the minds of all who were interested in her scheme the intention of the founder that graduates of the Nightingale School were not expected to enter the field of private duty which had been accustomed to absorb the best nurses, but were, rather, to spread over the hospital field throughout the world, as nurse missionaries, teaching the art of nursing, hygiene, and health.

The form of application blank to be filed with the Matron contained practically the same questions that have been asked candidates for schools of nursing down to the present day. One question, however, has been lost by the way, and this loss is significant of another reform already begun, that of education for all women. The question was, "Can you read and write well?"

Miss Nightingale drew up in minute detail, also, the form for an efficiency report. This was called the "Monthly Sheet of Personal Character and Acquirements," and it was to be filled in by the Matron who thus would provide a means of following up the student's character development and technical progress. Punctuality, quietness, trustworthiness, personal neatness and cleanliness, were to be graded with her ward work, according to the following schedule: Excellent, good, moderate, imperfect, zero. Similarly, the nursing practice was to be graded under fourteen main headings with subheadings to help the grader in deciding what went to make good nursing, for, up to this time, it had not been so analyzed.

Newspaper advertisements brought applicants for interview, and fifteen of these were selected for the first class. *On June 24, 1860, these fifteen young women became probationers in the Nightingale School for Nurses, St. Thomas Hospital, London, England.* The school was privileged to have the services of Mrs. Wardroper for more than twenty-five years, and during this period of service five hundred nurses graduated to take hospital positions in St. Thomas' and elsewhere. Fifty of this group belonged to the "paying pupil" group, and had become Matrons or superintendents, some of them far away from the homeland and their school. *Modern nursing was founded.* As all new ideas do, so this one met with considerable opposition from conservative hospitals and medical men. Its success, despite such opposition, proved the value of a definite plan of education for nursing, and the idea spread throughout the world.

Florence Nightingale, deeply religious herself and living in days when a rabid sectarianism tore people apart, had found a way to end nursing's "Dark Period" by providing an efficient nursing service outside of the control of any religious group. Her success marks the beginning of a complete secularization of nursing. She had a means to prepare for a useful, suitable occupation many women who were seeking to use their talents outside of the home circle. The early

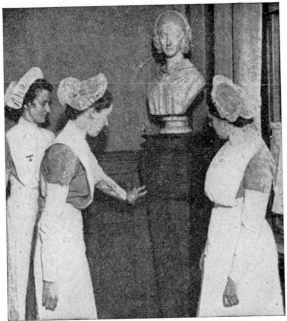

STUDENT NURSES OF TODAY AT THE LIVERPOOL ROYAL INFIRMARY

They are inspecting a bust of Florence Nightingale which she presented to their school. (From Nursing Times, August, 1941.)

nurses of the Nightingale School she was accustomed to refer to as her "daughters." She prepared annual letters for them, which have been gathered together in the book, "Florence Nightingale to her nurses." Fitly, these successors in every corner of the world acknowledge her the "Mother of Nursing."

MODERN DISTRICT NURSING

Experience of nursing, at Lea Hurst as well as at Kaiserswerth and with the Sisters of Charity, had shown Miss Nightingale that there was a great field for nurses' work lying almost neglected beyond the walls of hospitals. Home nursing had been always of supreme interest to her, and she had longed to find a way to get into it in her own country. Now, in 1861, a rich resident of Liverpool, *William Rathbone*, had written several times of his desire to secure nurses trained in her new school, to undertake this type of nursing among the poor of his city. He was coming to see her about it. The students of St. Thomas', however, had no special training for district work, and, in any case, none of the new graduates were available, nor was there a nurse to be had at King's College Hospital where the Sisters of St. John's House did such excellent work. She would have to suggest to him that it might be a good thing to start a school for nurses similar to the Nightingale School, at the big Royal Infirmary of Liverpool.

This Mr. Rathbone is not entirely a stranger to us. He will be remembered as the kind friend who, with his wife, gave refuge and care to Miss Dorothea Lynde Dix, the American reformer, when she found herself alone and sick in England. Mrs. Rathbone had passed away in 1860, and her husband, during her illness, learned to appreciate deeply the dependence of sick people on nursing. He wanted to use some of his wealth thereafter to make it available to those who needed it as she had, and lacked means to pay for it. At his request *Mary Robinson*, an untrained but capable nurse who had cared for Mrs. Rathbone, gave up private nursing in order to nurse the sick poor in the great industrial and seaport city of Liverpool, and Mr. Rathbone paid her a salary. He supplied, too, the needed sickroom appliances, and made arrangements for any special diets required. Popularity soon brought her more work than she could do, and a search for other nurses to help showed that none were to be had. It was then that Miss Nightingale's welcome suggestion of a school offered its great possibilities.

By 1862 necessary school buildings, built and equipped by Mr. Rathbone, had been added to the Royal Infirmary. *Miss Merryweather*, a graduate of the Nightingale School, was secured for the position of Superintendent of Nurses. It was arranged to train student nurses on the Infirmary wards, after the manner of the School at St. Thomas' but in addition to this training they were to be sent to nurse in the homes of the poor. Liverpool was divided into eighteen districts, with a nurse in each, her supervision to be the responsibility of a group of volunteer lady visitors. Mr. Rathbone himself followed up the work closely, and personally accompanied nurses on their visits to the sick.

London, too, developed a district nursing service, details of which were worked out by another Nightingale nurse, *Florence Lees*. Experience of the Liverpool system of placing in the district students educated solely in the hospital, brought another reform. A school for the teaching of home nursing as a specialty was part of this new organization. It was planned to build up gradually a national system of like Schools and Homes for district nurses. Instead of a course which had really been a preparation for hospital work, the students of district nursing entered upon a course that included, with one year of hospital work, a six-months' period of special instruction on the district by teachers of home nursing.

This principle of a special type of instruction for a special kind of nursing was new. Another innovation was the limiting of admission to the course. Only ladies were permitted to become district nurses. This was a further step toward raising the general status of nursing. Englishwomen of this class had education in those days while few of the class below them enjoyed its privileges. It was a problem destined to vanish before the spread of educational facilities. Meanwhile, district nursing homes were developed through Great Britain and Ireland.

To William Rathbone and to Florence Nightingale is due the introduction of a new phase in nursing history, for out of her idea and his pioneering grew the modern schools for public health nursing.

WORKHOUSE INFIRMARY REFORM

While he made the unusually close contact with the poor which the district nursing work made possible, William Rathbone stumbled upon something else about Liverpool's care of her sick that led him still further into the field of nursing and its reform.

This discovery was in connection with the city Workhouse and House of Correction, one of those institutions already seen to be popular at the time, and combining in their functions a hospital for incurable and chronic cases among the destitute. Mr. Rathbone found that poor citizens of Liverpool dreaded the Workhouse, and especially its Infirmary. Crowded into it were over a thousand patients cared for by inmates of the Workhouse, who were rough, often drunken paupers, women and men. Officials of the institution, wearing kid gloves to keep their hands clean, made rounds by day, supposedly, to supervise. By night, a policeman kept order in convalescent wards, but sick patients were locked in their rooms and left alone. Nobody did anything for them all night long. Infirmary and patients, too, as might be expected, were dirty beyond present-day conception. Food was indeed poor. It seemed to Mr. Rathbone that Miss Nightingale was the very one to turn to again if this truly terrible place was to be made better. He went to London to suggest that he would maintain for three years a staff of trained nurses if she would find for him another Superintendent of Nurses.

The outcome of his visit and much correspondence was that in 1864 *Agnes Jones*, Nightingale nurse, and twelve other certified nurses from the same school essayed the task of organizing a better nursing service for the twelve hundred patients then confined to the Liverpool Workhouse Infirmary. Some pauper nurses had to be retained for the time being. Eighteen probationers were secured for a first class. It was a meager staff, and certainly the work that confronted this young woman in her first executive position must have been discouraging.

Miss Jones found it difficult to stay in spite of the fact that Mr. Rathbone, thoughtfully, had seen to it that she had a pleasant apartment to offset the wards in which she must spend so much of her day. She was, after all, still quite young, and, in spite of religious zeal, rather frightened as she came to find out the kind of people that lived in a Workhouse. Only a few years before, she had been an eager young girl, disappointed because she could not go to work with the famous Florence Nightingale in the Crimea. She had been told that she must know how to do nursing, and she had gone to Kaiserswerth in 1860 and studied it for a year. Returning, the next step had not been plain until Miss Nightingale herself had advised her to enter the new Nightingale School. This she had done, and now that she really was a nurse, it seemed almost impossible to cope with a situation where people and things were so filthy, and little sick children had to be piled seven or eight in a bed, while their elders, too, had to be persuaded to sleep together. It was all very unlike Kaiserswerth or the hospital in which she had been trained. To encourage her, Miss Nightingale had written that it was "Scutari all over again." She pulled herself together, and went on.

In due time Miss Jones had gathered together a staff that included fifty nurses and probationers. The pauper nurses had been organized into a cleaning staff. It was all so strenuous, however, that her physical resistance fell, and after three years, Agnes Jones, reformer of Workhouse Nursing, died of typhus fever contracted in her ward contacts. That short time proved the success of Mr. Rathbone's second experiment. London followed suit and, again under the sympathetic direction of Florence Nightingale, the nursing in forty workhouses was changed. By 1874 English workhouse infirmaries were changed places, and there were no longer any pauper nurses in them.

Once more the leadership of William Rathbone, the citizen, of Florence Nightingale, the nurse educator, had changed the course of nursing history, this time by transforming the infirmaries of public workhouses.

BIRTH OF THE RED CROSS IN 1864

While all this reform of military and civilian nursing was going on, another seed planted by Florence Nightingale as she worked in the Crimea had not only matured, but already was bearing fruit. In 1859 Europeans were again at war. Italy was trying to free herself from Austrian rule, and France and Sardinia were helping her. In June of that year, a great battle took place near the little town of Solferino, in Lombardy, a province of northern Italy. About forty thousand men were killed or wounded. Both armies had trampled down fallen friends as well as foes. A traveler from Geneva in neighboring Switzerland, who had managed to get near enough to see what a battle was like, wrote this about it:

"In the burning midday heat still more furiously, the battle rages. . . . Drunk or mad with blood, the butchery goes on. Over the field of slaughter dashes the wild cavalry charge, the horses' iron hoofs beating down the wretched men. . . . Back of dark, threatening clouds, the sun is lost. A tempest of wind and lightning arises; icy rain sweeps across the field. As the shadows of the night begin to fall the tumult of the battle dies away. Exhausted men sink down to sleep where they stand, or search for some missing comrade. The silent darkness is broken by the groans and cries for help of the wounded men."[1]

The stranger moved among them, helping where he could, and shaming cruelty in men who still went about killing enemies as they

[1] Quoted in "Under The Red Cross Flag at Home and Abroad" by Mabel T. Boardman. Philadelphia, J. B. Lippincott Co., 1915, p. 33.

came across them. "We are all brothers," he cried. Preparation for care of the wounded soldier had been as poor as it was at the Crimea five years before. An inadequate medical service was again overwhelmed. But something had to be done. Suffering men shouldn't be left lying on a freezing field. Springless village carts arrived to torture them still further as they jolted back toward neighboring villages. There churches, convents, soldiers' barracks, and private homes were being turned into makeshift hospitals. Verandas and the streets had to take the overflow.

The curious traveler followed when he could do no more on the field, and, being a man of initiative, gathered together a group of volunteers among the women of one of the villages. Under his direction, they helped him to give what nursing care was possible. To wounded men of any nationality *Henri Dunant* and these women gave water to drink, or soup, put on warm covering or wound dressings, or just comforted, if that was all that they could do. The Italian mothers, who readily understood what it meant, took up his cry, "We are all brothers," and, as they worked, kept saying over and over, "Tutti fratelli." After the great emergency was over, Dunant wrote letters for survivors, bought little luxuries for them, sent money to their families from their pay, did all the little things which Florence Nightingale had found to mean so much to wounded and homesick men.

In a town, not far away, were other thousands of wounded. Monsieur Dunant went to see what was being done for them, and witnessed operations being performed without anesthetics, although the use of both ether and chloroform had been demonstrated more than ten years before. More and more he realized how much could be done to improve conditions for soldiers wounded while fighting for the safety of those at home, who, surely, could not understand or they would not permit the things that he knew to be true. Improvements in the implements of war might make it possible to do away with more enemies, but they also made wounds worse and more painful. He was aware of the very recent work of English nurses during war; in fact, he wrote:

"The picture of Miss Florence Nightingale, during the night, going through the vast wards of the military hospitals with a small lamp in her hand, noting the condition of each sick man, will never be obliterated from the hearts of the men,

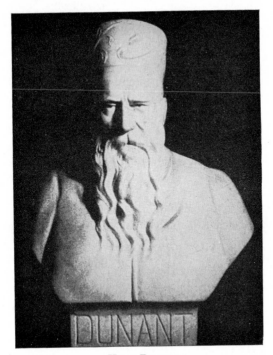

HENRI DUNANT

(Sculpture by Ernst Durig, in the National Headquarters of the American Red Cross, Washington, D. C.)

who were the objects or the witnesses of her admirable beneficence, and the memory of it will be engraven in history."[2]

Speaking in London, years after, he referred again to Miss Nightingale's influence in these words: "What inspired me to go to Italy during the war of 1859 was the work of Miss Florence Nightingale in the Crimea."[3] His hope fixed itself on finding a way to make war less horrible. With Solferino fresh in his mind, Henri Dunant embodied this hope in the following question put to his readers among

[2] From The Origin of the Red Cross ("Un Souvenir de Solferino") by Henri Dunant, translated from the French by Mrs. David H. Wright. The John C. Winston Co., 1911, pp. 81–82.

[3] Cooke, Sir Edward: A Short Life of Florence Nightingale, 1925, p.240. By permission of The Macmillan Company, New York, publishers.

the public: "Would it not be possible to found and organize in all civilized countries permanent societies of volunteers which in time of war could render succor to the wounded without distinction of nationality?"[4] This was the great idea born of his sad experience. It is the germ idea which has given us all of our familiar Red Cross Societies, but its development consumed the rest of Dunant's life and used up all of his funds. He wrote a pamphlet entitled "A Remembrance of Solferino" from which has been quoted his description of the battle. What he described awoke Europeans to a realization of the truth that lay behind the glamour of glory with which horror and cruelty had been veiled. This story was followed by visits to many countries where he enlisted the support of kings and influential citizens.

After five years of work, Henri Dunant had the satisfaction of seeing a national congress gather at Geneva to consider ways and means of raising volunteers to serve in the event of another war. In 1864 fourteen countries signed what is known as the *Treaty of Geneva* in which they agreed that military hospitals were to be respected by armies as zones of safety, while *their staffs of doctors and nurses were to be neutral*, and serve the wounded of any nationality without prejudice. Suffering, in a very practical sense, was to make the whole world kin, "Tutti fratelli," as Dunant had dreamed.

In its own way, each country was to develop its own separate volunteer society. All of these societies would use the same design for their flag, and set it up over all the hospitals in which they were called upon to serve during war. It would be a sign of neutrality and indicate readiness to care for the wounded of all countries involved. Such a flag, in itself, would go a long way toward facilitating early treatment, for hitherto the injured who were able to walk had been compelled to search for a field hospital flying their own national flag. A field hospital under another flag would refuse to take them in. The design selected for the new common flag of the various national Societies was that of the flag of Switzerland with its colors reversed, a red cross on a white background instead of a white cross on a red background. This was a gesture conferring public honor on

---

[4] From The Origin of the Red Cross ("Un Souvenir de Solferino") by Henri Dunant, translated from the French by Mrs. David H. Wright. The John C. Winston Co., 1911, p. 78.

both Henri Dunant and his native country. England signed the treaty in 1870, and, as time went on, other countries did the same. In line with its established policy of avoiding all entanglement with European countries, the United States refrained from confirming it until 1882.

NURSING IN THE AMERICAN CIVIL WAR (1861-65)

When the next war came, only two years after the battle of Solferino, it was a civil war in the New World. By 1861, however, many of the people of the United States had learned of the work of Florence Nightingale, and probably a lesser number had heard of the efforts of Henri Dunant to form a neutral organization of volunteers to serve the combatants of all armies at war. That they profited by adopting some of the ideas of both of these notable persons, is evident from the system of relief which they developed. Although they did not form one of the Red Cross Societies advocated by Dunant, an organization similar to these grew out of an early and widespread development of women's circles or soldier's aid societies aiming to provide clothing or dressings for army use. Every village town and city had a group of this kind. In the north, alone, there were seven thousand of them.

WORK OF THE SANITARY COMMISSION

It soon became evident that a central organization through which supplies might be distributed was very desirable. New York sent a group of representatives to Washington from its women's societies, and also from an association made up of local physicians. The government was asked to appoint a body to be known as a "Sanitary Commission" which would act as advisor to the Medical Department of the Army. Its aim was set forth as "a simple desire and resolute determination to secure for the men who have enlisted in this war, that care which it is the duty of the nation to give them."[5] The usual opposition, governmental and military, was met but, in spite of it, the idea was put over, and a *Sanitary Commission* was appointed.

An arrangement then was made for the relief work of the scattered

[5] Boardman, Mabel T.: Under the Red Cross Flag at Home and Abroad. Philadelphia, J. B. Lippincott Co., 1915, p. 53.

circles to become tributary to the Commission which thus became the center of relief activities. Among its first activities was an inspection of army camps in the vicinity of Washington. These were found lacking in drainage, in bathing facilities, and in adequacy of space. Crowding, cold, and lack of ventilation forced the men to spend much of their time in foul air. Clothing and bed coverings were not only shoddy but filthy. Food and cooking were poor, and rations lacked fresh vegetables. Scurvy and dysentery were present. Troops arrived in these camps without rest or a chance to clean up after a trip in ordinary freight cars that might have carried them all the way from the far west. On the basis of findings such as the above, recommendations were made, but they fell upon barren ground. The usual number of conservative souls in authority were satisfied with things as they were.

Then something happened, and government and army were jogged into action. The northern forces suffered defeat at the battle of Bull Run. An inquiry into the reason for this showed that it lay in conditions already exposed by the Sanitary Commission. The health of the men had not been conserved. They had gone into battle unfit. From now on, preventive medicine readily held its own against the theory of producing physical endurance through rough treatment. The interrelation between health and morale had been plain enough for all to see.

Hospitals for sick and wounded became the next object of consideration from the Sanitary Commission. Inspection showed the buildings to be often unsuitable, even after some adaptation, while the nursing service was in the hands of untrained men and women. A recommendation was made that army hospitals assume a temporary form and, through a pavilion system of construction, afford opportunity for expansion of their facilities. Other recommendations dealt with the need for better inspection of bedding, clothing, drinking water, food and its preparation, and better methods of transporting the wounded to the institutions.

The activities of the Sanitary Commission continued to grow apace with the progress of the war. It became a source of such volunteer assistance to the army as Dunant had been suggesting, an efficient agency of relief for the soldier. Supplies began to flow through central distributing offices. Enormous amounts of money were raised and deposited in its treasury. When shortage of vegetables showed its effect in scurvy, the Commission remedied the condition by enlisting the help of the only too-willing farmer. Great soup kettles, mounted on wheels and with a base so contrived as to permit carrying their own fire beneath, were moved to follow the battle lines. It was the Sanitary Commission, too, that arranged for fitting up hospital trains by installing swinging beds in freight cars, and seeing that doctors and nurses were assigned to these traveling hospitals which were to become a permanent feature of army equipment. Their patients also were given the comfort of good bedding, necessary clothing, and nourishing food.

The Sanitary Commission established itself also as a connecting link between the individual soldier and his family. It kept his name on a roster of the patients spread over two hundred hospitals, and reported his condition. When the war ended, it provided temporary maintenance for thousands of discharged men, got their discharge papers for them, paid their way home. The sum of its activities and the spirit of neutrality which characterized the Commission, gave it the character, without the name, of those Red Cross Societies that were being talked of abroad. During the years in which it strove to meet the demands made upon it, Florence Nightingale, from London, kept in touch with its leaders, enthusiastically sharing with them her knowledge of European moves toward improved care of army health, as well as the lessons learned from her own war experience. In her sympathetic eagerness she offered to cross the Atlantic to give personal assistance, but was restrained from doing so by recurring illness.

As there was no Red Cross Society ready to step into relief and social work in 1861, so there was almost no organized nursing. What there was existed solely among Catholic and Protestant Sisterhoods, and the governments of both sides naturally turned to them for help. All of these women were disciplined to institutional life, and some of them devoted themselves wholly to care of the sick. As soon as the need for their service was known, the nuns led the way in nursing both north and south. Their established hospitals became crowded with patients, their convents were turned into emergency hospitals, the devoted sisters served at the front or were to be found on battlefields throughout the war.

VOLUNTEER NURSING

Everywhere throughout the country there were young girls who had thrilled to the story of Florence Nightingale and her nurses in the Crimea. There were thousands of Louisa M. Alcotts pining for "something to do," and war was offering to women in America the same opportunity for useful occupation that it had offered Florence Nightingale in the same dissatisfied state. They found it in making dressings, in rolling bandages, in stitching uniforms, in nursing.

The circles of northern women had their counterpart in the south, and the fact must not be overlooked that the south had to find another way of managing its relief work without benefit of established government backing. A centralized organization was here lacking, it is true, but the spirit of cooperation was notably strong. Hospitals were opened in homes and in tents. There were convalescent homes established. Southern women ploughed the fields and harvested the crops. Money became so scarce that even those who had been richest among them found their families nearing privation. Everywhere, American women were leaving the home for a life in public, with public responsibilities. As they did so, they inevitably passed beyond old ways of thinking and old satisfactions.

It was not long before there was a rush of womankind into nursing. In the great need, they were seldom refused; but, as time went on, they were not always welcomed. Some talked inadvisedly, stirring up trouble; some gave splendid service throughout the war. Among leaders in relief work were those who urged training for women who wanted to do this particular work. *Dr. Elizabeth Blackwell*, one of the earliest of the "new women" in America, as well as the first woman to receive the degree of Doctor of Medicine anywhere in the world, understood this need probably better than most. On terms of intimate personal friendship with Florence Nightingale, she had but recently made a visit to her, and was very familiar with her views. Professional contact with New York's hospitals enabled her to arrive at further conclusions of her own.

Through the cooperation of Bellevue and other of these institutions, a course of one month of practical experience in their wards was arranged for those wishing to enlist for war nursing. One hundred women took advantage of this preparation. Other women here and there throughout the country also fitted themselves for nursing by varying periods of hospital practice. The majority of volunteers, however, were like *Louisa M. Alcott*, who has described graphically in her "Hospital Sketches" the experiences of one who went to war without it. Not a few of them, in that period of woman's emergence to a larger life, must have known occasions when they felt as she after one precious day had gone in futile effort to get settled a little matter of transportation that put itself in the way of her ambitions.

"I am a woman's rights woman, and if any man had offered help in the morning, I should have condescendingly refused it, sure that I could do everything as well, if not better, myself. My strongmindedness had rather abated since then, and I was now quite ready to be a 'timid trembler,' if necessary."[6]

In describing her initiation to war nursing, she must have spoken, too, for many a raw recruit:

"My three days' experience had begun with a death, and owing to the defalcation of another nurse, a somewhat abrupt plunge into the superintendence of a ward containing forty beds, where I spent my shining hours washing faces, serving rations, giving medicine, and sitting in a very hard chair, with pneumonia on one side, diphtheria on the other, two typhoids opposite, and a dozen dilapidated patriots, hopping, lying, and lounging about, all staring more or less at the new 'nuss,' who suffered untold agonies . . . and blundered through her trying labors with a Spartan firmness."[6]

All was "hurry and confusion," and an army nurse-in-the-making found her way to a great ward that once had been a gay hotel ballroom. Not knowing what to do, and filled with an unexpected longing to hide, she took stock from a sheltered corner.

"Round the stove was gathered the dreariest group I ever saw—ragged, gaunt, and pale, mud to the knees, with bloody bandages untouched since put on days before."[7]

Yearning to serve, but not knowing how, she stood in her refuge until some one

"put basin, sponge, towels, and a block of brown soap into my hands, with these appalling directions. 'Come my dear, begin to wash as fast as you can. Tell them to take off socks, coats and shirts, scrub them well, put on clean shirts, and the attendants will finish them off, and lay them in bed.' "[7]

6 Alcott, Louisa M.: Hospital Sketches. Boston, Roberts Brothers, 1885, pp. 11, 26.
7 *Ibid.*, pp. 28, 29, 33, 36, 37.

This job accomplished, somehow the ward machinery carried her on:

"Great trays of bread, meat, soup, and coffee appeared; and both nurses and attendants turned waiters, serving bountiful rations to all who could eat."[7]

"All having eaten, drunk, and rested, the surgeons began their rounds; and I took my first lesson in the art of dressing wounds. Dr. P., whose aid I constituted myself, fell to work with a vigor which soon convinced me that I was a weaker vessel, though nothing would have induced me to confess it then."[7]

"The amputations were reserved until tomorrow, and the merciful magic of ether was not thought necessary that day, so the poor souls had to bear their pains as best they might. . . . Their fortitude seemed contagious, and scarcely a cry escaped them, though I often longed to groan for them, when pride kept their white lips shut, while great drops stood upon their foreheads, and the bed shook with the irrepressible tremor of their tortured bodies."[7]

The work had not stopped since that dusky evening more than twenty-four hours ago, and Louisa M. Alcott had learned a few things about war nursing. No day would ever be so hard again, and a succession of days made it possible for her to express very beautifully for all nurses one of the satisfactions that few among them have missed:

"More flattering than the most gracefully turned compliment, more grateful than the most admiring glance, was the sight of those rows of faces, all strange to me a little while ago, now lighting up, with smiles of welcome, as I came among them, enjoying that moment heartily, with a womanly pride in their regard, a motherly affection for them all."[8]

Individual or local accomplishment has been lost sight of in the years that have passed since women made history by adapting meager but womanly knowledge to public service. Only a few stood out from the mass for conspicuous action. One who understood the hardships of adjustment vainly tried to establish a school for war nurses. One, at least, rode on to the field to rescue the wounded. Some braved official rules, as had Florence Nightingale, that the men dependent upon them might have what they needed. At night, big-hearted, famous *Mother Bickerdyke* searched the lines of the dead, to make sure that none who might be living had been laid there by mistake. A daring free-lance by the name of *Clara Barton* went where she pleased, nursing friend and enemy, using her own

[8] *Ibid.*, p. 41.

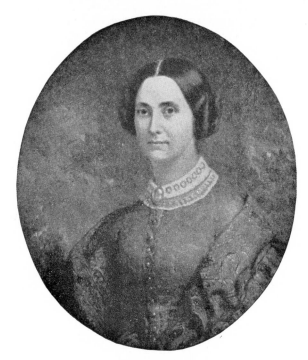

CLARA BARTON
(Courtesy of "The Trained Nurse and Hospital Review," May, 1938.)

resources to furnish necessities. Northerner and southerner, white and black, man and woman, gathered to render service, but, just as in the Crimea, of all the nurses of the Civil War a small proportion only could be gifted with outstanding qualities and leadership.

ORGANIZATION OF ARMY NURSING

It took only about six months of this uncertain type of nursing service to bring the authorities in Washington to the point of seeing that it would be unwise to depend upon it too much. To organize army nursing, a woman was put in charge of it whom the country adored for her unselfish public work toward reform of prisons, poor houses, and asylums for the insane. *Dorothea Lynde Dix* was a volunteer nurse herself, in Washington, when she was appointed "Superintendent of Female Nurses." *She proceeded to gather together the first nurse corps of the United States Army.*

The regulations which Miss Dix outlined were suggested by difficulties experienced by Miss Nightingale who, among many trials of similar nature, was once confronted by six of her nurses bent upon immediate marriage. The flavor of her ideas will be recognized without difficulty. No nurse was to be less than thirty years of age, and all must be as homely as possible. Youth or beauty of noticeable degree was enough to bring refusal. Hair dressing must be of the plainest style. Ribbons, jewelry, and the wearing of any ornament were forbidden. While no uniform dress was designated, sombre brown or black were the colors insisted upon, partly to sober charm, partly as an acknowledgment of difficulties in matters of warmth and washing. An allowance of twelve dollars a month was arranged for accepted applicants, although Miss Dix herself served without remuneration throughout the war.

At no time, however, did these nurses enlisting directly through the governmental agency solve the whole problem of nursing during the Civil War, even in the north. Large numbers of men served as nurses, some as members of the army, others as auxiliary volunteers, and some as representatives of a society then rather new, the Young Men's Christian Association. Before the war ended, there were thousands of women nurses throughout north and south, constituting a varied mass of intelligence, diplomacy, daring, and experience. All levels of society were represented. The predominant spirit was one of great courage and self-sacrifice, while nursing methods savored mainly of the home and the Middle Ages, and often must have failed to achieve results.

When peace was made, the smaller, restricted group of women war workers with talents of leadership found other public tasks to which they turned. Dr. Elizabeth Blackwell, Dorothea Lynde Dix, Louisa M. Alcott, and Clara Barton continue to stand out as progressives in feminine ranks. Dr. Blackwell bent her energies once more toward improving the opportunities for women in the field of medicine. Dorothea Lynde Dix, whose war service had been a sequel to years of effort to improve mental hospitals, took up that work again. Louisa M. Alcott resumed her literary work where she had left off, and spent the rest of her life entertaining young America, while imparting to it her own happy philosophy. Clara Barton, for the time being, applied herself to tracing missing soldiers, and with characteristic hard work and persistence ran down records of fully one quarter of many thousands left unaccounted for. She remained the spectacular, isolated figure that she had been, destined to know great publicity, and to win an acknowledgment of womanhood in public affairs that was international.

FOUNDING OF AMERICAN RED CROSS SOCIETY (1882)

In 1870 the world saw the Franco-Prussian War break out and Clara Barton at work with the Red Cross Society which Germany, among other European nations had developed. As she helped in German hospitals she learned of the superior nursing done by deaconesses trained after the manner of Kaiserswerth, and of Red Cross nurses trained in the specialized Red Cross hospitals that were springing up everywhere along the trail of Henri Dunant. The efficiency of his Red Cross Society as an agent of relief was thrilling to one who so fully understood its need, and she burned with enthusiasm to get a Red Cross Society for the United States. As it happened, this problem had been troubling the United States government, at intervals, ever since the Civil War. At home and abroad for nearly a decade, there had been pressure brought, and resisted. The new country wanted to maintain its political isolation, and, jealous of its independent political organization, was determined to take full advantage of a geographical location that put an ocean between it and Europe's squabbling kings. When Miss Barton came home, full of her plan to push formation of an American Red Cross Society, her ardor was not killed by a warning that this was a project to leave alone. Nevertheless, for three years more, "outwardly, the subject slept."[9]

Meanwhile, by writing and talking about it, Miss Barton did her best to bring the idea of a Red Cross Society before a widening public audience. Several times after that she ventured personally to enlist presidential or congressional influence. The number of nations with such societies had by this time risen to thirty, but her country was convinced that there would be no more wars, and its leaders with-

---

[9] Epler, Percy H.: The Life of Clara Barton, 1927, p. 231. By permission of The Macmillan Company, New York, publishers.

held their support. The usefulness of a Red Cross Society in other forms of disaster became her talking point.

"None is more liable than our country to great overmastering calamities. Seldom a year passes that the nation from sea to sea is not brought to utter consternation by the shock of some unforeseen disaster and stands shivering like a ship in the gale, powerless, horrified, despairing. Plagues, cholera, fires, floods, famine, all bear upon us with terrible force. . . . What have we in readiness to meet these emergencies save the good heart of the people and their impulsive gifts?—Certainly no organized system for collection, reception, distribution, no agents, no nurses."[10]

Finally, reward for her labor could be seen as it approached. In 1882 the American Red Cross Society became a fact, and Miss Barton its first president.

REFORM OF NURSING IN AMERICA

Shortly after the Civil War, representative citizens of New York— men and women who had taken part in relief activities—determined to find out through personal visits what kind of care was provided for the prisoner, the mentally ill, the poor, and the sick by tax-supported institutions in their state. Prevailing methods of hygiene and sanitation, of nursing and administration constituted the basis of their observations. The findings of Liverpool and of London, of Elizabeth Fry, John Howard, William Rathbone, Dorothea Lynde Dix, and Florence Nightingale were repeated wherever they went.

Actual reform of nursing in America, however, began with a group of women which followed this first group and was known as the *New York State Charities Aid Association.* Again, the majority of members had seen some kind of service during the Civil War. A committee was appointed to concentrate its investigation on Bellevue Hospital, New York City, and make report of a careful study of conditions there. The story was the same—inefficient management, bad nursing, and miserable, neglected patients. A soapless laundry in an institution admitting the dirtiest of city slum dwellers was indicative of conditions throughout. One of the new schools for nurses was recommended as the first and biggest step to be taken toward transforming the situation.

Meantime, the fame of the Nightingale system of preparing nurses

10 *Ibid.*

had spread among medical men, who were meeting changes brought into their practice by the science of Pasteur, Koch, Lister, and others. as well as by the advent of ether as a general anesthetic. They felt the need of better assistants in the care of their patients and, through the American Medical Association, advocated formation of modern schools throughout the United States. America was getting interested and looking about for some of those missioners of health being graduated from the Nightingale School in London. She was on the threshold of a period of pioneering in nurse education during which the Nightingale system would be the basis for development of new methods in her nursing.

PRE-NIGHTINGALE REFORM

It was not America's first experience in training nurses for their work, for already two schools existed. As early as 1860 the *New England Hospital for Women and Children* in Boston, Massachusetts, had attempted the teaching of nurses, but had no success until it introduced the Kaiserswerth method. When this change was made, the first student to enroll was a young woman named *Linda Richards*, who graduated in 1873, and ever after was known as the "first trained nurse in America." According to her own account, her course of one year involved both patriotism and considerable physical endurance.

"My desire to become a nurse grew out of what I heard of the need of nurses in the Civil War."[11]

"We nurses did very different work from that done by pupil nurses nowadays. Our days were not eight hours; they were nearer twice eight. We rose at 5:30 A.M., and left the wards at 9 P.M. to go to our beds, which were in little rooms between the wards. Each nurse took care of her ward of six patients both day and night. Many a time I have got up nine times in the night; often I did not get to sleep before the next call came; but, being blessed with a sound body and a firm resolution to go through the training school, cost what it might, I maintained a cheerful spirit. We wore no uniforms, the only stipulation being that our dresses should be washable."[12]

In 1861, one month before the beginning of the Civil War, a group of Quaker ladies of Philadelphia established the *Woman's Hospital*, and announced their intention of opening a school for

11, 12 Richards, Linda: Reminiscences of America's First Trained Nurse. Boston, Whitcomb and Barrows, 1911, pp. 5 and 10.

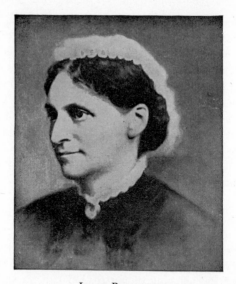

LINDA RICHARDS

(From a painting given to the New England Hospital for Women by its alumnae.)

training of a superior class of young women. In 1864, their records showed that "one thoroughly qualified nurse had left the institution to follow her profession in the community." In 1876 *Martha M. Waldron* was graduated. Both she and Miss Richards, neither of them Nightingale nurses, were yet trained in nursing, and valuable as superintendents for some of the new schools. Side by side with them, in the first attempts to implant ideals in American nursing, was Sister Helen of the Protestant Sisterhood of All Saints of England and acquainted with the system at St. Thomas', who inaugurated the school at Bellevue Hospital. In addition, several Nightingale nurses were imported by Canada.

NIGHTINGALE REFORM

The stimulation to see the need for schools for nurses on the pattern of the renowned Nightingale School in London, in the light of urgency, came from the Civil War, which had exposed the need for better nursing in America, just as the Crimean War had exposed it to England and Europe. The following list of some among the early

American schools based on the Nightingale system, will serve to illustrate the rapidity with which the idea spread, the breadth of geographical area touched, and the scope of a social movement which envisioned service for all the people.

1873—Bellevue Hospital Training School, New York
　　　Massachusetts General Hospital Training School, Boston
　　　Connecticut Training School, New Haven Hospital, New Haven
1874—General Marine Hospital Training School, St. Catherines, Ontario, Canada. Later known as the "Mack Training School"
1875—Montreal General Hospital Training School, Montreal
1879—Spellman Seminary Training School for Colored Nurses, Atlanta, Georgia
1880—Children's Hospital Training School, San Francisco
1881—Toronto General Hospital Training School, Toronto
1884—Blockley Hospital Training School, Philadelphia
1887—Winnipeg General Hospital Training School, Winnipeg
　　　St. Luke's Hospital Training School, Denver
　　　California Hospital Training School, Los Angeles
1888—Mills Training School for Men, Bellevue Hospital, New York
1889—Johns Hopkins Hospital Training School, Baltimore
1890—Royal Jubilee Hospital Training School, Victoria, British Columbia, Canada
　　　Good Samaritan Hospital Training School, Portland, Oregon
1891—Harper Hospital Training School, Detroit, Michigan

Inevitably, the complete story of this development of nursing schools would show deviations from the original plan, and be colored by national or economic circumstance springing from conditions of growth in young lands. Two Nightingale principles were always kept in view. Women, as expert in nursing as the times allowed, were placed in charge of the schools. Courses stressed continued practice in nursing over a long period of time. In the beginning, one year of training was to be followed by one year of practice, supposedly supervised.

As it turned out, America tried and failed to make a successful adaptation of that system of apprenticeship known to the manual arts. It was unfortunate that in these days of imitation the importance of clinical and bedside instruction as stressed by Miss Nightingale was apt to be overlooked. There was a tendency, too, to a let-down, as time went on, in the matter of care in selection of applicants. In the real apprenticeship system the apprentice learns under the personal direction and supervision of a master in an art. He is

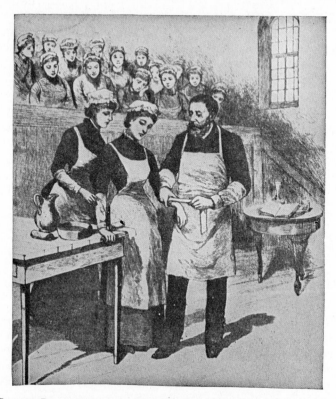

A CLASS IN BANDAGING AT THE PHILADELPHIA GENERAL HOSPITAL ABOUT 1890
(Courtesy of "The Nursing World," February, 1939.)

given time also to observe the master as he works in skilled fashion. In the face of an obvious lack of artists to teach nursing, this was difficult, and a crucial point in nurse education was soon lost. Student nurses in their second year often were given a major share of responsibility for instruction in nursing procedures of first-year students. Schools were organized as departments of hospitals, and, naturally enough, became tools of the institution.

It did not take long, either, for these institutions to recognize the profit in a subsidiary organization that provided more efficient care for patients than had been procurable hitherto, and at surprisingly low cost. The graduate head nurses eventually placed in charge of wards accepted remuneration slightly above that allowance which Miss Nighingale had advised for the student. Students in their second year began also to take special duty cases in and out of the hospital, the hospital augmenting its own funds with the fee charged for their service. It is not strange that student nurses frequently did not complete their course, but, as free-lance nurses, seized an opportunity for themselves in this remunerative field of private duty nursing. There were long days ahead when these mistakes of early days must be paid for. The responsibility which nursing then was forced to shoulder was that of getting schools started that there might be even inadequate response to the sudden public demand for more and more of the new luxury—trained nurses.

Throughout the whole period from 1860 to 1893, the eyes of the world were focused on the Nightingale system of training women for nursing as exemplified in the Nightingale School. British possessions and Protestant countries first sought its help, then came Germany where the empress, a daughter of Queen Victoria, sponsored its reception. Holland followed, but in neither of these countries was there the same need for good nursing that existed in the others. They had deaconesses, Red Cross nurses, Beguines, and others. Catholic countries were well supplied with nursing sisterhoods or brotherhoods. Probably the most extensive movement, and one which ran almost parallel with that in America, began in Australia in 1868.

When it is considered that the city of London alone started eight schools, that the first and natural thought of all who wanted to share in this great reform was to get a Nightingale nurse to show the way, it is clear that the school in such a short time could not supply all the demands upon it. As soon as possible after they were set going, therefore, the young schools sent forth a proportion of their own graduates to shoulder part of the burden of pioneering. This proved to be, in the end, a most desirable way of meeting a problem which entailed not only development of schools, but very often demanded radical personal adjustments to people and surroundings. Inability to meet these demands is thought to have been a chief reason for failure of one of the earliest groups of Nightingale nurses, which eventually returned to England. Unfortunately for the progress of nursing, this maladjustment meant delay and a loss to America of the constructive power represented by trained women. To them had been given an opportunity, perhaps not fully unrealized, to sow seeds for development of an art necessary to a new country. The Montreal General Hospital Training School, which they might have established, grew from a later planting.

Other Nightingale nurses in remote lands had greater success. In 1868 *Lucy Osborn* took to Sydney Hospital, Australia, a group of five nurses. A school was organized and, as the need for their service came to be met by the nurses whom they trained there, these Nightingale nurses, with the help of a few more St. Thomas graduates, raised a line of nursing schools throughout Australia and New Zealand. In Edinburgh, Scotland, *Miss Barclay* and a group of Nightingale nurses reorganized the nursing at the Royal Infirmary. In 1873 *Miss Money*, with the help of two English nurses, successfully organized the Mack Training School in St. Catherines, Canada, and in 1884 *Alice Fisher*, another Nightingale nurse, performed a task of conspicuous difficulty in the establishment of a school for nurses at Blockley Hospital, now the Philadelphia General Hospital.

New York Graduates *Graduates of Bellevue Hospital Training School*. The Bellevue Hospital school in New York was the first to establish itself as an outstanding exponent of the Nightingale plan in America, and this school naturally supplied many pioneers of reformed nursing on this continent. Some of them established schools which they served for many years; others assumed what was to them the more appealing role of traveling reformers who laid foundations for various schools. Outstanding among this brilliant group of Bellevue graduates was *Isabel Hampton*. She had been a young school teacher in Canada when she decided to change her profession. She was only twenty-six years old when, in 1886, she was made superintendent of the Illinois Training School which supplied a nursing staff for Cook County Hospital, Chicago. In this difficult situation, her constructive influence and educational insight brought into effect something that was quite new—a *graded system of theory and practice*. In 1888 she succeeded also in arranging for an *affiliation* by which the course taken by her students could be rounded out to a desirable completeness through experience in care of private patients, although the abuse of special duty which had crept into this and other schools was no longer permitted.

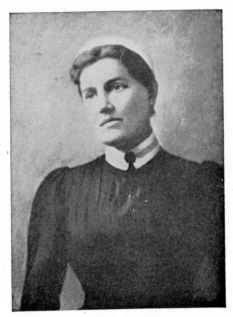

ISABEL HAMPTON ROBB
(League pamphlet, "Nursing Leaders.")

In 1889, Miss Hampton left the Illinois Training School and went to Baltimore to organize a new school in connection with the Johns Hopkins Hospital. It was a thrilling opportunity, for the school, like the hospital, was planned to have a place in America as a model for American institutions. It was to avoid those unfortunate deviations from the Nightingale plan which pressure so far had forced upon American schools for nurses, and was to assume a leadership in nurse education. Significantly, the title chosen for the head of such a school was "Principal," rather than "Superintendent." During her years at Johns Hopkins Training School, Isabel Hampton arranged for a regular period of two-hours' free time during a day which was limited to twelve hours, and which she would have liked to have limited to eight. Definite recreation periods, time allowance for meals, and even the limit placed on a day's work were innovations.

Miss Hampton strove to demonstrate nursing education as a balanced development, intellectual and manual. Women of mental abil-

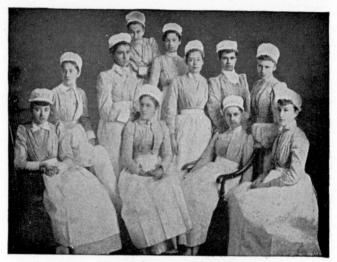

BELLEVUE HEAD NURSES, 1891
(Courtesy of "The American Journal of Nursing," November, 1940.)

ity drew about her as students and as head nurses. Recognizing the dearth of books written especially for nurses, she wrote one which came to be recognized as a standard text in American schools: "Nursing: Its Principles and Practice for Hospital and Private Use." Another text, "Nursing Ethics" followed after Miss Hampton had married Dr. Robb in 1894, and had given up the project which she made so successful. By that time, one of the pupils in her first class at Johns Hopkins was ready to assume her role in American nurse education through the medium of Johns Hopkins model school. This was *Mary Adelaide Nutting*, another young woman from Canada, who went on to establish a course of training preliminary to the actual ward practice. Miss Nutting also succeeded in reducing the student's day to eight hours, in a course lengthened to three years.

When Isabel Hampton was in her second year at Bellevue, another Canadian school teacher arrived to enter the school as a probationer. This was *Mary Agnes Snively*, who, curiously enough, had grown up only a few miles away from the home of Miss Hampton. In 1884, on completion of her course, Miss Snively returned to Canada to

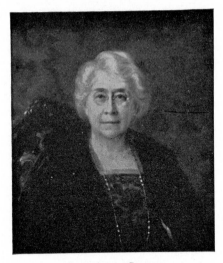

MARY AGNES SNIVELY
(Courtesy of "The Trained Nurse and Hospital Review.")

take charge of the training school for nurses which had been started two years before at the Toronto General Hospital. For twenty-five years from that time, she was destined to carry on the development of this school. From here, she sent trained nurses wherever Canada needed them, for the story of hospital and nursing school growth in the United States was being repeated across the border. At the same time, Miss Snively bore a large share of responsibility for the direction of Canadian nursing organization, and the general advancement of its nursing education.

Another distinguished graduate of Bellevue in these early days was *Lavinia L. Dock*, who held executive positions in Bellevue, was assistant to Isabel Hampton at Johns Hopkins, and Superintendent of the Illinois Training School. It was while she was night superintendent at Bellevue that Miss Dock made time to write a textbook on materia medica. Her whole professional life shows her to have been an adventurer, delighting to get off the beaten path, performing brilliant service in her own way. Not the least brilliant part of this was her joint authorship with Miss Nutting of a standard text on the history of nursing, in four volumes.

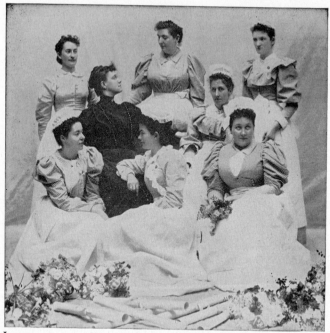

MISS LOVERIDGE AND AN EARLY GROUP OF STUDENTS, GOOD SAMARITAN HOSPITAL,
PORTLAND, OREGON

As early as 1890, the graduates of Bellevue had found their way to communities far from the home school, and *Emily L. Loveridge* had crossed a continent to establish the training school for nurses at Good Samaritan Hospital, Portland, Oregon. Upon arrival, she found herself to be one of three nurses in the city. Her first entering group consisted of five students, for whom she held classes in her room in the evening. For fifteen years, Miss Loveridge remained as head of this school, and then for twenty-five years longer as superintendent of the hospital, leaving behind her an enviable record of achievement.

Jane A. Delano was another school teacher among Bellevue's nurses who leaned toward the excitement of emergency and the far-off unknown. Miss Delano graduated in 1886, saw service with the Red Cross in Florida's epidemic of yellow fever in 1888, and had charge of a mining hospital in Arizona before she settled down to nursing

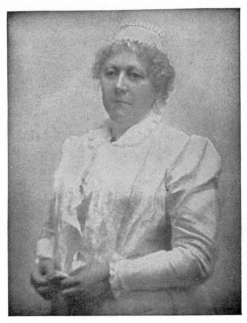

NORA LIVINGSTONE

(From "Pioneers of Nursing in Canada," published by the History of Nursing Society of McGill University, Montreal, under the auspices of the Canadian Nurses' Association.)

education work as superintendent of the training school at the University of Pennsylvania Hospital in Philadelphia. Later she served in similar capacity at her alma mater.

Graduates of the New York Hospital Training School. There was another school in the city of New York which was sending out an almost parallel group of graduates who would gain distinction too, as they helped to lift New World hospitals out of the traditional darkness of their administration and their care of patients. The New York Hospital Training School produced *Nora Livingstone* who, for thirty years after completing her course, guided nursing instruction at the Training School of Montreal General Hospital. At the New York Hospital, too, was graduated *Clara Weeks* (Shaw), author of what was known always as the "Clara Weeks" textbook of nursing, one of America's first, and for many years a favorite.

Two young graduates of the New York Hospital also discovered a new field of pioneering. Thousands of sick people were still without benefit of the new nursing. Where nurses were being trained, institutions had profited by a growth of order and hygiene. The sick within their walls were getting much better nursing than would have been possible only a few short years before. The rich knew the luxury of the trained nurse on private duty. The poor in their homes had little or no nursing although it was fairly customary for hospitals to try to send nurses to them. Thirty years before, in a similar situation, William Rathbone and Florence Nightingale had planned a district nursing service for Liverpool. To carry the skill of the trained nurse where it was still unknown in an American city, *Lillian D. Wald* and her friend, *Mary Brewster*, ventured into New York's slums. In 1893, these two went to live where the poor lived. Their new home on an upper floor of a tenement in Henry Street grew by a very simple process into the Henry Street Settlement, now famous as a center of public health nursing.

The poor brought all sorts of problems besides illness to their kind neighbors, and the nurses tried to solve them as best they could. What they heard and saw, while nursing the sick or sharing the family troubles, taught them the life of the poor man as a whole. They learned to recognize social causes lying behind those bacterial causes that the nursing school and the hospital had brought to their attention. They tried to prevent the things that harmed these unfortunate people, helpless through their complete ignorance of how to protect themselves. The nurses had, indeed, stumbled upon the road to public health, and, from this time on, visiting nursing had a new outlook.

School Nursing. It was natural that school nursing should follow in the wake of visiting nursing, as the latter developed. With knowledge of the plan in operation in England, Miss Wald visited some New York public schools, observing the pupils and conferring with the teachers. She made a report to the health officers concerning the symptoms of communicable diseases that she discovered. A medical inspection of the schools was made soon thereafter, with recognition of the possibilities for improvement through gaining the services of school nurses.

In order to demonstrate what could be done to conserve the health of school children, Miss *Lina L. Rogers*, graduate of the Toronto Hospital for Sick Children, was loaned for a month in 1902, on salary from Henry Street Settlement. So much was accomplished by this capable and tactful nurse during the time allotted that the institution of school nurses on a permanent basis followed. Later, Miss Wald and Miss Rogers were requested to visit schools of other communities to tell them of the experiment, with the result that school nursing was added to the visiting nursing of a number of large cities. School nursing and visiting nursing became, very soon, a wedge for participation by the school and hospital in a social service that reaches into the homes of the school child and the discharged patient, and removes factors in the way of their adjustment to society.

Boston Graduates   Boston as well as New York contributed her share towards supplying leaders for nursing schools. *Linda Richards*, *America's first trained nurse*, interpreted the role of nurse missioner quite literally, and far beyond New England. She carried the Nightingale message west to Kalamazoo, Michigan, and in 1885 to Japan where she founded the first training school for nurses in that country. In all, Miss Richards must have taken opportunity to inject reforms through the medium of nursing into at least twelve important hospitals. Some of these were specialized mental hospitals in which she followed up the work of Dorothea Lynde Dix by organizing nursing staffs, and sometimes, by initiating training schools in which students of mental nursing received a period of training in general hospitals. *Sara Parsons*, graduate of Massachusetts General Hospital and of McLean Hospital for the Insane, carried this idea into mental hospitals along the eastern coast in succeeding years.

From Boston City Hospital Training School in 1874 came *Anna Caroline Maxwell*. Miss Maxwell served in the position of superintendent of training schools for nurses at Montreal General, Massachusetts General, St. Luke's, and Presbyterian of New York. From the last-mentioned school she continued to radiate a helpful influence on nursing affairs for twenty-nine years.

English Graduates   While the pioneers in America were building up schools for nurses, two other young women had taken places

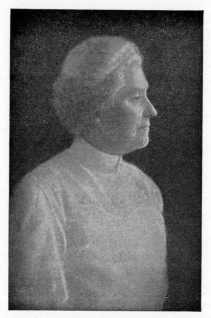

ANNA CAROLINE MAXWELL
(From "Early Leaders of American Nursing," published by the National League
of Nursing Education.)

among leaders of nursing in England. *Mrs. Bedford Fenwick,* start-ing at the early age of twenty-four, had organized in the ancient St. Bartholomew's Hospital of London a school which became sister in importance to the one at St. Thomas'. Mrs. Fenwick was not a Nightingale nurse, but a graduate of the Training School of the Royal Infirmary at Manchester. Then, after six years of building, she resigned to be married. *Isla Stewart,* a Nightingale nurse of 1879, succeeded her. For the next twenty-five years, Miss Stewart was to give generously of many talents, not only to the school at "Bart's" but also to the building of a new profession.

FIRST PRELIMINARY COURSES

In the early days of training schools for nurses, a common criti-cism on the part of their students seems to have been the dearth of instruction. Sometimes it was bedside instruction, sometimes the non-

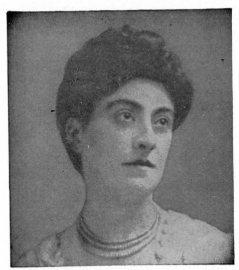

MRS. BEDFORD FENWICK
(Courtesy of "The Trained Nurse and Hospital Review.")

explanation of why things were as they were. Inquiring minds like those of Isabel Hampton Robb or Lavinia L. Dock were apt too often to feel a lack of mental satisfaction in the hurried nursing practice that was theirs. A course of preliminary instruction would have helped, but Kaiserswerth had not been imitated in this respect. It was in 1893 that *Mrs. Rebecca Strong*, a Nightingale nurse of Glasgow, Scotland, devised a plan of having such a preliminary course of instruction given to her students at St. Mungo's Medical College before they entered training. Here, under the same regulations as other college students, they were taught all classroom subjects, and the training which followed was confined to the realm of nursing practice. In 1901, the first preliminary course in America was introduced by Miss Nutting at the Johns Hopkins Hospital in Baltimore. Three years later, Simmons College in Boston undertook a course in sciences applicable to nursing for students preparing to enter the Massachusetts General Hospital Training School for Nurses, Boston. These appear to have been among the very earliest attempts to assure for the infant school of nursing the advantage of methods of general education.

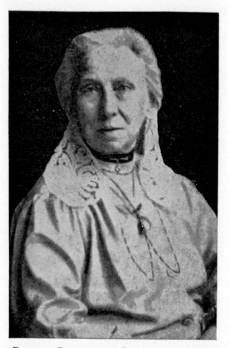

MRS. REBECCA STRONG, THE CENTENARIAN (1843–1944)
Graduated from Nightingale School in 1867. (From American Journal of Nursing,
August, 1927. Also in Nursing Times, May 6, 1944.)

FIRST TEXTBOOKS

Textbooks and manuals of nursing meanwhile were appearing.
The Connecticut Training School published in 1878 "A Handbook
of Nursing" written by a Committee. Bellevue soon had its own
manual. Some that had been written in England after Florence Nightingale's "Notes on Nursing" were also in use. There was a text
available on midwifery, and one on the care of the mentally ill.
There were the texts on Nursing, Nursing Ethics, and Materia
Medica referred to as written by Clara Weeks Shaw, Isabel Hampton
Robb, and Lavinia L. Dock. Huge medical books quite often were
presented to the schools, especially if they were antiquated, and some
ambitious nursing students personally invested in Gray's "Anatomy"
and Osler's "Practice of Medicine." Classroom work, where it

existed, centered around procedures, ethics, anatomy, physiology, materia medica, and hygiene. Schools were extremely individual in teaching method, although in daily routine they were not.

PREVAILING METHODS

Applicants for training were required to show evidence of refinement, youth, and vigor. The preferred age was between twenty-five and thirty-five. Educational requirements were consistent with times when the ideal accomplishments for a woman were a little music, a little painting, and a considerable knowledge of how to adorn herself, charm men, and manage a home. Private schools or convents gave finishing touches to a mother's careful rearing. Public schools, it was feared, might damage a refined personality. The high school was available, a few colleges were opening their doors, but as yet it was mainly the "strong-minded" who sought education beyond that of the grades. A great many students in the nursing schools began their careers as teachers, or had sought to avoid entering this traditional gateway to genteel employment. The schools in distant great cities had a mysterious attraction. To thousands of girls of high intelligence the flight between was toward freedom. It was the first time since the Middle Ages that women of the better classes had left their homes in such numbers to care for the sick.

Students were admitted to the schools, not in classes or in groups, but one at a time, to take the place of graduates as they left the school. Courses covered one year, in many instances, but gradually were lengthened to two, and finally to three years. Some schools were administered by hospitals specializing in the care of one type of patient only, and having a very limited number of beds. Some hospitals were entirely under the control of a small group of people. Accommodations, when provided, as they occasionally were, in a nurses' home, were monastic in simplicity. Emphasis was set on care of the patient and self-sacrificing service on the part of the nurse. The more worn-out her physical appearance, the better she could overlook personal discomfort or fatigue, the nearer did she approach the ideal of a good nurse.

British traditions of discipline were carried to other countries, and the life of the nurse came to be regulated by a curious mixture of military rule and custom inherited from the army and military orders, and combined with a good deal of that asceticism which the monastery fostered. Much deference for authority had to be learned. Youthful or high spirits must be crushed to uniform and unquestioning obedience. The student nurse must *do*. She was not asked or expected to *think*. If she could not learn to take an order, carry it out, and talk not at all when doubts or desire for knowledge overcame her, she went home. If her knowledge of housekeeping failed her, she was apt to take the same road. Punishment for lack of precision in filling medical orders was severe. In America, the nurse who succeeded in graduating was free to follow her own bent, and the private duty field, which attracted her most, expanded more quickly than trained nurses could be found to fill it. The building up of a capable supervisory group for the schools was, consequently, a slow process.

ADOPTION OF UNIFORMS

The military and the religious order did not immediately influence, by their dress, the outward appearance of the new nurse in America. She wore no uniform in the beginning, and, strange to say, was opposed to wearing one. At Bellevue, very early in the history of the school, the authorities were in sympathy with the idea of adopting a uniform mode of dress for motives of economy and cleanliness, as well as for that psychic influence which moves a group in uniform toward loss of self-consciousness and improved morale. As early as 1875, some type of cap was worn in the hospital since the minutes of their Board Meeting of December 1st stated that, ". . . it should be impressed upon our nurses that the caps were intended to cover the hair and not to be simply coquettish ornaments, also that long dresses in the Wards are most objectionable."

Finally, in 1876, it was decided to ask one student to wear the cotton dress proposed, and see what effect her appearance would have on the prejudice of the others. Happily, there was in the school an exceptionally good-looking girl, *Euphemia Van Rensselaer*, member of the socially elect of New York. The matter was broached to her, and she agreed to go home for two days' leave during which she would have a uniform made for herself. When Miss Van Rensselaer came back to the wards, her tall and elegant figure was arrayed in blue and white striped seersucker, with white apron, collar, cuffs, and cap. Of course, all the girls wanted uniforms after that.

Other schools soon wanted uniforms too, and cotton dresses, aprons, cuffs, fichus, caps, took on variety as they became badges of distinction between schools. Until the meaning of the word *uniform* was understood in its literal sense, distinctive individual touches were apt to be added. Prevailing fashions had their influence. A dress common to particular groups of women was often the inspiration for the uniform's design. The garb of Catholic and English Episcopal religious orders, the dress of Quakers and other Protestant sects, Deaconesses—all contributed ideas. The long full skirts were spread out by several layers of starched petticoat beneath them. Frequently they were lined as well to a depth of eighteen inches from the bottom, and for modesty's sake they escaped the floor by not more than two inches. Waists were fitted tightly to the figure, and also lined. The popular apron followed European peasant style, being similar to that worn by Sisters of Charity. It was made of several widths of sheeting gathered into a belt that was sometimes tied behind by a huge bow made of ruffled strings, and had a bib to cover the front of the waist.

The lineage of the cap goes back to medieval, and even to those earlier times when woman's humility and obedience were signified by her assumption of a bridal veil. The nurse's cap was the symbol of her service to humanity. It tried with varying success to fulfill, also, another purpose demanded of it by an age awakening to consciousness of germs. Caps were intended to promote hygienic care of patients by covering up heads adorned with more or less complicated arrangements of hair that might reach far below the waist when let down. In the general absence of the beauty parlor, as known today, hair washing was a long and tedious function, not undertaken oftener than could be helped. What ultimately evolved as the typical American cap bears an interesting resemblance to the one worn by Sister Helen, and the high bib which became so popular appears to be related to her wimple.[13] The cap selected for the Bellevue school, however, and that adopted by the school at the Massachusetts General Hospital are more like the one worn by Nightingale nurses at St. Thomas' Hospital. They savor of Kaiserswerth, British and continental schools, and generally appear to have followed even more

13 See illustration in "A History of Nursing," by Dock and Nutting, Vol. 2, p. 394.

closely traditions inspired by the deaconess and the nun; and the veil in different forms commonly was featured in their headgear.

School uniforms came to be worn in the home by the graduate on private duty. Patient and doctor learned the particular virtues concealed beneath each school costume. Pride in individual achievement lost itself in school pride which gradually assumed an intense form. Inevitably, the barrier raised grew higher, and symbolized itself in devotion to a school uniform which assumed a fixity that made any future modification very difficult. At the same time, the uniform caught the imagination of the public, for the lure of spotless simplicity and soothing uniformity enhanced the lure of the nurse's youthful charm, enthusiasm, and kindly service.

OTHER EVIDENCE OF SOCIAL REFORM

Between 1860 and 1893 the Florence Nightingale reform of nursing and attendant regeneration of hospitals had started in Canada, Australia, New Zealand, Scotland, Ireland, Sweden, Germany, India, Holland, United States, and Japan. It was one among many social reforms that were now beginning to take the place of the lost monastery. All were based on religious ideals, but were outside of church authority. In them women as well as men were taking part, the share assumed by the former being generally important. Many world-wide organizations, existing in great power today, had their origin during this time. Especially was the condition of the poor, dumped and left neglected by industry in its great centers, an incentive to these beginnings of organized social work.

SALVATION ARMY

Outstanding among the new leaders was *William Booth* who began a mission among the poor of London. By 1877, his group of associates became known as the "Salvation Army" and its organization on a military basis went on from that time. By 1893, this army of peace had invaded a goodly part of the world. Under its protection it gathered the poverty stricken, the discharged prisoner, the old, the young, any that were miserable, and those who had fallen from the grace of orthodox living. Its founder wrote a book, "In Darkest England and the Way Out," and raised a sum of money to forward the plan that he had in mind.

SETTLEMENT HOUSES

Other social organizations started and soon were flourishing, each in its chosen area of misery. A typical one of these was the "settlement house" which frequently developed as an offshoot of the university. It was an answer to the interest being taken by the intellectual group in investigating conditions, bringing help or consolation, and trying to find a remedy for distress among the poor in old lands, or the unadjusted alien immigrant to the new land. It was a means of reestablishing the old idea of human brotherhood. *Toynbee Hall* in London was one of these settlement houses which arose to prominence. It was founded as a memorial to a social worker among the poor, and began as a residence for a few students from the neighboring university of Oxford. Under a clergyman director, these young men studied community problems and devoted some time to helping, in whatever way they could, the people who lived in its sordid neighborhood.

It was Toynbee Hall in which *Jane Addams* found answer to a long quest for means to express her own urge to know intimately, and socially uplift, all who were held back by difficulties that might be removed. By 1889, she had found a large house in Chicago which she furnished as her home, then invited all her neighbors to visit. Among these neighbors were representatives of over thirty nationalities—people who clung to their own customs and, at the same time, wanted for their children the education and the opportunity that they felt America had to offer. Many of the mothers worked in factories. Some of them worked for meager pay in their homes. A day nursery, a kindergarten, a library soon answered very obvious needs. In any time of distress there was some remedy to be found at Hull House, and the community learned to look to Miss Addams as its standby. Her settlement, like the one at Toynbee Hall in England, came to be typical of many others developed about this time in America.

Y.M.C.A. AND Y.W.C.A.

Even before the Civil War, another social organization had transferred itself from England across the Atlantic. The *Young Men's Christian Association* had been organized in Canada and the United States. It had also gone into Europe, for Henri Dunant was a member of it, and some of his enthusiasm for humanity is traceable to this influence. The work of the Y.M.C.A. grew in popularity and in efficiency. Character building, body building, recreation, education, relief, sick visiting, employment, gradually took their place among its growing functions. In 1894, a corresponding movement among women culminated in the world's Y.W.C.A.

MEDICAL MISSIONARIES

A unique phase of social work in America which had its beginnings about this time found a setting in Labrador. Here, in a region of icebergs and arctic cold, fishermen and trappers lived with their families under the most primitive conditions. They were English subjects on a far-off frontier; the barren land which they called home attracted no one else. Their lives were passed in such hazardous work, their food supply so uncertain and so unbalanced in quality, that disease no less than accident levied heavy toll among them. They were without any medical care.

In 1892, an English physician who had chosen the missionary field as his sphere of work, procured a small ship, had it fitted up as a hospital, and set out to see what need existed in Labrador for the medical service that he was prepared to give. *Dr. Wilfred T. Grenfell* found work for life-time effort—work that has been appreciated the world over. Beginning with one small hospital, "Grenfell of Labrador" undertook to develop a chain of hospital centers along the coast of Labrador and the northern part of Newfoundland as well. No person in need of care was ever refused for lack of money, and those who could, paid according to their means. Doctors and nurses, as well as college students, gave volunteer service to the Labrador mission. Land travel in winter was made possible through use of dog teams, and in summer the hospitals could be reached by boat. A complete health service to cover physical and spiritual needs was developed as the years went by.

The honor of knighthood made the missionary doctor "Sir Wilfred Grenfell." Always, to him, the need of Labrador stood as a challenge to the "chivalry of the Christ service." The way in which he and his associates met that challenge seemed to a contemporary, "one of the most simple, direct, and vital applications of the Gospel of Christ to human needs that modern times have met."[14]

---

[14] The Challenge of Labrador, p. 15. (A pamphlet issued in 1928 by the International Grenfell Association, Boston, Massachusetts.)

Sir Wilfred Grenfell's work was a part of that great expansion in the foreign missionary field which took place during the latter part of the nineteenth century. Medical missionaries in great numbers were spreading Christian teachings into the heart of India, Africa, China, Japan, and other countries sorely in need of their influence. Hospitals, schools of nursing, and dispensaries were established as pivotal points of friendly contact where nurses and doctors, some of whom were of international reputation, devoted their lives to adding a share toward making the world a better and happier place in which to live.

Salvation Army, settlement houses, Christian associations of young people, missionaries, nursing of the poor in great public hospitals—all these and many others are only examples of a tremendous stirring socially that was going on everywhere. After a Dark Period of more than three hundred years, the idea of human brotherhood was asserting itself again under new forms, and to suit changed ideas of the meaning of a church. Both churches, old and new, were experiencing the need of proving Christianity to be something that was to be lived rather than argued or fought about. Wars, revolutions, religious differences which had kept men bound had also released them. Business grew apace. The west of America was being settled. Transportation was changing. Inventions were increasing. The tide of immigration to the New World from Europe had few restrictions. Hospitals and nursing, of necessity, followed the people to every new frontier.

THE NEW NURSE

The nurse of this period was, typically, a bedside nurse whether in the hospital or in the home. In both fields she gave unstinted devotion to her work, and radiated an unaffected enthusiasm. Hundreds of attractive young girls, immaculate and eager to please, were replacing the Sairey Gamps who had so long held sway. Here and there, too, were head nurses with natural aptness for teaching, who delighted in their ward housekeeping, enjoyed the scope that nursing offered to their ingenuity, and delighted in developing efficient duplicates of themselves. There were superintendents of nurses in the new schools who faced and solved problems without the aid of precedent. A few only of these earnest pioneers have been carried along in historical records, but institutions and local communities had honor in their hearts for many more. Among "career girls" in this transition time, the nurse stood out as particularly attractive. Here was one form of "new woman" who could be loved, who needed not to defend herself against public opinion, and who, in consequence, had nothing masculine about her and was led into no strange forms of behavior. Her virtues were those admired in the old kind of woman, while familiar skills took on a new efficiency under trained hands. Her public lavished praise on her.

It was an age in which the great cobweb of organization, which gathers all into itself today, was in its initial stages. The new woman was showing that she intended to stay to do her part in the world's work, and make use of organization as another tool. It was natural that the next phase of nursing development should see its various groups drawing together in small units for friendly reasons, for consultation, and ultimately, as we shall see, for protection.

MEDICINE ENTERS A REVOLUTIONARY PERIOD

We have seen that, in spite of medical schools and the work of many individual scientists, medicine in its actual practice had so far changed little. Medical men had stumbled on ways of preventing smallpox by inoculation or vaccination, scurvy by avoiding an unvaried diet and by using citrus fruits, or of curing malaria by use of quinine. They did not owe their success in these treatments to scientific method. They did not know what action took place in the body to bring about the effects observed, and, aside from a few specific measures, applied medieval methods to diagnosis and treatment, too. There were favorite cures that covered an amazing number of ailments, treatment of which would vary with their number today.

Sydenham, it is true, had re-directed the doctor's attention to study of symptoms and observation of differences in the pictures of disease. Experience had shown that segregation of some diseased persons permitted healthy persons to remain healthy. There was more accurate knowledge of anatomy and physiology. Many diseases had been described. Individuals here and there gave out ideas on how the microscope might be used to examine tissues, on the value of cleanliness in surgery and midwifery, on military and naval, as well as municipal, hygiene, and even on the prevention of illness, but few had a true scientific basis. Medicine remained cluttered with unscientific practices.

By the middle of the nineteenth century the slow-working leaven of science began to show more clearly. Its precise methods, invading the medical field, brought into common use a number of precision instruments that offered means of accuracy. *The stethoscope, the mercury thermometer, the microscope, and the Roentgen ray* would change the whole face of medical examination and medical care. After 1860 came great scientific minds to make discoveries that set up, for all time, a dividing line between past and present in medicine and surgery.

The pathway toward understanding of causes and means of transfer of contagious diseases was disclosed by a French chemist, *Louis Pasteur* (1822–1895). His conception of living bacteria as the source of infection seized upon professional and popular imagination. The eagerness of both physicians and surgeons for germ elimination contributed toward a change in medicine more rapid than any it had known hitherto. Through experiments with chicken cholera and anthrax, Pasteur also clarified the process of vaccination, and established a principle on which vaccines could be produced for use in preventing disease. His contemporary, *Robert Koch* (1834–1910), a German doctor who spent his spare time with the microscope, discovered the causes of tuberculosis and cholera, and published methods of laboratory technic that enabled him to prove them.

By this time great improvements had been made in travel, and young physicians from the world over gathered at classes conducted by Koch. Science and invention now contributed to more rapid spread of knowledge, when it was discovered, than had been possible in any previous age. Many men followed Pasteur and Koch, and the laboratory became of world-wide use and importance in scientific medicine. Today a new disease no sooner sticks its nose above ground than the laboratory pounces upon it to discover the means by which mankind may be rid of a danger. In these times when humanity is constantly on the move the laboratory has become indispensable, and its benefits reach far places in a short space of time.

Surgery was a field that offered the bacteriologist dramatic possibilities. For long centuries wounds had had close association with death. The germs which the laboratory was busied in disclosing had easy access to the body, for there was little in the treatment of wounds to keep them out. *Lord Joseph Lister* (1827–1912), another contemporary of Pasteur, happened upon a paper written by the latter. He set about finding means to destroy germs while they were still on the hands, instruments, and dressings that came in contact with broken tissues. His method was the use of antiseptics, and on carbolic acid the choice fell. His success marks the beginning of a long line of scientific surgeons, and of the preventive procedure used in operating rooms today. Although asepsis has almost wholly superseded antisepsis, both technics rest on principles established by Louis Pasteur and Joseph Lister.

The treatment of disease was revolutionized speedily as men found out its causes and cooperated in devising means to rout them. After 1880, the germs of many infectious diseases were discovered according to principles laid down by Koch. About 1894, *Emil von Behring* introduced a new principle, that of using serum from immunized animals to prevent diphtheria. The year 1898 saw *Pierre Curie* and his wife, *Marie Curie*, isolating the precious radium now applied to treatment of certain types of cancer. It was the ethical spirit of true science that moved its discoverers to put radium at the service of mankind. No fault of theirs was the accident of commercial monopoly that has hampered the interpretation of this spirit and set the price of radium too high for common use.

Soon after 1900 the responsibility of being transmitters of some of those microorganisms that produce disease was pinned on certain insects. It was proved that yellow fever is transferred by a species of mosquito, and that the common housefly is a source of many dangers. It was logical to investigate the carrying facilities of other insects, so that now it is possible to control even the typhus transferred by the body louse which once, unhampered, carried a trail of epidemics through ages of European history. In 1910 came a cure for syphilis in the form of arsphenamine introduced by *Paul Ehrlich*. This is but a small part of the contribution of science to the advance of medicine. Many, many are the men who have devoted their lives to developing its resources, offensively and defensively, for the service of humankind. Others have been organizing their resources for the science of preventive medicine which, with the help of bacteriology, chemistry, and other laboratory functions, is coming to supersede curative medicine, once the end of medical endeavor. Efforts in this direction have received the encouragement of popular contribution and private wealth.

It was appropriate that the people of France should subscribe to the foundation, in 1888, of an institute for research in application of preventive methods in the control of infectious diseases. Louis Pasteur became director of the *Pasteur Institute*, and thousands of cases of rabies alone have been prevented through this center from which scientific medical knowledge radiates to all the world.

In 1901, millionaire John D. Rockefeller gave to America a corresponding institution which likewise has international significance. *Simon Flexner*, eminent in the field of bacteriology and pathology, as director of this *Rockefeller Institute for Medical Research* was enabled to gather about him men whose names stand for fame in medical science. Human knowledge and protection in the presence of communicable disease were further advanced. Here *Noguchi* made his investigations on syphilis, yellow fever, and trachoma, and *Alexis Carrel* found opportunity to conduct studies of cancer and to develop histology. Other brilliant minds have helped to dispel some of the obscurity that surrounded other infectious diseases or contributed to improvement of laboratory method.

In order to keep up with the sudden change in the tempo of medical events, both Europe and America found it necessary to increase educational facilities for students of medicine. Attempts to reform the schools by introducing higher requirements for education and by requiring better preparation of students who entered them were not lacking. About 1870 public recognition of the problem was secured by organized medicine in America, and in the next twenty years State Boards of Medical Examiners were built up. Still it was hard to make people understand what constituted a good school. Although many were eliminated by failure of their graduates to pass the state examination, and commercial schools were given up as added requirements became too expensive for profit, improvement of remaining schools was slow. What seemed to be needed was a concrete model to go by. A large endowment made it possible to establish, in 1893, the Johns Hopkins Medical School in Baltimore, Maryland, on lines worthy to be followed. Some schools reorganized according to its pattern.

By 1908 the number of medical schools in the United States and Canada had been considerably reduced, and it was decided to grade them in order to have a basis for determining the requirements of a satisfactory school of medicine, and to permit schools to see in what measure they attained these requirements. The Carnegie Foundation commissioned an educator, *Abraham Flexner*, brother of Simon, to make a study of medical schools in the United States and Canada. Mr. Flexner, in his travels, visited one hundred and fifty-five schools, recording his observations. Both good and bad facts were uncovered, with suggestions for improvement, and published in a general report in 1910. Many schools soon closed their doors, and ever since his grading the work of making better medical schools has gone on. Improved buildings, improved facilities for instruction, better instructors, and fewer schools have been the result. The standards of requirement in preliminary preparation of incoming students have been raised, and a long step has been taken toward coordination of school and hospital in the teaching program. The success of this radical move by the medical profession toward self-understanding and self-improvement has especial interest to nurses. Its success, doubtless, influenced similar gradings of nursing schools in the United States, begun under similar provocation only a few years later.

SUMMARY 1860-1893

During the latter part of the nineteenth century considerable progress was made in the development of social agencies that would replace the work of medieval monasteries. The sick benefited through establishment of the Nightingale School at St. Thomas' Hospital in London, by Florence Nightingale, in the year 1860. The guiding principles set by Miss Nightingale were to be careful selection of well-bred young women, a course of training covering a period of either three or four years, and close supervision by well-qualified nurses. There was to be a prescribed course of instruction with lectures, classes, and bedside instruction, and supervision in the nurses' residence as well as in the hospital.

In 1862, with the encouragement and assistance of Miss Nightingale, modern district nursing was inaugurated by William Rathbone in the city of Liverpool, England. It was through Mr. Rathbone's influence, too, that reform in the management and nursing of English workhouse infirmaries came about.

Aware of Miss Nightingale's work in the Crimea, Henri Dunant, a native of Switzerland, directed his energies toward establishment of a neutral society that would render aid to all combatants in time of war. Beginning in 1864, many national Red Cross societies were organized, but it was not until 1882 that one appeared in the United States, through the untiring efforts of Clara Barton. Nevertheless, the functions of such a society were assumed by the Sanitary Commission of the Civil War.

During the early part of the Civil War, nursing services were rendered by Protestant and Catholic Nursing Orders and by many men and women volunteers. Noteworthy among the latter group were Louisa M. Alcott, Clara Barton, and Mother Bickerdyke. In an effort to improve the situation, a course of one month was arranged in several New York hospitals by Dr. Elizabeth Blackwell, first woman graduate of any medical school, and other leaders, to prepare women for army nursing. Later, Dorothea Lynde Dix was appointed Superintendent of Female Nurses by the authorities in Washington, and the regulations set by her for selection of nurses were aimed at securing a group that would give their undivided attention to nursing.

Before the advent of the Nightingale System in the United States, schools of nursing along the new lines were established at the New England Hospital for Women and Children of Boston, and the Woman's Hospital of Philadelphia. The former was modeled after the Kaiserswerth institution, and the latter expressed the ideals of a group of Quaker ladies. Linda Richards graduated from the School of the New England Hospital for Women and Children in 1873, and is known as the "first trained nurse of America." Miss Richards, Miss Waldron, and Sister Helen of England, although not Nightingale nurses themselves, became able organizers and administrators of some of the first schools to be established along Nightingale lines in the United States.

After the close of the Civil War, the women of America assumed a new interest in public affairs. Reform of Bellevue Hospital by a group of these philanthropists was followed by the recommendation that one of the new training schools for nurses would further improve the situation. In 1873, three such schools based on the Nightingale System were established, as follows:

Bellevue Hospital Training School, New York
Massachusetts Hospital Training School, Boston
Connecticut Training School, New Haven

Other schools followed, and soon their graduates were ready to establish similar courses of nurse instruction in other hospitals. The familiar names of many of our nursing leaders appear during this period, as their owners initiated movements that have extended to the present time. It was in 1888 that Isabel Hampton arranged the *first affiliation* in order that her students of Cook County Hospital might learn the care of private patients. The first nursing textbooks and the first uniforms for secular nurses to be used in the United States appeared during this period.

Renowned among early British nurses were Mrs. Bedford Fenwick who as a young graduate became matron of St. Bartholomew's Hospital of London, and Isla Stewart, a Nightingale nurse, who assumed the responsibilities of this position when Mrs. Fenwick married. Mrs. Rebecca Strong, also a Nightingale nurse, is best known for her achievement of instituting the *first preliminary course of instruction* at St. Mungo's Medical College in Glasgow, Scotland, in the year 1893. The first preliminary course in America appeared at the Johns Hopkins Hospital in Baltimore in 1901, under the guidance of Adelaide Nutting.

The young women who were to benefit from the courses of instruction worked out by their early nursing leaders became essentially bedside nurses. They learned to devote their energies conscientiously to the welfare of their patients, and to work long hours in so doing. In the minds of the public, viewing with considerable misgiving those women entering lines held exclusively as man's work, the nurse stood out as particularly feminine and attractive. The skilled service that she was prepared to give was new to them, and great adoration and praise were lavished upon her.

In addition to schools of nursing and Red Cross societies, other social agencies to develop during the latter half of the nineteenth century were the Salvation Army, Settlement Houses, the Young

Men's Christian Association, the Young Women's Christian Association, and Christian missions in foreign lands. Among the last named, the work of Sir Wilfred Grenfell in Labrador stands out as particularly impressive.

Medicine, stimulated by contributions to scientific knowledge made by Pasteur, Lister, Koch, and others, was making revolutionary progress. The stethoscope, mercury thermometer, microscope, and x-ray came into general use as important instruments of diagnosis. The introduction of ether and chloroform as general anesthetics greatly aided the practice of surgery. The modern era of medicine and surgery, based on the science of bacteriology, had been ushered in. It was necessary to devise new technics for the practice of nursing that would be in accord with recent discoveries. More and more well-prepared nurses would be demanded.

The Pasteur Institute and the Rockefeller Institute were established for the advancement of medical science. The Johns Hopkins Hospital was founded in Baltimore, with a large endowment, to serve as a model institution. In 1908, a general survey of medical schools in the United States and Canada resulted in a reduction in their number, and considerable improvement in the standards of those remaining.

TOPICS FOR DISCUSSION

1. (*a*) Where, when, and by whom was modern nursing established?
   (*b*) How was the new school financed?
2. Explain the general principles that Miss Nightingale had in mind when founding this model school for nurses.
3. For what special work were the nurses of the Nightingale School prepared?
4. Name some prejudices of the time that had to be met and overcome.
5. (*a*) What biblical character is credited with being the first district nurse? (*b*) What events led to founding of district nursing of the modern era?
6. Describe the beginning of reform in workhouse infirmaries.
7. (*a*) What experiences of Henri Dunant led him to devote much time and energy to founding of Red Cross societies? (*b*) In what way did Florence Nightingale influence him in this work?

8. Where, and in what year, did fourteen countries first sign the Treaty of Geneva?

9. (a) Compare date of founding the Nightingale School with that of the beginning of the American Civil War. (b) Was it possible for trained nurses for army service to be procured at this time?

10. Compare activities of the Sanitary Commission of the Civil War with those of a national Red Cross society.

11. (a) Discuss the problem of nursing care for soldiers during the Civil War. (b) Name several of the women who gave volunteer nursing service.

12. (a) What influences led to founding of the American National Red Cross? (b) Who is now its president?

13. (a) Why were women of America restless after the Civil War? (b) Name some of the public services in which they engaged.

14. Who is regarded as the first trained nurse of America and where and when did she graduate?

15. Name several women, not Nightingale nurses, but familiar with the Nightingale system, who were of value in founding early schools in America.

16. (a) What "trio of training schools" was founded in 1873 according to the Nightingale plan? (b) Name and locate several other early schools to be established. (c) Collect data in regard to the founding of your school of nursing.

17. Name several outstanding problems of early schools of nursing in America.

18. Give the history of the following:
   (a) First preliminary courses of instruction
   (b) First affiliations in nursing
   (c) First textbooks

19. Trace the transfer of the Nightingale System for training nurses from England to other countries.

20. Make an outline of a number of early nursing leaders, with their schools and outstanding achievements.

21. Where, when, and by whom was district nursing introduced into America?

22. How does district or visiting differ from public health nursing?

23. (a) Where, and by whom, was the first nurse's uniform worn in

America? (*b*) Discuss the advantages and disadvantages of wearing a uniform.

24. (*a*) What were the entrance requirements of nursing schools in the late nineteenth century? (*b*) At what times did new students enter, and how long was the course?

25. Describe the "new nurse" of the time.

26. How did the new type of nurse agree with the popular conception of the "new woman"?

27. Name a number of social agencies other than nursing that showed rapid development in this period between 1860 and 1893.

28. (*a*) What revolutionary changes were taking place in the practice of medicine? (*b*) Show how they inevitably affected the practice of nursing.

REFERENCES

Alcott, Louisa M.: Hospital Sketches. Cambridge, Mass., University Press, 1869.

Baker, Nina Brown: Cyclone in Calico. (Mother Bickerdyke). Boston, Mass., Little Brown and Co., 1952.

Baker, Rachel: The First Woman Doctor (Elizabeth Blackwell). New York, Julian Messner, Inc., 1944.

Boardman, Mabel T.: Under the Red Cross Flag at Home and Abroad. Philadelphia, J. B. Lippincott Co., 1915.

Breckinridge, Mary: Wide Neighborhoods: A Study of the Frontier Nursing Service. New York, Harper and Brothers, 1952.

Cooke, Sir Edward: A Short Life of Florence Nightingale. New York, The Macmillan Co., 1925.

Dock and Nutting: A History of Nursing. New York and London, G. P. Putnam's Sons, 1907, Vol. IV.

Dock and Stewart: A Short History of Nursing, 4th edition. New York and London, G. P. Putnam's Sons, 1938.

Dubos, Rene J.: Louis Pasteur: Free Lance of Science. Boston, Little Brown and Co., 1950.

Dunant, Henri: "Un Souvenir de Solferino," translated from the French by Mrs. David H. Wright, The Origin of the Red Cross. Philadelphia, The John C. Winston Co., 1911.

Epler, Percy H.: Life of Clara Barton. New York, The Macmillan Co., 1927.

Goodnow, Minnie: Outlines of Nursing History. 8th edition, Philadelphia, W. B. Saunders Co., 1948.

Gumpert, Martin: Dunant: The Story of the Red Cross. New York, Oxford University Press, 1938.

Nightingale, Florence: Florence Nightingale to Her Nurses. London, The Macmillan Co., 1914.

———: Notes on Nursing. New York, D. Appleton & Co., 1929.

Pavey, Agnes: The Story of the Growth of Nursing. London, Faber and Faber, 1938.

Pennock, Meta Rutter: Makers of Nursing History. New York, Lakeside Publishing Co., 1928.

Richards, Linda: Reminiscences of Linda Richards. Boston, Whitcomb & Barrows, 1924.

Seymer, Lucy Ridgely: A General History of Nursing. New York, The Macmillan Co., 1949.

Seymer, Lucy Ridgley: Florence Nightingale. New York, The Macmillan Co., 1951.

Trattner, Ernest R.: Architects of Ideas (Louis Pasteur and others). New York, Carrick & Evans, Inc., 1938.

Woodham-Smith, Cecil: Florence Nightingale. New York, McGraw-Hill Book Company, 1951.

Woolsey, Abby Howland: A Century of Nursing (1876 report edited by the N.L.N.E.). New York, McGraw-Hill Book Co., 1951.

Group Consciousness Develops with Growth of Schools

1893-1920

The latter part of the nineteenth century was one in which a long-evident tendency for society to draw together once more into small units showed gathering speed. Support had slipped away with the patriarchal rule of feudal lords, guilds, and church. Sectarian grouping had not restored it, while changing times and individualism were bringing new reasons for wanting companionship or protection. An expanding and ever more crowded world made necessary the getting together of those who had interests in common, and encouraged personal or group ambitions. Although *clubs*, even among women, had existed for a long time, the club as a social movement began now. All kinds of organized units sprang into being—industrial, professional, social—many of them devoted to the uplift of those whom industry had trodden down.

After the Civil War, women of the United States were very eager to secure for themselves greater opportunities for professional education, for positions in trade and industry, for equality with their men. Even before the war, they had discovered the relationship between voting power and such advancement. By 1865 women's suffrage was also a national movement. The importance of women's clubs as units of their organization became more and more apparent. By 1889 the strength of these units scattered over one nation was consolidated in a *General Federation of Women's Clubs*. Logically, the young profession of nursing would be influenced by these trends toward grouping which affected other countries as they did the United States.

The need for concerted action among nurses was felt in England first. Here, as in America, the schools were growing up in isolation from one another. No bond was felt other than the common purpose of developing Miss Nightingale's plan for giving a better type of nurse to the sick. No legal difference had been established between the new nurse and the old. The educational basis of distinction between them had not been defined by accepted standards of curriculum. The result showed in exploitation of the public by women who claimed to have had training when they had not, and the recognition of trained and untrained on equal footing by hospitals. It was *Mrs. Bedford Fenwick* who, in 1887, proposed an association of trained nurses. The purpose of this *Royal British Nurses' Association* was to bring together all trained nurses for protection of their interests, to promote measures for improvement of training, and ultimately to have graduates of nursing schools registered by the government as educated, skilled workers of definite, officially accepted preparation. In less than a decade, a group of nurses working in opposition to this registration movement nullified efforts to bring it about. To this group Miss Nightingale gave her sympathy. Nursing, to her was a calling, and could not be regulated by law. It was in 1894 that the *Matrons' Council of Great Britain and Ireland* was organized, and Isla Stewart became its first president.

On the other side of the Atlantic corresponding trends toward grouping of nurses were to be observed. Individual schools interpreted, in their own way, the general outline of the Nightingale plan and brought considerable variance into the constituents of a nurse's training. Isabel Hampton (Robb), endeavoring as she was to arrange a model curriculum for a model school which would be as a light for others to follow, had been disturbed by the lack of uniformity in their conception of nursing among the head nurses that came to her from different schools. To a few like her, the need for a move toward attaining similarity of training courses for nurses was apparent.

GROWTH OF NURSING ASSOCIATIONS

New World Organizations   The earliest organization of New World nurses took the form of the *alumnae association*, which arose from the simple need of companionship. If she assumed charge of another training school when she left her own, the graduate, whether in Canada or the United States, was likely to move far, and work alone. If she became a private duty nurse, even in the same city as her alma mater, there was no bond to hold her to old and pleasant associations. She was a free lance, and she was alone. In 1888 the Training School of the Woman's Hospital in Philadelphia formed an alumnae association, Bellevue followed with one in 1889, the Illinois Training School of Cook County Hospital in Chicago in 1891, the Johns Hopkins in 1892, the Massachusetts General Hospital in 1895, and the Boston City Hospital in 1896.

About this time, there occurred an event of international moment which ultimately was to cement trained nurses of old and new worlds in professional union. Civilization had been moving west and, to celebrate its astounding development, the city of Chicago undertook to hold a World's Fair. This was in 1893, and the Fair buildings, significantly, were to include a Woman's Building. Among exhibits in this building was to be one arranged by the nurses of Great Britain, and placed by them under the charge of Mrs. Bedford Fenwick. Naturally, Mrs. Fenwick was interested in meeting other trained nurses wherever they might be, and was thoroughly aware, too, that the difficulties which had induced organization in England were likely to affect those of other lands.

Mrs. Fenwick suggested to World's Fair officials that there be a space provided in the Woman's Building for American nurses to meet. She also planned her own trip so that she might travel by way of Baltimore and make the acquaintance of Isabel Hampton at the Johns Hopkins Hospital. The upshot was that a nursing section was arranged at the Fair in connection with a group meeting of people interested in hospitals and dispensaries. Eighteen superintendents of training schools gathered to discuss their problems, and Miss Hampton was made chairman of the section. The facts elicited showed a need of united effort to keep the standard of work done in training schools as uniformly high as possible. A definite established course of instruction formulated by the educators for all the schools was indispensable toward this end. To work out such a course, discussion and planning would be required and it would be necessary to get together the nurses in charge of schools.

To this end, a private meeting of superintendents was arranged, and held after the convention ended. At this meeting, initial steps were taken toward organization, and a committee appointed to draft a constitution. *The American Society of Superintendents of Training Schools for Nurses* came into existence in 1893, and included nurses from the United States and Canada. In 1907 the Canadians withdrew to form their own association, the *Canadian Society of Superintendents of Training Schools*, with Mary Agnes Snively as first president. In the beginning, only those at the heads of schools of large, general hospitals were admitted, but later on the policy became more liberal.

Since their beginning in 1888 the alumnae associations had been spreading themselves over the United States and Canada. Their influence would remain a restricted one unless they found a way to work together for the nurses of their respective countries rather than for the graduates of their respective schools. In 1896 the tide of consolidating organization reached them, and under the guidance of Sophia Palmer and Isabel Hampton Robb they bound themselves together in the *Nurses' Associated Alumnae of the United States and Canada*. This group, too, had a policy of excluding graduates of small or special hospitals, but later found that their work would be more effective if it covered a larger field. The two countries functioned together in this association for the next twelve years. These various groupings of women were responsible for producing skilled nurses to protect the public from the unskilled, and mark the beginning of setting up standards which could be made a legal distinction between them.

International Council of Nurses   Nurses of Great Britain, Canada, and the United States by now were reaching a national viewpoint on their affairs. Finland, in 1898, and Australia and Denmark achieved the same end through their new national councils. Holland and Ireland followed in 1900, Germany in 1903, and New Zealand, China, and Cuba in 1909. National associations of Sweden and India were organized in 1910, that of Norway in 1912, and South Africa in 1914. The evolution of ideals in organization going on within the woman movement helped them to the attainment of a still broader ideal. Women in different countries already had gathered together as members of national councils, of the numerous clubs and associations that we have seen them forming. These national councils had combined to form an *International Council of Women*. Its delegates carried back to their respective clubs news of woman's progress in many fields besides their own. Through her club's membership in a national organization which was affiliated with an international one, the individual woman learned prevailing trends in her own and other women's affairs.

In 1899 this International Council of Women was to hold a meeting in London. At this meeting, nurses from different countries were present. Mrs. Bedford Fenwick was one who saw the advantage to nursing of its representative organizations being grouped similarly in international federation. She placed the idea at once before the Matrons' Council of Great Britain. Representatives from those countries where nurses were organized were formed into an executive committee to arrange a plan by which an *International Council of Nurses* might be formed. Before 1899 was over they had it ready. Two years later, the International Council of Nurses met for the first time at the World Exposition in Buffalo, New York, and Mrs. Bedford Fenwick was elected president.

Membership was not yet through national associations, but individual, and so it remained until the Congress in Berlin, Germany, in 1904. After that, national associations of nurses constituted the membership, which numbers about thirty at the present time.

Organization in nursing now had a substantial framework on which to build, and the building has gone on ever since. It continued immediately with the establishment in England of groups of nurses corresponding to the alumnae associations in America. These began in 1899 under the sponsorship of the Matrons' Council. The first to form such organizations were the graduates of St. Bartholomew's and those of St. John's House. In 1904, these alumnae associations were affiliated in the *National Council of Nurses of Great Britain and Northern Ireland*, which is the British nurses' representative in the International Council of Nurses. Mrs. Bedford Fenwick became once more the first president, and, consequently, the chief motive power of this new organization.

The year 1908 marks the formation of a *National Association of Colored Graduate Nurses*, an organization separate from the American Nurses' Association by request of a group of nurses who felt that by working alone they could further the nursing cause and their own special interests more readily. And so it has gone on in all countries to which the flow of nursing organization penetrated, and difficulties of one kind or another have been met. In England, especially, where doctors and hospitals were intent on maintaining their control over nurses, the opposition was particularly strong.

It is necessary to learn to distinguish between the professional type of organization into which nurses had begun to gather, and a corresponding movement that was evidence of grouping among industrial workers. Labor unions had replaced the ancient guilds, their mode of organization and their ideals developing under the influence of the Industrial Revolution. The union aimed at exacting from industry shorter hours, increased pay, and better working conditions for its members. The professional organization, on the other hand, aimed to give ever better service to the public through constant improvement in methods of education for service, together with protection of public, doctor, and nurse from invasion of its field by unqualified workers.

When the professional organization takes hold of similar problems of shorter hours, increased pay, and better working conditions, it sees these as contributing factors in the solution of that greater problem of improving its social service. This service, in the final analysis, must depend on the professional fitness of individual nurses, an ideal unattainable without health, professional growth, and that financial security which is a deep-felt human need.

First Journals and Registration   In America there was felt a need for a journal to establish a means of communication between scattered groups of nurses, and interpret the activities of the Nurses' Associated Alumnae to the public. On October 1, 1900, the first copy of the *American Journal of Nursing* appeared, under the editorship of *Sophia Palmer*, a graduate of the Massachusetts General Hospital and, at that time, superintendent of the Rochester City Hospital. Individual nurses and alumnae associations bought shares of stock to finance the enterprise, and interested nurses donated their services to keep it going. Serving as editor until her death in 1920, Miss Palmer was succeeded by *Mary M. Roberts*, who maintained and then gradually raised the already high standards of the journal until 1949 when she was made Editor Emeritus. Representative of the

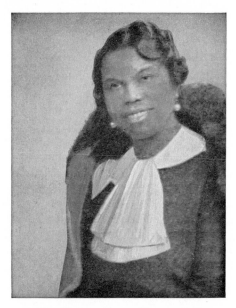

MRS. ESTELLE MASSEY RIDDLE, R.N.
Active in organization work among Negroes. (American Journal of Nursing.)

nursing associations of Great Britain and Canada are the two official organs, the *British Journal of Nursing* established in 1893, and the *Canadian Nurse* established in 1907.

The new magazines were begun while national associations were in the midst of a struggle to protect the public and the nurse from unqualified workers. The first journals gave considerable space to a proposed program of legislation, chief objectives of which were to improve the actual practice of nursing and, by improving educational standards, to raise nursing to the level of a profession. Opposition was surprisingly strong, even though *Cape Colony, South Africa, had succeeded in passing the first law requiring registration as early as* 1891. Throughout the United States the formation of state societies lent dignity and strength to the campaign.

The first *state* to enact a registration law was North Carolina in 1903. The first province of Canada to obtain registration was Manitoba, in 1915; but it was not until 1919, after a struggle commonly

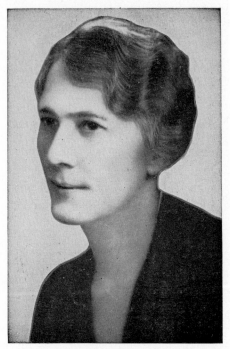

MARY M. ROBERTS
Editor Emeritus, American Journal of Nursing.

referred to as the "Thirty Years' War," that the nurses of England could get a law to regulate their practice. Wherever adopted, registration has had positive results, among them the accrediting of, and a movement toward uniformity in, nursing schools.

WARS OF LATE NINETEENTH CENTURY

Two wars now intervene to add their influence to the trend of nursing development. They brought another type of organization, that of practicing nursing in groups to increase efficiency. In army nursing, this system now replaced the old system of dependence on the work of individual nurses. Early in 1898 the United States entered upon the Spanish-American War; late in 1899 Britain began her war against the Boers of South Africa. The soldier of either nation had a better chance for good care than had been his in previous wars. National Red Cross Societies stood ready to assist both armies, although in the United States the weight of organization stood on the side of disaster relief. The United States, Britain, and her Dominion of Canada had schools in which nurses were being trained and through which skilled graduates could be secured. None of these countries, however, was wholly aware of its opportunity in this respect, or of the fact that nurses could be reached through their associations, the Royal British Nurses' Association of England, and the Nurses' Associated Alumnae of the United States and Canada. Epidemic disease, especially typhoid, turned out to be the particular scourge of the armies, and one which demanded an unusually large number of nurses to combat it.

NURSING IN THE SPANISH-AMERICAN WAR

In the early days of the Spanish-American War, care in selection of nurses was inadequate. The volunteer nursing group represented the trained, the partly trained, and the untrained, and men as well as women. There was confusion arising from the fact that system was lacking in supplying them, and a condition of emergency arose which forced itself upon the attention of both government and people. The latter were loud in their demands for better care of troops. The Nurses' Associated Alumnae of the United States and Canada was disturbed by avoidable conditions, and took them under its consideration at an annual meeting. In bringing these conditions before the members, the president, Mrs. Isabel Hampton Robb, suggested that the society offer itself to the government as the agent through which more and skilled nurses might be reliably secured. When, however, she and another official had been empowered to visit Washington for this purpose, they were disappointed to find the department of army nursing already under the direction of the Daughters of the American Revolution. This society had chosen as director of the service a successful young woman physician, *Dr. Anita Newcomb McGee*, who was busy with the enrollment of nurses, and was setting up her own standards for their selection. Fortunately, in addition to the requirement of recommendations as to health and character, she insisted upon a certificate of graduation from a training school for nurses. The nurses thus chosen were given over to the Red Cross which assisted with their expenses while in service. This system of cooperation between Army and Red Cross held for the remainder of the war.

Several superintendents of training schools volunteered to share in the organization of camp nursing, among them *Anna C. Maxwell*, who had leave of absence from the Presbyterian Hospital in New York. Miss Maxwell was made Chief Nurse at the camp hospital of Chickamauga Park, Georgia—one in which the nursing situation offered very difficult problems, not the least of which was the fact that fourteen of her nurses contracted typhoid fever. Her own description gives some insight into the causes of these difficulties and shows how they bore comparison with those encountered by Miss Nightingale about forty years earlier:

"The laundry work for the camp was contracted for by a firm in Chattanooga, and so little conception had they of the work before them, that they sent a boy with a mule and cart to remove a tent full of soiled linen. I personally listed these clothes (over eight hundred pieces), the condition of which was indescribable.

"Only one pound of carbolic was found, chloride of lime was secured at Chattanooga, and linen was much damaged by its use. The trenches between the tents, and the ground, saturated with typhoid bacilli, where the buckets stood, were finally disinfected, but not until the entire camp has been exposed to the infection from the millions of flies that gathered about these spots."[1]

NURSING IN THE SOUTH AFRICAN WAR

In South Africa, as in the United States, war had emphasized the need for greater preparedness for efficient army nursing through permanently organized groups of nurses, certified as to character, health, and experience, selected from the ranks of those trained in the schools. The Boer War had drawn into it contingents of Canadian soldiers and Canadian nurse volunteers who went to assist the British Army Nursing Service, which had been organized in 1881 as a result of Crimean experience, coupled with the post-war efforts of Miss Nightingale. These nurse volunteers for South African service were assembled under the direction of *Georgina F. Pope*. On their return, the Canadian Government gave them placement on a Reserve list in the active militia, and from this beginning, Canada, too, built up a *Permanent Army Medical Corps Nursing Service. When, in 1904, she*

[1] Quoted in "A History of Nursing" by Dock and Nutting, 1907, Vol. III, pp. 207–208. G. P. Putnam's Sons, New York and London, publishers.

also gave to these first reserve nurses the relative rank of "Lieutenant," she was the first country to accord military rank to women. Miss Pope ultimately was awarded the relative rank of "Captain."

The bestowal of rank on nurses proved to be a move of high importance. Rank in armies is a system of designating the position and power to command of its holder. Without it, the nurse could be classed only with the private soldier, and had no authority to direct his work on the wards where he served as orderly. With it, she could be assured that her directions in regard to care of patients would be carried out, not only by him, but, when necessary, by those non-commissioned officers whose status was relatively below her own.

Britain also had learned that it did not do to depend on any set number of army nurses to meet the exigencies of war, and reorganized her Army Nursing Service to include a Red Cross reserve that could be called upon in an emergency. The name was changed to that by which it goes today, *Queen Alexandra's Royal Army Nursing Corps.* The United States, Canada, and Britain henceforth looked to their Red Cross and their nursing schools to supply an efficient nursing service in time of war.

ARMY AND NAVY NURSE CORPS ESTABLISHED

After the Spanish-American War was ended, leading nurses all over the country began to use their influence to procure legislation that would ensure an efficient army nursing service—one that would not limit itself to wartime emergency but would be effective also in times of peace. Women who had been prominent in relief work met with committees from the American Society of Superintendents of Training Schools and the Nurses' Associated Alumnae of the United States and Canada. A joint committee was chosen to draw up a bill for the establishment of an *Army Nurse Corps*, to be presented to Congress. After many difficulties had been overcome, the bill was passed in 1901, outstanding among its sponsors being Dr. Anita Newcomb McGee, Isabel Hampton Robb, Anna C. Maxwell and Adelaide Nutting. To the ability of the latter as chairman was due, in great part, this final success. In 1908, following the example of the army, a *Navy Nurse Corps* was established.

AMERICAN RED CROSS NURSING SERVICE ESTABLISHED

What had thus far been accomplished was provision of a staff of nurses to serve the army and navy during times of peace. This was only a preliminary step. It took no account of the elasticity which an Army Nurse Corps and a Navy Nurse Corps would require to show to meet the emergencies inseparable from war. By this time, the new nursing organizations had had an opportunity to learn the power inherent in united effort, and to understand the value of a recognized position for the trained nurse in public service. They did not stop, but began to work towards an affiliation with the national Red Cross Society, which had demonstrated its efficiency as a medium of enrollment when additional nurses were needed. Meantime, affairs moved toward a complete reorganization of the Red Cross.

Mabel T. Boardman, a resident of Washington and later the author of "Under the Red Cross Flag," took active part in outlining plans for the policies to be embodied in the new charter of 1905. Miss Boardman was an authority on Red Cross organization, having given much time to its study at home and abroad. She was in sympathy with the nurses' movement to establish a *nursing service* as one of the needed reforms. About this time, Mrs. Robb was enabled to bring before the Red Cross a plan representing the ideas of the nurses' associations and herself for development of a *nursing department within the Society*. This department would enroll, through the office of the Director of such a nursing service, a nursing staff adequate to meet the demands of any emergency. The volunteer system would give way to a system providing salaries.

Unfortunately, the plan seemed too costly to be undertaken immediately, and it was laid aside. However, *Jane A. Delano*, who was then Superintendent of the Army Nurse Corps, proved herself a valuable coordinator of Army, nursing, and Red Cross interests when, in 1909, she decided to devote herself wholly to the work of the Society. To Miss Boardman she confided the idealistic motive that prompted this decision,

"I have a little means of my own, and I would rather serve the Red Cross than do anything else in the world. I will gladly give my services to the Red Cross if it desires them, to organize and develop its nursing department."[2]

[2] Official History of American Red Cross Nursing, 1922, p. 97. By permission of The Macmillan Company, New York, publishers.

Miss Delano, in a service which ended with her death in France at the close of World War I in 1919, did not receive a salary. Under her capable administration, the *American Red Cross Nursing Service* developed step by step, and in close harmony with the ideas of Mrs. Robb and the Associated Alumnae. Everything was done to make clear to all nurses her aim of building up, by enrollment through the office of the Red Cross Society, a list of those ready to serve their country in time of war or other disaster. Qualifications would be set to determine acceptance, the accepted nurses would continue with their regular work until needed, *would not be compelled to give service*, and when on duty with the Red Cross would be paid a salary. This method of maintaining a roll adequate to meet any emergency was in force until late in World War II; when full responsibility for recruitment and maintenance of a Reserve Nurse Corps was assumed by each of the federal nursing services. The Red Cross continues to enroll nurses, but it is now for service with the Red Cross itself.

ADVANCED EDUCATION FOR NURSES

An early opportunity to demonstrate the usefulness of their organization, as well as its professional quality, came to the nurses of America about the time of the Spanish-American War. There was growing dissatisfaction with the haphazard trend of nursing education. Apparently, only two attempts had been made to link the nursing school with an institution of higher learning. In Scotland, Mrs. Strong's arrangement with a college, in 1893, was for a preliminary course only. About the same time, the University of Texas established a university hospital with the nursing school as part of the medical department, although it was not placed on a strict university basis. These college courses were designed solely to meet the needs of student nurses.

In 1898, the American Society of Superintendents of Training Schools for Nurses decided that the problem was one the solution of which depended on advanced education of the graduate nurse. Just as was the custom in the field of general education, so, in the nursing field, special preparation should be expected of those nurses who were responsible for the education of students in hospital schools. A committee, on which Mrs. Robb served as chairman and Miss Nutting as one of the members, found that a promising ar-

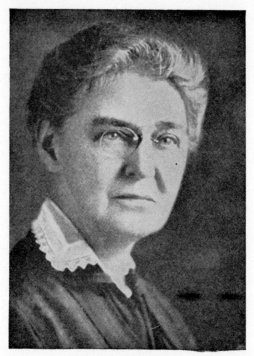

M. Adelaide Nutting
(Courtesy of "The American Journal of Nursing.")

rangement for this instruction of the graduate nurse might be made with the new Teachers College at Columbia University, New York City. Here, regular courses in psychology, science, and household economics would be made available to students accepted through the Society, while such special courses as dealt with nursing school and hospital work would be financed by the Society of Superintendents. The step was taken, and, in 1899, a course in *hospital economics* was offered. Mrs. Robb, Miss Nutting, and a promising young graduate of the New York Hospital, *Annie W. Goodrich*, and others lectured on special subjects, often without remuneration. Two students formed the first class.

Growth was seen in the gradual addition of courses and students. In 1907 Miss Nutting resigned from her position of Superintendent

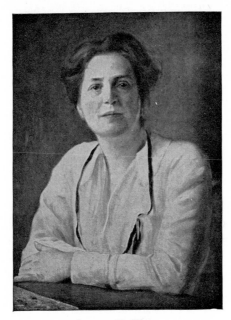

LILLIAN D. WALD

of Nurses at the Johns Hopkins Training School for Nurses, to give her full time to developing this first school for graduate nurses. The College honored her with a professorship, the first to be held anywhere by a nurse. Other illustrious nurses were added to the teaching staff, including Lillian D. Wald of Henry Street and *Clara D. Noyes*, a graduate of Johns Hopkins. Miss Goodrich became an assistant professor. By 1909, Miss Nutting needed an assistant, and *Isabel M. Stewart*, a Canadian graduate of the Winnipeg Hospital and also a graduate of Teachers College, came to fill this position. Miss Stewart was able to arrange special courses for nurse teachers, but it was even then apparent that courses would be needed for visiting nurses, head nurses, and other specialists appearing in the nursing field. The need for financial assistance was met by Mrs. Helen Hartley Jenkins, a trustee of Teachers College, who endowed the department to the amount of two hundred thousand dollars.

Time has proved the judgment of the members of the Society of Superintendents to have been wise. The vital factor in improving edu-

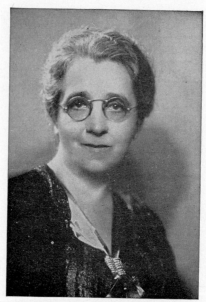

ISABEL M. STEWART
(Photograph by G. Maillard Kesslere.)

cation has been shown to be the educator, and results of the work done at Teachers College to prepare the educator for her task are to be seen all over the world. By 1919 its graduates had gone home to make practical application of their wider knowledge and to demonstrate its usefulness in England, Canada, Denmark, Finland, Japan, India, Germany, the Philippines, Puerto Rico, France, and Italy. The influence of the college department that started with two ambitious students in 1899 has been international.

The principle of giving the student in the nursing school an *education* designed to fit her for giving good nursing to the public has been used to displace the overemphasis once placed on practice. Her increasingly intelligent work has improved the status of nurses generally, and brought them greater opportunity with greater satisfaction in their work. The Department of Nursing Education at Teachers College has led the way to "a broader conception of nursing as an art which requires intelligence, knowledge, and social vision, as well as a high degree of practical skill, and which includes the prevention of disease as well as the care of the sick, the nursing of the community as well as of the individual, and the nursing of the mind as well as of the body."[3] Oftentimes, its graduates have been called upon to develop corresponding departments in universities of the United States and Canada, and even farther afield.

The plan of raising the level of teaching in nursing schools through collective opportunity bore early fruit. Mrs. Robb had hardly dared to consider as more than a dream the possibility of some day seeing students of nursing accepted on the level of college students, and taught in college classes. As early as 1909, however, a brief ten years since it had been made possible for graduate nurses to enter Teachers College, nurses in training in one school were being placed on a college level. The University of Minnesota, under the leadership of *Dr. Richard Olding Beard*, was first to institute a plan by which nurse education became a branch of college work. Thus, a new emphasis was placed on knowledge. In the years following this radical move, in line with the thought of Mrs. Robb and progressive co-workers in the nursing field, many and varying types of university affiliation have been brought about.

Nursing had thus made considerable progress in its first fifty years. It was not behind those varied humanitarian efforts which had influenced so much the life and work of Florence Nightingale. Her girlish choice among them all was bearing fruit with the others, and she, by this time, had seen more than ninety years of life. On August 13, 1910, she passed away, and by her own wish was laid to rest in the churchyard of St. Margaret's, East Wellow, near her old home at Embley Park, although England gladly would have placed her with those whose fame gives reason for their burial in Westminster Abbey. Monuments have been built to her memory in her own country, in Florence, Italy, where she was born, and in far distant places as well. The nurses of the world through their International Council proposed, as a living memorial, some form of nursing education work that would bring to all peoples, through their nurses, the treasure of ever better nursing. This was done in 1912, on the instance of Mrs. Bedford Fenwick, seconded by Miss Nutting, but years were to pass before a plan for an international graduate school was completed.

3 Teachers College Bulletin, February, 1926, p. 3.

As Miss Nightingale's life was coming to a close, a period of new developments in nursing organization was opening. In Canada and the United States, nursing groups were reorganizing, forming plans to set professional standards and improve existing methods of nursing education. In 1907 the American Society of Superintendents of Training Schools divided into two groups, one eventually to become the *Committee on Institutional Nursing of the Canadian Nurses' Association*, and the other, whose province was the United States, the *National League of Nursing Education*. Both continued to work for improved methods of instruction in their respective countries. An alteration of rules of the National League of Nursing Education permitted the membership of those who served in any teaching capacity in a school of nursing, directors in public health work, members of State Boards of Nurse Examiners, and others actively concerned with education. Its curriculum for schools of nursing, first published in 1917 under the leadership of Mary Adelaide Nutting, afforded a new basis for educational standards.

In 1908 legal complications which interfered with the smooth functioning of the Nurses' Associated Alumnae of the United States and Canada induced the Canadians to withdraw and form their own *Canadian Nurses' Association*. The remaining group, with a membership no longer restricted to alumnae, adopted in 1911 the title of *American Nurses' Association*, and persisted in its efforts to support legislation affecting the profession.

In the United States, a pioneer organization in the field of visiting nursing was the *National Organization for Public Health Nursing*, founded, like the League, in 1912. Its first president, Lillian D. Wald of Henry Street Settlement, was already famous for her interest in community health and social uplift. Under her direction the new association laid down a broad program of action. It undertook, first of all, to draw into itself the increasing numbers of those who were filling the demand for a new type of nursing. It arranged for special courses in Public Health Nursing, set up standards, and stimulated group interest in this rapidly-expanding field.

In the United States there were, therefore, three major national associations, the American Nurses' Association, the National League of Nursing Education, and the National Organization for Public Health Nursing. The single Canadian Nurses' Association, made up of three Service Committees: the Committee on Institutional Nursing, the Committee on Private Duty Nursing, and the Committee on Public Health Nursing, carried on activities corresponding to those of the three separate associations in the United States. The history of this organization and reorganization may be expressed in outline form as follows:

1. *The American Society of Superintendents of Training Schools* was founded in 1893, separated into Canadian and American groups in 1907, the latter taking the name of *National League of Nursing Education* in 1912.
2. *The Nurses' Associated Alumnae of the United States and Canada* was founded in 1896, separated into Canadian and American groups in 1908, the latter taking the name of *American Nurses' Association* in 1911.
3. *The National Organization for Public Health Nursing* was founded in 1912.

NURSING DURING WORLD WAR I, 1914-1918

Events in Europe were creating the great occasion to test the workability, under strained conditions, of modern developments in nursing. Precipitation of World War I occurred in 1914 when Austria declared war on Serbia, Germany invaded Belgium, and France and England became involved in the conflict. Warring countries soon faced shortages of doctors and nurses, medical supplies, and other means of relief for the suffering. The Red Cross of still neutral America responded by organizing units of doctors, nurses, and other social workers to be sent out to each belligerent country. Until exhausted funds and the imminence of America's entrance into the war caused their recall, men and women of these units did much to express the spirit of the Red Cross as they worked amid the fire and bombshells of large-scale war.

British Nursing Services   Contact of American units with British nursing services showed the latter to be impressive in size and efficiency. At the beginning of the war, three English nursing groups were prepared to meet the emergency. *Queen Alexandra's Royal Army Nursing Corps* offered its thousands of nurses for the relief of sick and wounded soldiers. *Dame Ethel Hope Beecher* served as matron-in-chief, her headquarters in close contact with the British

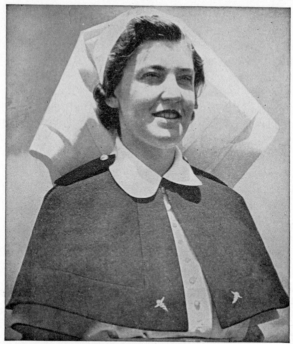

A Member of Princess Mary's Royal Air Force Nursing Service
(From Nursing Times, London, England.)

War Office. *Queen Alexandra's Royal Naval Nursing Service*, small at the outbreak of the war, was soon enlarged. *The Territorial Nursing Service*, organized for service within the Empire, soon embraced foreign fields of activity. For the purpose of supplying nursing care for the newly organized Royal Air Force, the *Princess Mary's Royal Air Force Nursing Service* came into existence in 1918.

The entire British nursing service was well administered, and enjoyed the respectful cooperation of the British Army and Navy. Although the "Q. A's," as English Army and Navy nurses were called, had no official rank, their authority within the field of nursing was unquestioned. *Dame Maude McCarthy*, Matron-in-Chief of the British Expeditionary Forces, like Dame Beecher, had offices close to those of the Director General of the Medical Department, and worked on terms of equal authority with the other officials.

As in all warring countries, English foreign service drew so many patriotic volunteers that civilian hospitals were left in painful need. To meet the insistent demand for more assistance, the British Red Cross, which had already supplied great numbers of nurses to hospitals, now became engaged in organization of a *Voluntary Aid Detachment*. Throughout the Empire, laymen and laywomen took the short emergency courses offered, and many of these "V. A. D.'s" served as assistant nurses in hospitals at home and overseas. Others worked in hastily set up dispensaries and rest stations, temporary havens for tired, sick, and wounded soldiers.

Nurses of the dominions of Great Britain, in Canada, South Africa, Australia, and New Zealand, expressed in many ways their desire to be of service. In Canada, nurses of the Permanent Army Medical Corps Nursing Service were placed a second time under the direction of Matron Georgina F. Pope of South-African War fame. Matron Pope was stationed at Canadian hospitals, first in England and later in France. After a little more than a year of service, failing health caused her return to Canada. The vacancy created by her withdrawal was ably filled by *Nursing Sister Margaret Macdonald*, who was promoted to a matronship with the rank of captain.

Edith Cavell   An undoubted inspiration to many volunteers was *Edith Cavell*, whose untimely death in 1915 stirred deep feeling throughout a troubled world. Miss Cavell, an English nurse, had organized the first school for nurses in Brussels, Belgium. Here, following the occurrence of several battles in its vicinity, school and hospital offered care to soldiers of all armies. By the Germans arresting her, however, Miss Cavell was charged with another activity, that of complicity in the escape to neutral territory of able-bodied Allied soldiers who had been separated from their companies and were in hiding nearby. Pleading guilty, Edith Cavell was sentenced to death, and executed at dawn of the following day, October 12, 1915. After temporary burial in Belgium, her body was returned to England in 1919, and buried near the Cathedral at Norwich, her home town. At the same time her memory was honored by impressive ceremonies in Westminster Abbey.

American Nursing Services   America's sudden entry into the war on April 6, 1917, caught many agencies unprepared. This was not true of the American Red Cross Nursing Service. Through the

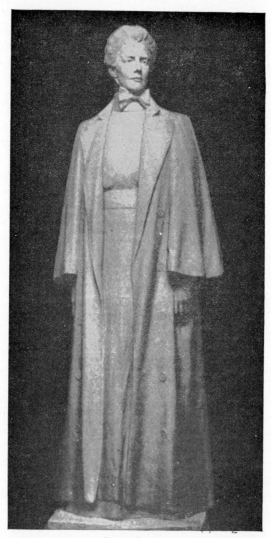

EDITH CAVELL

This figure of Edith Cavell, the martyred British nurse of World War I is a part of the Edith Cavell Memorial in Trafalgar Square, London, donated by a grateful people. The sculptor was Sir George Frampton, R. S.

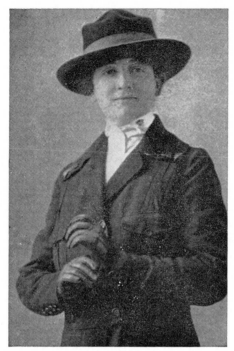

A MEMBER OF THE U. S. ARMY NURSE CORPS DURING WORLD WAR I
(From Red Cross Magazine, January, 1947.)

efforts of Jane Delano and her assistants, a stable and efficient organization had developed. Great numbers of carefully selected nurses had been enrolled and could now be turned over for service with the expanding Army Nurse Corps and Navy Nurse Corps. Other able and experienced nurses were soon enlisted, and new recruits were actively sought and obtained.

To aid in the supply of a long-term demand for nurses, the *Army School of Nursing* was organized in 1918 with *Annie W. Goodrich* as dean. The course she organized covered three years, with a special credit of nine months to college graduates. Army hospitals and affiliating civilian hospitals offered their facilities for instruction. Applications poured in from thousands of enthusiastic women who wanted to make use of this opportunity to give service.

Another opportunity for a selected group of women was offered by the American Red Cross and Vassar College when the *Vassar Training Camp* was formed. It gave a special three months' course of preliminary instruction to four hundred eighteen college graduates, one hundred sixty-nine of whom graduated from cooperating nursing schools.

In civilian hospitals and private homes, the absence of enlisted nurses created a serious problem which resulted in a new development in health education. Jane Delano's varied experience had led her to believe that women in the home could be taught to safeguard the health of their families. She advocated the establishment of classes, conducted by well-prepared nurses, in which the fundamentals of health protection and nursing care of the sick would be taught to wives and mothers.

However, this new plan for spreading health education was vigorously opposed. One objection was that such classes would draw partially trained women into the profession. Another cited the old adage: "A little knowledge is a dangerous thing." Undaunted, Miss Delano, with the help of Isabel McIsaac, had already put her ideas for a course of the type suggested into a textbook now known as "The American Red Cross Home Nursing Textbook." The book, the classes, and Miss Delano's building proved so successful that providing classes in American Red Cross Home Nursing has continued as an important peace-time activity of the American Red Cross.

In spite of continuous efforts to supply nurses in civilian as well as army hospitals, the scarcity became more marked as time went on. Enemies of public health, such as pneumonia throughout the war, typhus spreading over Serbia and Poland, and the great influenza pandemic of 1918, made their appearance, each claiming some doctors and nurses among its victims. In the field of sanitation, typhoid fever presented a less serious problem than during previous wars because of control by vaccination and better provision for water supply.

The complexity of problems, the unending work, and the strain on all attempting to alleviate human suffering was very great. At no point could there be a slowing up. As far as any one knew, the circumstances which called for ever-increasing numbers of nurses might continue indefinitely. The following quotation illustrates the

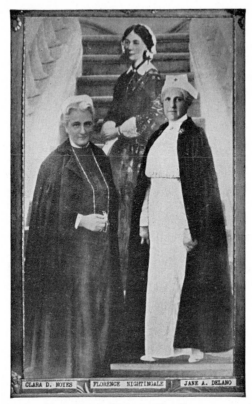

CLARA D. NOYES   FLORENCE NIGHTINGALE   JANE A. DELANO

THREE PIONEERS OF THE RED CROSS

An imaginary grouping on the marble staircase of the American Red Cross National Headquarters Building, Washington, D. C. (Courtesy of League of Nursing Education.)

expenditure of energy, the undivided interest, and the persistence which in many instances met the emergency:

"Miss Delano worked early and late, Sundays and holidays. She lent her great organizing ability to obtain larger numbers of applicants for civilian hospitals so that if the war should be protracted through many years, there would always be enough graduate nurses for every need. It was not an unusual occurrence for Miss Delano, after working in her office until nine at night, to investigate emergency calls, and, it is known, that on more than one occasion she rolled up her sleeves in order to give nursing care."[4]

[4] Gladwin, Mary E.: The Red Cross and Jane Arminda Delano. Philadelphia, W. B. Saunders Co., 1931, pp. 62, 63.

On November 11, 1918, the Armistice became effective and actual fighting ceased, but the ills of war continued and new problems arose. Among the ranks of the fighting men, injured and sick were still to be cared for and transported with as much comfort as possible to their homes. In addition, an underfed, discouraged civilian population offered its plea for help. War orphans, refugees, and throngs of the sick overflowed understaffed hospitals. Finally, emotional strain associated with the violent catastrophe of war had left all Europe sick in mind and spirit. At the same time, the field of nursing suffered several setbacks. While new demands were being created, its ranks were greatly depleted by departure from nursing schools of those who lost interest as the war closed. Also, within this period, the American Red Cross Nursing Service lost its energetic and unselfish leader.

Shortly after the Armistice, while studying emergency problems and planning a program of relief activity, Jane Delano sailed for France to make a tour of inspection of nursing in military hospitals. While there she became concerned about the working conditions of her nurses, and was greatly impressed by the need for public health work in devastated Europe. Heavy work and responsibility had lessened her vitality. She contracted mastoiditis, and underwent several operations at the Base Hospital in Savenay. When she passed away, March 15, 1919, the last words of this "Great War Nurse" were, "My work, my work, I must get back to my work." Burial, at first, was at Savenay, in the plot of ground set apart for American soldiers; later her body was interred with the nation's famous dead at Arlington Cemetery.

Clara D. Noyes, whose ability and experience were well suited to leadership in this era, had acted as assistant to Miss Delano, and she took up her friend's burden as the new Director of the American Red Cross Nursing Service. She, too, visited military hospitals in France, studying their problems, and planning for concerted action among nurses to benefit the many distressed nations of the world. Another inspector of conditions surrounding patients and nurses in France was *Julia C. Stimson*, Superintendent of the Army Nurse Corps. Observations were made of nursing under war-time conditions that would be useful in future planning.

ROYAL COLLEGE OF NURSING

While thousands of their number were giving active service in military and civilian hospitals, English nurses became acutely aware of need for creating an organized body to work toward more uniform professional standards, as well as to deal with other serious problems. To accomplish this end, the *Royal College of Nursing* was founded in 1916. A committee was appointed to seek financial backing for the new institution, and so generous was the response of the English people that the College has been able to sponsor many progressive activities relating to nursing education.

As a means of providing for inspection and accrediting of nursing schools, compulsory registration of nurses became of immediate concern to the Royal College of Nursing. Through its influence, in 1919, more than thirty years after founding of the Royal British Nurses' Association, the long-hoped-for legislation was procured. Other accomplishments of the College have been establishment of special courses in hospitals and universities for sister tutors, nurse administrators, midwives, industrial nurses, and health visitors.

The Student Nurses' Association was organized by the Royal College of Nursing in 1925. Her Royal Highness, The Princess Elizabeth, graciously became first president in 1944, which office she faithfully and conscientiously filled until her accession to the throne in 1952 as Queen Elizabeth II.

POSTWAR RECONSTRUCTION
LEAGUE OF RED CROSS SOCIETIES

Acutely aware of the necessity for continuing into peace time the activities of national Red Cross societies in war-torn Europe, delegates of a number of these societies met in conference at Cannes, France. The outcome of this *Cannes Conference* was the organization, in 1919, of the *League of Red Cross Societies*, its original membership the Red Cross societies of France, Great Britain, Italy, Japan, and the United States. The League, representing the greatest international agreement so far in history, outlined its objectives as follows:

1. Encouragement of the development of national Red Cross societies in all countries

2. Placement of all the benefits of modern science in the field of health within reach of all the people
3. Provision for means of cooperating between national Red Cross societies, especially during international disaster

Along with other pressing problems, it was soon evident that immediate plans must be made for instituting advanced courses to prepare a large proportion of the public health nurses that would be indispensable in the effort to combat post-war suffering. During the war it had been disclosed that although nurses with three years' basic training proved capable within the limits of hospitals, as public health nurses their work had been less successful. Fast-moving events and a far-reaching Red Cross program had shown them to be highly trained in hospital technics, but lacking in knowledge of those fundamentals of public health work that could be acquired only through advanced preparation.

In the effort to meet quickly its overwhelming responsibility for the alleviation of human misery, the League of Red Cross Societies set up temporary courses in Public Health Nursing in London, in connection with the Royal College of Nursing and Bedford College for Women, a branch of the University of London. Similar courses were established in other places, and systems of scholarships promoted. Schools of nursing were established in countries where none had existed.

What is known as the *International Red Cross* is made up of the League of Red Cross Societies, the various national Red Cross Societies, and the International Committee of the Red Cross. The last named is composed of a group of Swiss citizens who, since inception of the first Red Cross societies, have been guarding and maintaining the fundamental principles for which the Red Cross stands.

LEAGUE OF NATIONS

While Europe was acutely conscious of the painful effects of wholesale destruction, and attempting to heal the wounds of war, plans were being directed toward securing a lasting peace. World leaders, prominent among whom was *President Woodrow Wilson* of the United States, expressed their faith in a *League of Nations* which would act as a body of arbitration between nations.

On all matters of dispute, member nations of the League were to be committed to arbitration and to postponement of hostilities until three months after a decision had been reached. Representatives of twenty-four countries set to work with the new objectives, January 10, 1920. With organization of a Permanent Court of International Justice consisting of fifteen judges, the first effort of man toward international control of nations of the world came into being.

Although many citizens of the United States were strongly in favor of adding their country's influence to the League of Nations, America's traditional policy of remaining clear of foreign entanglements prevented her from ratifying its Covenant.

The new organization for world peace soon proved its value by preventing a number of conflicts. For a while it enjoyed considerable prestige, and worked with increasing confidence on other problems of social significance. In time, however, lack of adequate means for enforcing decisions weakened its influence considerably.

Among the contributions of the League of Nations to public welfare were encouragement of commerce and transportation facilities, solution of national financial problems, promotion of scientific progress, and efforts toward improvement of the life of working people everywhere. Its Health Section carried out surveys of hygienic facilities and requirements of backward countries, of national food consumption and adequacy of diets. It directed its efforts toward suppression of traffic in opium and women, and reduction of child labor. It set standards for the manufacture of certain drugs, and endeavored to check, on an international scale, the spread of communicable diseases.

To reach desired goals, the League of Nations sought and gained the cooperation of the League of Red Cross Societies. Meanwhile, heavy demands on the latter had emphasized the necessity for an aggressive campaign to secure greater numbers of public health nurses. Through its influence, the national Red Cross societies of western Europe and America made every effort to attract competent young women into the field of nursing, while daily newspapers depicted the misery and disease which former war activities had served to eclipse.

Many people were becoming conscious, on the one hand, of the horrible conditions existing in stricken areas, and, on the other, of a declining interest in nursing as war-time enthusiasm waned. In the beginning, lure of overseas service had attracted great numbers of young women into schools of nursing. Now that the war was over, new business opportunities which it had caused to be opened up, acted as a counterattraction. In spite of drawbacks, emergency preparation for public health nursing now became an important part of national Red Cross programs, and scholarships for university courses were provided.

GENERAL TREND IN NURSING FROM 1893 TO 1920

The general long-time trend in nursing from the beginning of its organization in 1893 to the end of World War I was considerably influenced by rapid expansion in the establishment of hospitals with a corresponding number of schools dependent upon them for support. The following figures[5] of the Federal Bureau of Education indicate this sharp increase:

Years	Number of Schools
1899–1900	432
1904–1905	862
1909–1910	1,129
1914–1915	1,509
1919–1920	1,755

Schools increased in size as well as in number. As a matter of economy, hospitals depended upon them to carry the chief load of the nursing care of patients. In line with this policy, greater and greater numbers of young women were accepted for entrance. At the same time there appeared a growing tendency toward less careful selection which culminated in the peak of the war-time emergency. Not only was little emphasis placed on educational backgrounds, but, in some cases at least, applicants with college training were suspected of being impractical and so discouraged.

Following the examples of the University of Pennsylvania and the Johns Hopkins hospitals, the length of the course, in most instances, had been increased to three years although the eight-hour day originally intended to be associated with it was less quickly adopted.

[5] Committee for Study of Nursing Education: Nursing and Nursing Education in the United States, p. 188. By permission of The Macmillan Company, publishers.

While the Farrand Training School of Detroit had set up the short-ened day in 1892, and Miss Nutting had instituted it at Johns Hop-kins Hospital in 1895, other schools did not follow. To make up for deficiencies in education, post-graduate courses had been offered since 1890, but were still inadequate. Improperly financed and con-trolled, they offered little in the way of instruction.

Certain developments, however, were promising. The plan for a preliminary course of instruction introduced by Mrs. Rebecca Strong in Glasgow, Scotland, in 1893 and by Miss Nutting at the Johns Hopkins Hospital in 1901, was gradually put into effect in other schools. Affiliations with institutions offering experience of types lacking in the home school increased in number after Isabel Hampton arranged for her students of the Illinois Training School in Chicago to become familiar with the care of private patients at the Presby-terian Hospital of the same city. Many hospital authorities, however, were reluctant to part with their senior students at a time when they considered them of greatest value to themselves, and no law required them to do so.

The apprenticeship system of educating nurses was coming under the fire of criticism. The efficiency of the nurse herself as a teacher of nurses was becoming apparent, and Teachers College, Columbia University, New York, offered a special course to prepare her for this work. By 1920, all states except Nevada had passed laws provid-ing for the registration of nurses. The World War, the influenza epi-demic, and post-war confusion were showing the need for a full program of public health nursing and preparations for this program were under way.

BROADER AIMS IN MEDICINE

Beginnings of Health Education   Following the achievements of Louis Pasteur, the public health movement made great strides toward the prevention and control of communicable diseases. Emphasis was placed first upon public sanitation, extended to enforced isolation and quarantine, and later came to include the use of sera and vac-cines. By the close of World War I, a new aim, that of *popular health education*, was developing. The medical profession was coming to recognize the patient, not merely as an individual who needed assist-ance, but rather as a member of family and community groups, all of whom might be taught the principles of healthful living. At the same time, as the services of the hospital extended into the home with development of public health nursing, more and more families were seeking advice on health subjects.

Medical Social Service   Along with advances in public health thinking, gaining in acceptance had been the belief that knowledge of the relationship between the patient and his home environment strongly influences successful diagnosis and treatment. In an effort to improve and extend the services of the out-patient department of the Massachusetts General Hospital in Boston, *Dr. Richard Cabot*, working at first with *Garnet Pelton*, and later with *Ida M. Cannon*, began an investigation of home influences surrounding their patients. Among other things, it was disclosed that, in many instances, there were causes for emotional disturbance that would contribute to illness. To ensure a knowledge of whole situations with consideration of patients as human beings with relationship to home, job, church, school, and community, a social worker was added to the staff of the out-patient department of the Massachusetts General Hospital. *The beginnings of Medical Social Service had been established.*

So convincing was the evidence brought forth by Dr. Cabot and his co-workers in regard to the necessity for knowledge and control of the environment of patients that today many hospitals operate a social service department. In this way a link is maintained between the patient and his home, both before and after his stay in the hospital. Through pre-hospital contacts factors contributing to the patient's condition are brought to light. Upon his dismissal, the social service department concerns itself with provision for special diets, obtaining surgical and orthopedic appliances, types of work that can be safely undertaken and other means of safe restoration to society.

As time went on, health experts came to recognize in the patient and his family their greatest allies in the struggle against ill health, and sought by means of education to gain their support. Public health departments accepted popular health education as a major responsibility. Hospitals, clinics, and health centers assumed a new importance as educational institutions. In addition to providing facilities for the education of physicians, nurses, and dietitians, they now also guide patients toward more satisfying ways of living. In the role of health missioner, the nurse now plays an all important part. Finally, in support of the new objective, the *American Medical Association*, the *American College of Surgeons*, and the *American Hospital Association* directed their energies toward developing programs to stimulate interest in all phases of health teaching.

The American Medical Association, founded in 1847, is the largest medical organization in the United States, with headquarters at 535 North Dearborn Street, Chicago.

The American Medical Association is composed of the combined membership of the various county and state associations. Through membership in his county association, a physician automatically becomes a member of state and national associations. National conventions are held annually. Activities of the A.M.A. are made known through the *Journal of the American Medical Association*, published weekly. Another of its many publications is the magazine, *Nation's Health*, which is written in popular language and intended primarily for education of the public.

Among numerous activities, it maintains *a Council on Medical Education and Hospitals* and also *a Council on Pharmacy and Chemistry*. Functions of the former include maintaining a register of hospitals conforming to established standards, and their approval for the education of interns and residents in certain specialties. The latter investigates new drugs appearing on the market with the aim of protecting the medical profession and the public from any fraudulent claims made by dispensers. It also publishes yearly the book, *New and Nonofficial Remedies*, in which is listed pertinent information concerning drugs too new to be admitted to the United States Pharmacopoeia, and includes also some proprietary preparations of established value.

The American College of Surgeons   To improve the practice of surgery, the *American College of Surgeons* was formed in 1913 by practitioners of the United States and Canada. In order to accomplish desired ends it was found necessary to initiate a campaign of hospital standardization. Institutions now meeting standards of the College must have an organized staff of licensed physicians who are graduates of approved medical schools, and hold staff meetings monthly. They must have diagnostic and therapeutic facilities which include specified types of x-ray and laboratory departments. An admitting diagnosis is to be submitted with each entering patient, and an accurate and complete history of the patient placed on file with a medical record librarian for future reference. Expert surgeons are to perform all operations.

Today, in order for a school of nursing to be accredited by the State Board of Nurse Examiners, a first requirement is that it must be connected with a hospital that is on the register of the American Medical Association and approved by the American College of Surgeons.

The American Society of Dental Surgeons and the first dental college, opened in Baltimore, had their beginnings in 1840. Each gave evidence of the fact that dentistry was attaining recognition as a science and a profession. Today, as an oral specialty of medical practice, it plays an essential part in the health services. The subject of anesthesia has always been of considerable concern to dentists. Dr. W. T. G. Morton of ether fame was one of their number.

The American Hospital Association, with a membership of both hospitals and individuals, is international in character. At the disposal of all hospitals, nonmembers included, its information and consultation service furnishes the latest information relating to hospital construction, equipment, administrative methods, and other factors basic to successful operation of these institutions. It also reviews all proposed legislation affecting hospitals, and takes action in support of that which is beneficial, and in opposition to that which is prejudicial, to their interests.

Hospitals are now a reflection of the health consciousness of a community, with doctors and nurses as expert advisers, interested in the whole life of man. As emphasis on physical, mental, and spiritual health continues to increase, the possibility of health education for each individual increases also. More and more, the world of today works toward this end as it does toward general and effective education for all. Medical centers are an expression of the ideals of preventive medicine which science, in combination with improved education, brings ever nearer to man's realization.

SUMMARY (1893-1920)

In the latter part of the nineteenth century many types of organized units sprang into being. Women's clubs grew in importance and, in the United States, were consolidated in the General Federation of Women's Clubs. On a larger scale was the International Council of Women. The feeling of need for concerted action spread to nursing, and was especially strong in England where, in 1887, through the efforts of *Mrs. Bedford Fenwick*, the *Royal British Nurses' Association* was organized. Seven years later, the *Matrons' Council of Great Britain and Ireland* was formed.

In the New World, the earliest form of organization for nurses was that of the *alumnae association*, which spread through the United States and Canada. Another organization, admitting to membership superintendents of training schools in the United States and Canada, was the outcome of a conference held by eighteen superintendents in the Woman's Building at the World's Fair in Chicago. Organized in 1893, it was known as the *American Society of Superintendents of Training Schools*. The objective was to improve courses of instruction, and bring about greater uniformity in them.

Three years later, in 1896, the scattered alumnae associations bound themselves together in the *Nurses' Associated Alumnae of the United States and Canada*. Other countries soon followed with national associations. In order to give publicity to the principles for which the new associations stood, nursing magazines were soon published. The *British Journal of Nursing* was established in 1893, the *American Journal of Nursing* in 1900, and the *Canadian Nurse* in 1907. That the gaining of registration as a legal distinction between the old nurse and the new was a major objective is attested by the number of articles on this subject in the early copies of these magazines. However, it was in none of these countries, but in Cape Colony, South Africa, that the first registration law was obtained, in 1891. This was not entirely a nursing law, but was incorporated as part of a Medical and Pharmacy Act. The first purely nursing act was obtained by the nurses of New Zealand in 1901. The first state of the United States to reap the benefits of such legislation was North Carolina, in 1903.

Glimpsing the broader benefits to be derived from international fellowship, Mrs. Bedford Fenwick of England directed her energies toward organization of the *International Council of Nurses* in 1899. In the beginning, membership was of individual nurses, but, as national associations developed and came up to prescribed standards, these became the basis of affiliation.

At the beginning of the Spanish-American War of 1898, no arrangement existed between the national nursing organizations and the Federal Government for the provision of nurses for war service. In order to get the backing of an organized group, army officials in Washington turned this responsibility over to the Daughters of the American Revolution. When standards were finally set they included character, health, and, for the first time, graduation from a training school for nurses. *Anna C. Maxwell*, on leave of absence from the Presbyterian Hospital of New York, did notable work at a camp hospital in Georgia, and became known as the "Florence Nightingale of America."

As a result of experiences in this war, a permanent *Army Nurse Corps* was established in 1901, and a *Navy Nurse Corps* in 1908. A later development was organization, in 1912, of the *American Red Cross Nursing Service*, under the leadership of *Jane A. Delano*. Through it was maintained a roll of selected nurses who, in event of emergency, stood in readiness to serve with the Army Nurse Corps or Navy Nurse Corps, or wherever needed.

In 1902, after the close of the South-African conflict, Canada placed her army nurses on a Reserve list of the active militia. When, in 1904, she also gave to these first Reserve nurses the relative rank of "Lieutenant," she was the first country to accord military rank to women. *Georgina F. Pope*, under whose direction the nurses had assembled for war service, received the relative rank of "Captain."

With growing disapproval of haphazard trends in nursing education came realization of need for special preparation for those responsible for the education of nurses in hospital schools. Sponsored at Teachers College, Columbia University, in 1899, by a committee of the American Society of Superintendents, a graduate course in Hospital Economics took shape, with Mrs. Robb, Miss Nutting, and Miss Goodrich as special lecturers. In 1907 Miss Nutting accepted a professorship from the college, and, in 1909, with Miss Stewart as her assistant, inaugurated the first course for nurse-instructors.

In 1909, under the leadership of *Dr. Richard Olding Beard*, the University of Minnesota was first to institute a plan for making nursing education a branch of college work. Since then many and varying types of university affiliations have evolved. At this stage in development of nursing, on August 13, 1910, fifty years after the founding of the Nightingale School in London, Florence Nightingale was laid to rest in the churchyard of St. Margaret's, East Wellow, near her old home at Embley Park.

Meanwhile, changes were developing in the nursing organizations of the New World. With them a number of new names appeared, and there emerged the *Canadian Nurses' Association* in 1908, the *American Nurses' Association* in 1911, and both the *National League of Nursing Education* and the *National Organization of Public Health Nursing* in 1912.

In contrast to previous wars, World War I found the belligerent countries provided with great numbers of nurses ready for service. The American Red Cross Nursing Service was able to supply immediately several thousand of its enrolled nurses. Students were recruited, and classes larger than usual were admitted to schools of nursing. Other war measures included the founding of the *Army School of Nursing* with *Annie W. Goodrich* as dean, and the Vassar Training Camp at Vassar College which gave a special preliminary course for college graduates, a number of whom later graduated from schools of affiliating hospitals. Women in the home were provided with classes in *Home Nursing* by the American Red Cross.

In 1919, to meet the needs of a period of social reconstruction, the *League of Red Cross Societies*, an international organization, was created to continue the humanitarian work of national Red Cross societies in times of peace. Also, with the aim of assisting in social uplift and bringing about lasting world peace, the *League of Nations* was established. Its *Health Section* undertook the gigantic task of promoting mental and physical health among all peoples.

Greatly influencing the general trend in nursing during this period extending from the World's Fair in Chicago to the close of World War I was the demand for students to carry the nursing load of a rapidly increasing number of hospitals. This demand, which culminated during the war activity, resulted in less careful selection of applicants. Emphasis was placed on getting work done rather than on nursing education.

By the close of World War I, the aim of medicine had shifted from treatment of the individual patient to that of health education for all citizens. The movement toward consideration of the patient in relation to his social background began in the out-patient department of the Massachusetts General Hospital of Boston when *Medical Social Service* was instituted by Dr. Richard Cabot, Garnet Pelton, and Ida M. Cannon. To support the new viewpoints, medical and hospital associations came forward with measures that would maintain a high level of medical practice.

TOPICS FOR DISCUSSION

1. Compare the first form of organization among nurses to appear in England with that in the United States.
2. Why is the World's Fair of Chicago, held in 1893, of significance in the history of American nursing?
3. Make a list, with dates of founding, of the first nursing organizations to appear in your country.
4. When, and through whose influence, was the International Council of Nurses founded?
5. Differentiate between a labor union and a professional organization.
6. Give reasons for the fact that soldiers of the Spanish-American and South African wars had better provision for nursing care than had soldiers of previous wars.
7. Show how problems encountered by Anna C. Maxwell during the Spanish-American War resembled those of Florence Nightingale during the Crimean War.
8. What circumstances led to organization of the U. S. Army Nurse Corps? The U. S. Navy Nurse Corps? The American Red Cross Nursing Service?
9. (*a*) What country was first to grant military rank to women? (*b*) Does your country grant such rank?
10. At what institution in the United States was a program first developed to provide graduate study for nurses expecting to fill educational and administrative positions?

11. At what institution in the United States was the education of students in a school of nursing first placed on a college level?

12. To what stage of development had nursing progressed when Miss Nightingale's life ended?

13. Add to your list of early nursing organizations the names later assumed.

14. How did provision for nursing during World War I differ from that of any previous war?

15. What nurse was shot, and for what reason, during World War I?

16. In what ways was the problem of shortage of nurses for home duty met?

17. What were the chief problems to be dealt with during the post-war period of reconstruction?

18. What two new organizations of international importance developed about this time?

19. What field of nursing was making great strides by the end of the war?

20. The emphasis in medicine was shifting in what direction?

21. What factors led to the beginning of hospital social service?

22. Make an outline of the headquarters and activities of the American Medical Association, the American College of Surgeons, and the American Hospital Association.

23. Who is now president of the American Red Cross?

24. Using the Official Directory of the American Journal of Nursing, make an outline of the names of nurses now at the head of each of the following federal services, with titles of their positions:

    (a) American Red Cross Nursing Services
    (b) U. S. Army Nurse Corps
    (c) U. S. Navy Nurse Corps
    (d) U. S. Air Force Nurse Corps
    (e) Veterans Administration—Nursing Service
    (f) U. S. Public Health Service—Nursing Service
    (g) Bureau of Indian Affairs—Nursing Service

25. Which of the above services were inaugurated during the period just studied, and which are of more recent origin?

26. Discuss the general long-time trends in nursing education from the time of beginning organization in 1893 to the period of reconstruction beginning about 1920.

REFERENCES

Boardman, Mabel T.: Under the Red Cross Flag. Philadelphia, J. B. Lippincott Co., 1915.

Breckinridge, Mary: Wide Neighborhoods: A Story of the Frontier Nursing Service. New York, Harper and Brothers, 1952.

Cabot, Richard C.: The Goal of Social Work. Boston and New York, Houghton Mifflin Co., 1927.

Cannon, Ida M.: Social Work in Hospitals. New York Survey Associates, Inc., 1913.

Clarke, Ida Clyde: American Women and the World War. New York and London, D. Appleton & Co., 1918.

Cushing, Harvey: The Life of Sir William Osler. London, Toronto, and New York, Oxford University Press, 1940.

Dock and Nutting: A History of Nursing. New York and London, G. P. Putnam's Sons, Vol. III, 1907.

Dulles, Foster Rhea: The American Red Cross: A History. New York, Harper and Brothers, 1950.

Gladwin, Mary E.: The Red Cross and Jane Arminda Delano. Philadelphia, W. B. Saunders Co., 1931.

Hampton, Isabel, and others (N.L.N.E., editor): Nursing of the Sick—1893. New York, McGraw-Hill Book Co., 1951.

Hayes, Moon, and Wayland: World History. New York, The Macmillan Co., 1941.

Judson, Helen: Edith Cavell. New York, The Macmillan Co., 1941.

Kernodle, Portia B.: The Red Cross Nurse in Action. New York, Harper and Brothers, 1949.

Koch, Harriet Berger: Militant Angel (Annie W. Goodrich). New York, The Macmillan Co., 1951.

Munson, Helen W.: The Story of the National League of Nursing Education. Philadelphia, W. B. Saunders Co., 1934.

Pickett, Sarah Elizabeth: The American National Red Cross. New York, Century Co., 1924.

Sigerist, Dr. Henry: American Medicine. New York, W. W. Norton & Co., Inc., 1934.

Stewart, Isabel M.: The Education of Nurses. New York, The Macmillan Co., 1943.

Werminghaus, Esther A.: Annie W. Goodrich: Her Journey to Yale. New York, The Macmillan Co., 1951.

Wyche, Mary Lewis: The History of Nursing in North Carolina. Chapel Hill, University of North Carolina Press, 1938.

XII

National Surveys of Nursing and Medicine

Medicine's new aim of teaching the principles of personal hygiene to as many citizens as possible raised the question of supplying teachers to meet the need. Were nurses equipped with the scientific background necessary for health teaching, or should this be the province of women with more specialized education but less professional preparation? Nursing leaders were of the opinion that the nurse should assume the new responsibility. She it was who entered homes of all types, cared for patients with many forms of disease, had excellent opportunity to teach the lessons of healthful living. With enough of her sisters in the field, the new movement could go forward rapidly.

Here again arose a problem for public health administrators. How could adequate numbers of such nurse-teachers be supplied? Now the war was over, no exciting cause attracted young women into nursing. At the same time, with many new hospitals springing up, all desiring schools, students were in great demand. Should entrance requirements be lowered in order to attract greater numbers of applicants? However, standards had already been appreciably declining for a number of reasons and, with them, interest in nursing was declining too. Obviously, further lowering was not the solution to the problem. Admittedly, conditions in hospitals were not such as to attract the best type of candidate.

THE ROCKEFELLER SURVEY (1920-1923)

To make a study of ways and means of providing well-qualified public health nurses, the Rockefeller Foundation called a special conference in December, 1918. Approximately fifty health leaders including doctors, nurses, and representatives of hospitals and health agencies, met, and after much discussion reached an opinion that the usual three-year course was inadequate preparation for public health work. To gain more information the delegates named a *Committee for the Study of Nursing Education*, whose efforts were to be financed by the Rockefeller Foundation. *C. E. A. Winslow*, of the department of public health of Yale University, was made chairman, while actually in charge of the investigation was the secretary, *Josephine Goldmark*, who was well known in the field of social research.

At a second meeting, called by the Rockefeller Foundation about a year later, the entire field of nursing was discussed, and the Committee requested to investigate all phases of nurse activity. The survey which followed covered public health groups, private duty nursing, and twenty-three representative schools connected with hospitals, large and small, public and private, over a wide territory. An educator from the field of nursing and another from the field of education, both experts, made detailed studies. The results of the survey, together with some definite conclusions, were published in 1923 in the volume, *Nursing and Nursing Education in the United States*, popularly referred to as the "Winslow-Goldmark Report."

Public Health Field   Findings in the *public health field* made clear the need for teaching personal hygiene in the home. Efforts to get the cooperation of parents of school children were a new development arising from the discovery that while communicable diseases were comparatively rare, physical defects that could be either prevented or cured were legion. Children too often had organic heart disease, hearing and visual defects, infected tonsils and enlarged adenoids, defects of joints and foot arches. Many of the undernourished came of families who, although able to provide a balanced diet, were ignorant of the subject of nutrition. In other directions mental defectives and drug addicts needed psychiatric guidance. Maternal and infant mortality rates offered yet another challenge to the ability of the public health nurse. Undoubtedly, it was she, health experts were coming to agree, who possessed the greatest opportunity for combating existing conditions. Longer contacts in the home than those of the private duty nurse, with fewer bedside responsibilities, were among her advantages.

Private Duty Field   Investigation of the *field of private duty* revealed a number of interesting facts. A nurse so engaged becomes acquainted with and cares for only one patient, and for a comparatively short period of time. Her opportunity for teaching principles of hygiene is thus limited to him and his immediate family. It is necessary, therefore, that she be a skilled bedside nurse rather than a health teacher. At the same time, some physicians regarded her as too expert and too high-priced for many of their patients. Nurses themselves were failing to recognize the need for a subsidiary type of worker whose preparation could be regulated by a system of grading comparable to registration. Through the services of such a group, it was believed by some, patients with less critical or chronic conditions could be spared considerable expense while still being guaranteed an attendant with a specific degree of preparation.

Still other facts of interest in the private duty field were disclosed by the survey. Although state registration afforded a means of differentiating the professional from the nonprofessional nurse, the standards set for such recognition were found to be inadequate. Among other deficiencies, affiliations for students in small or special hospitals were not generally required, and many nurses were practicing without sufficient knowledge of the care of patients with medical diseases or of the diseases of children. It was apparent also that skilled care was available only for those in comfortable circumstances and for the very poor. For the rich there were the services of the private duty nurse and the private hospital; for the poor, the visiting nurse and the free hospital. Those of moderate means were left unprovided for, although a few insurance plans for the benefit of this group were just coming into existence. It was the opinion of some that increased employment of the subsidiary worker might solve this problem. Others felt that reductions in the rates of graduate nurses were in some instances justifiable.

Nursing School Field   A study of *nursing schools* brought to light the fact that courses of instruction had received meager attention during the period of rapid expansion. Nearly one-half of such schools were connected with hospitals of less than fifty beds. Financial circumstances were largely influential in policy-fixing. Ancient traditions of asceticism and unquestioning obedience savored of the Middle Ages. Ideals emphasizing sacrifice of personal desires and the blind acceptance of authority had been carried over from the monasteries and military nursing orders. Moreover, many nurses in responsible positions had little preparation beyond that of the basic course. Senior students were often used as head nurses, or were kept for long periods on night duty. They were sent out on private cases, and the financial return made to the hospital.

Among other points of weakness was the dual responsibility of the director of nursing, who was expected to provide both care for the patient and education for the student. Full-time instructors were little known. Lecture rooms, demonstration rooms, laboratories, and libraries were generally inadequate. A great lack of uniformity in courses of instruction increased the general confusion. Such courses were often based on ward needs, and frequently modified to comply with pressure of work in the hospital. In relation to these deficiencies and those of the other two phases of nursing studied, the following recommendations of the Winslow-Goldmark Report stand out as significant:

1. "That as soon as may be practicable, all agencies, public or private, employing public health nurses, should require as a prerequisite for employment the basic hospital training, followed by a post-graduate course, including both class work and field work, in public health nursing.

2. "That steps should be taken through state legislation for the definition and licensure of a subsidiary grade of nursing service, the subsidiary type of worker to serve under practicing physicians in the care of mild and chronic illness, and convalescence, and possibly to assist under the direction of the trained nurse in certain phases of hospital and visiting nursing.

3. "Superintendents, supervisors, instructors, and public health nurses should in all cases receive special additional training beyond the basic nursing course.

4. "That the development of nursing service adequate for the care of the sick and for the conduct of the modern public health campaign demands as an absolute prerequisite the securing of funds for the endowment of nursing education of all types; and that it is of primary importance, in this connection, to provide reasonably generous endowment for university schools of nursing."[1]

As an immediate answer to the recommendation that nursing schools be independent of hospitals and on a college level, two en-

[1] Committee for the Study of Nursing Education: Nursing and Nursing Education in the United States, 1933. By permission of The Macmillan Co., publishers

dowed university schools of nursing were developed, one in connection with Yale University, New Haven, Connecticut, and the other with Western Reserve University, Cleveland, Ohio. The Yale School of Nursing was financed by the Rockefeller Foundation as an experiment to prove the feasibility of planning both classroom instruction and ward practice from the standpoint of educational needs of students. Patients of a type and number suitable for teaching were to be selected for care during the course in each special subject, and emphasis was to be placed on the social and health aspects of nursing.

Annie W. Goodrich, leaving her position on the faculty of the Department of Nursing Education at Teachers College, Columbia University, became dean of the Yale school. After five years the experiment proved so successful that it was put on a permanent footing with a large endowment by the Foundation. The school at Western Reserve University was made independent by endowment from *Frances Payne Bolton*, and with the able assistance of *Carolyn E. Gray* as dean, also proved successful. With the Yale School of Nursing, it has demonstrated the value of university standards and up-to-date educational practice in the field of nursing.

THE GRADING OF NURSING SCHOOLS, 1926–1934

A second and far-reaching result of the Rockefeller Survey was strengthening of a long-cherished determination on the part of the National League of Nursing Education to undertake a comprehensive study of nursing education which would lead to actual grading of nursing schools. Grading, it was believed, would set up standards to which all schools would be compelled to conform. Results within the medical profession, after a similar practice had been adopted, lent probability to this belief.

The first move toward securing support for this undertaking was made when the Education Committee of the National League of Nursing Education met with a committee which the American Medical Association had recently appointed for study of nursing education. The outcome of this interest in a common cause was appointment of a *Committee on the Grading of Nursing Schools*. Its purpose was to be a cooperative study of nursing practice in all its aspects. The following organizations, all vitally interested in the project, elected representatives to serve with the newly-appointed committee:

National League of Nursing Education
American Nurses' Association
National Organization for Public Health Nursing
American Medical Association
American College of Surgeons
American Hospital Association
American Public Health Association

In addition to these groups, there were representatives of university education and of the public at large. *William Darrach*, M. D., of the American Medical Association, was made chairman of the committee, and *May Ayres Burgess*, Ph. D., statistician, became director of the investigation. *Mary M. Roberts*, editor of the American Journal of Nursing, attended all meetings in order that, through the medium of the Journal, she might interpret proceedings. The services of Committee members were voluntary, while extensive studies and publications were financed by the following contributions:[2]

Nurses Committee for Financing the Grading Plan	$98,892
Mrs. Frances Payne Bolton	93,000
Rockefeller Foundation	30,000
American Nurses' Association	16,500
National Organization for Public Health Nursing	11,600
Commonwealth Fund	10,000
National League of Nursing Education	10,000
American Medical Association	5,000
American Hospital Association	4,000
American Public Health Association	1,100
Mrs. Helen Hartley Jenkins	1,000
Special Contributions	121
Total	$281,213
Bank interest	2,287
Grand total	$283,500

The general purpose of the Committee on the Grading of Nursing Schools was early defined as "The study of ways and means for insuring an ample supply of nursing service, of whatever type and quality needed for adequate care of the patient, at a price within his

[2] Committee on Grading of Nursing Schools: *Nursing Schools Today and Tomorrow*, p. 17.

reach."[3] In 1926 a five year program was adopted to cover three projects judged to be worthy of study over such a period, with varying degrees of emphasis on each. These were to be as follows:

1. Supply and demand for nursing service
2. Job analysis of nursing and nurse teaching
3. Actual grading of nursing schools

Nurses following with interest the proceedings of the group were desirous that the Committee publish a list of schools, graded according to their respective standards of education. Such a list, they believed, would serve the dual purpose of forcing poorer schools to raise their standards, and helping young women attracted to the profession in choice of a school. Experts in the field of higher education, however, argued drawbacks to an actual grading at this time. Unless each school could be visited personally, the value of the rating would be questionable, and for this the cost would be too great. To the disappointment of many, this advice was followed. Notwithstanding this change in program, the committee continued with its original name.

Supply and Demand for Nursing Service   For investigation of the first problem—*that of supply and demand for nursing service*—the questionnaire method was used. Replies from hospitals, public health directors, registries, patients, nurses, and physicians throughout the nation formed the basis of conclusions. *Nurses, Patients, and Pocketbooks* is the title of the book published in 1928 that contained the result of eighteen months' investigation. In it are given a variety of viewpoints on the many-sided subject of nursing economics. Opinions are expressed as to how much and what type of nursing service are necessary, as to urban and rural distribution of nurses, and as to costs associated with satisfactory care of patients. In all, the book covers a wide and interesting group of problems. After its publication, however, the American Medical Association withdrew from the Committee on the Grading of Nursing Schools, although its reasons for so doing were never clearly understood. Notwithstanding this alteration, Dr. Darrach graciously consented to remain as chairman.

[3] A Five-year Program for the Committee on the Grading of Nursing Schools (a pamphlet), p. 10.

Soon after publication of *Nurses, Patients, and Pocketbooks,* an article by May Ayres Burgess appeared in the American Journal of Nursing with the following startling disclosures on the distribution of nurses:

"Nurses are crowded into the cities far in excess of the needs of the population. Nurses are hard to find in the country and there are many parts of the United States where large areas are completely unreached by graduate nurses.

"Nurses are eager for private duty in hospitals and they are reluctant to fill calls for private duty service in the home. There are too many nurses waiting for calls on week days and often too few ready to work over the holidays. There are many nurses trained and interested in taking surgical cases and there are very few trained and eager to take special types of medical cases. There are thousands of unemployed nurses eagerly seeking for opportunities to become self-support-ing; but there are hundreds of unfilled positions which remain unfilled either because nurses are afraid or unwilling to undertake the work, or because there are not enough nurses with the specialized administrative or educational prepara-tion for which some of the unfilled positions call."[4]

Analysis of Nursing and Nurse Teaching   The goal of the second project—*a job analysis of nursing and nurse teaching*—was to discover all activities that constitute nursing, and then to determine the man-ner of instruction necessary to prepare for it. Such information was intended to approach a scientific basis from which a satisfactory revision of the national curriculum could be constructed. Results of studies made by nurse educators were gathered together in book form by *Ethel Johns and Blanche Pfefferkorn* and published, in 1934, in *An Activity Analysis of Nursing.*

"What is good nursing?" is the question raised in the first chapter. Opinions of patients, physicians, hospital administrators, and com-munity answer the question. Briefly, patients look for skill combined with kindness and willingness to adjust to their particular situations. Physicians expect skill, reliability in transfer of necessary information to them, and personal loyalty. The need of hospitals is for nurses who satisfy both patients and physicians. In addition, they seek em-ployees who will assume responsibility for smooth functioning of their departments, and who will learn and interpret the spirit of the hospital. Continuing the analysis of what the total field of nursing embraces, the authors listed the basic conditions calling for the

[4] "The Distribution of Nursing Service" by Mary Ayres Burgess. American Journal of Nursing, July, 1930, p. 857.

services of a nurse, and the many types of activities included in hospital, public health, and private duty nursing.

The Grading of Nursing Schools The interest of many hospitals in the third project, which proved to be that of a *comparative study of nursing schools*, was so great as to make the questionnaire method again feasible. Each school was encouraged to evaluate its own system with the help of monthly outlines provided by the Committee. All schools were identified by numbers rather than names. As the investigation proceeded, results were returned to each in printed form. The graphs included showed the relative standing of all schools on a given subject. The position of the individual school in the general picture was checked in red.

Those concerned frequently discovered their schools to be excelling in some particulars but lagging far behind in others. This opportunity to see how individual facilities compared with those of similar institutions provided the most valuable basis for self-evaluation that any school had ever possessed. All associated with a given institution, from nurses to trustees, could see how it stood in the whole scheme of American nursing education. Not only were deficiencies discernible by comparison, but new incentive was offered for removing them, and many schools took immediate steps in that direction.

Not all schools, however, were able to raise their standards of instruction. Those that were small or economically unsound found that any worthwhile attempt to improve conditions would put too great a strain upon the hospital. In many such cases, the trustees voted their discontinuance. Notwithstanding these evidences of cooperative spirit, the nursing group felt that to discover just how well nursing education had reached higher levels, further measurement would be necessary.

Second Grading In 1932, to determine what had been accomplished, *a second self-study* under supervision of the Committee on the Grading of Nursing Schools was undertaken. This *Second Grading of Nursing Schools* did not cover as wide a scope of investigation as the first, but was given more publicity. Boards of Nurse Examiners received data relative to all schools in their respective states, but without names of institutions. If they wished, however, they could get additional information.

That nearly all surviving schools which had participated in the first grading took part in this second study shows the widespread interest that the first had awakened. The information gathered was gratifying. Several hundred of the poorer schools had closed their doors. In the others, there was improvement in about three-fourths of the items investigated, two of which are shown in the graphs on page 443.

As a secondary result of the study, a new interest was focused on consideration of the school as a paying or nonpaying department of the hospital unit. A new study of costs was made by a number of progressive hospitals, in which their schools were evaluated as economic assets or liabilities. In a number of instances, results showing profit or loss were published for the benefit of others. A conclusive opinion on the subject was not reached.

The final report of the Committee on the Grading of Nursing Schools, along with specific suggestions for improvement, appeared in book form in 1934. This volume, *Nursing Schools Today and Tomorrow*, showed that the chief purpose of hospitals was the care of their patients, that nursing schools had been operated as paying service departments, with student nurses regarded in the same light as employees. It showed that the training offered provided efficient hospital workers, but gave little or no insight into the private duty or public health fields. It criticized the existent form of apprenticeship teaching, and emphasized the need for instruction on a college level. Recommendations were made also for providing opportunities for graduates to make up deficiencies of training, or to receive advanced instruction.

Certain absolute requirements for all schools of nursing were listed. They must be connected with an institution on the Hospital Register of the American Medical Association, approved by the American College of Surgeons, with a daily average of at least fifty patients. They must be accredited by the State Board of Nurse Examiners, and their entering students must have not less than high school graduation as preparation.

The report also disclosed the fact that while there were too many nurses in large cities, there was yet a dearth of those with sound professional preparation. It stressed the necessity for a more even distribution of nursing service, for its recognition as a public respon-

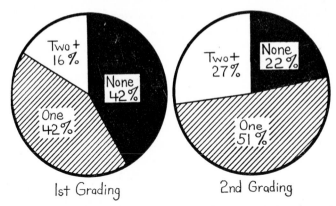

Per cent of schools having no instructor, one instructor, and two or more instructors, in the first and second gradings. (May Ayres Burgess in "American Journal of Nursing," June, 1932.)

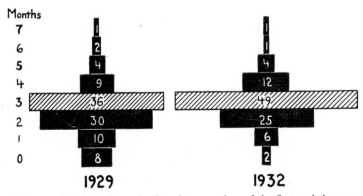

Per cent of students in graduating classes at time of the first and the second gradings who had spent each number of months on the Pediatric Service. (Ella A. Taylor in "American Journal of Nursing," November, 1933.)

sibility, with appropriation of public funds that would put nursing education on a level with other essential lines of education.

Organization of the Association of Collegiate Schools of Nursing
With a major interest of strengthening college relationships, a new organization of nurses, the *Association of Collegiate Schools of Nursing*, was organized, in 1933, to represent schools or departments

of nursing associated with universities. Members are pledged to promote research in their particular fields, and to evolve educational methods on a college level.

As time goes on, more and more nursing schools are finding means of associating themselves, in some manner, with colleges or universities. Also, with the rise of junior colleges, an increasing number of candidates enter with a background of one or two years of college work. Since these entering students are both older and better prepared than those of former years, it has been possible to eliminate some basic subjects from the nursing curriculum, and to put more stress on those of a professional nature. If, in addition, credit for a prenursing course has been received, the preliminary period of instruction in the hospital, in many cases, is shortened.

Other encouraging signs of progress are gradually appearing. In a number of schools more adequate budgets have been secured through tuition charges or other means. Employment of a larger graduate staff by hospitals has relieved much pressure of the nursing load from students. Better prepared instructors are providing education which stresses not only principles of healthful living, but assists the student to understand the whole patient in relation to his social, psychologic, and economic backgrounds. At the same time, increasing attention is being given to bedside care of patients, and treatment requiring ever greater knowledge and skill is being entrusted to the nurse.

In answer to the disclosures of the Rockefeller Survey and the Committee on the Grading of Nursing Schools that many areas suffered from lack of nursing care, the three national nursing organizations—American Nurses' Association, National League of Nursing Education, and National Organization for Public Health Nursing in 1928 appointed a *Joint Committee on the Distribution of Nursing Service*. The objective was to be "the attempt of organized nursing to formulate and execute a plan which will bring the well-prepared nurse in contact with those situations in which her services are needed, and in which her services will be available to all patients, under conditions which will allow for satisfaction in workmanship to the nurse."[5] This aim would serve the twofold purpose of supply-

[5] Quoted in Forty-sixth Annual Report of the National League of Nursing Education, 1940, p. 120.

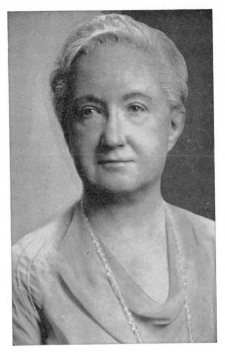

JEAN ISABEL GUNN, O.B.E., LL.D.
(Courtesy of Toronto General Hospital.)

ing each citizen with essential care, and of ensuring needed employment among nurses during a period of great financial depression.

Surveys of Nursing in Canada and Great Britain   While nurses of the United States were thus showing both a critical spirit and a disposition to right old wrongs, no less conscious of need for change were those of Canada and Great Britain. In 1927, three delegates from the Canadian Medical Association and three from the Canadian Nurses' Association made up a committee which proposed an investigation. Nurses on the committee were *Jean I. Gunn*, Superintendent of Nurses, Toronto General Hospital; *Kathleen Russell*, Director of the Department of Nursing, University of Toronto; and *Jean Browne*, Secretary of the Junior Red Cross Society of Canada. Chairman of the group was *Dr. G. Stewart Cameron*. All were in favor of studying educational conditions, but were agreed further that an expert from outside the two professions would be needed to visit and investigate schools. Such an expert was found in *Professor George Weir*, who secured a leave of absence from his work as head of the Department of Education of the University of British Columbia.

Work on the project began in November, 1929, and drew to a close July 31, 1931. The expense had been borne by the two professions: 70 per cent by the nursing group, and 30 per cent by physicians. Sufficient funds were furnished for Dr. Weir to cover every province, and make many visits to hospitals and schools. His investigations took in economic and sociological, as well as public health implications of the field, and a report was published in the volume, *Survey of Nursing Education in Canada*.

In England, the decline in numbers of students entering nursing schools and a corresponding decline in candidates for hospital positions led to a critical attitude toward prevailing methods. In 1930, an investigation of certain phases of nursing activities was conducted by the medical group through the *Lancet Commission*, which was made up of nurses, doctors, educators, sociologists, economists, and hospital trustees. The method followed was that of self-rating through the use of questionnaires. After studying the data returned, the Commission set down sixty-one conclusions in a published report. Among the deterrents to increased entrance into the profession, disciplinary problems, poor educational opportunities, long hours of work, and salary difficulties figured prominently.

REGISTRATION AND LICENSING

Following completion of the two national surveys of nursing education by the Rockefeller Foundation and the Committee on the Grading of Nursing Schools, interest became centered in revision of registration laws. By this time it had been discovered that existing laws afforded inadequate protection for the general public, the physician, and for the nurse herself. For some time, increasing numbers of "practical" nurses had been coming into employment when long-time care was needed in the home, or when housework was to be combined with nursing. In such a capacity, a reliable woman could be depended upon to work longer hours for less money than the graduate nurse. On the other hand, no standards had been fixed for the training of a practical nurse, and she bore no guarantee of adequate preparation for the tasks which she undertook. Those who employed her must discover for themselves her individual worth.

Even though the law set apart the Registered Nurse as one who had met certain educational requirements, anyone might call herself a nurse and accept remuneration from those who were willing to employ her. The law prohibited her from placing the letters *R.N.* after her name, but it did not prohibit her from nursing. While it had long been a requirement that all who practice medicine first meet certain fixed educational standards and become *licensed*, or legally permitted to practice, those who practiced nursing had been granted the privilege of obtaining state recognition as Registered Nurses, but were not legally required to make use of it. The unregistered nurse might practice provided that she could find anyone willing to employ her. In other words, laws were *permissive* rather than *mandatory*.

Upon critical examination of proposed legislation which would provide for *licensing* of all who practice as professional, graduate, or registered nurses, the question of responsibility for the training of practical or subsidiary nurses presented itself. Was the nursing profession to assume this new responsibility, making itself accountable for all types of nursing? Should subsidiary workers be required to have a specific type of preparation and be licensed also? Discussion brought forth much controversial opinion.

A pioneer in the movement to regulate all nursing practice, the State of New York enacted, in 1938, a law requiring licensing of all who nursed for hire. This law established two groups, one entitled to practice as professional nurses, the other as practical nurses. After July, 1940, it became unlawful for any person not so licensed to be employed in any capacity for the care of the sick in the State of New York. It was soon discovered, however, that the situation thus created was incompatible with the demands of World War II, and the law was suspended until 1950 when its mandatory provisions once more came into full effect.

Several other states followed the example of New York with the enactment of similar, but often less inclusive, legislation. From time to time the question of a *national* licensing system which would permit the nurse to practice in any state of the union was agitated, but met with stumbling blocks in the form of provision for "States' Rights" in the Constitution of the United States, and also in differing standards for state accreditation of schools.

Recognizing a need for revision of all nurse practice acts, the Joint Boards of Directors of the three major national nursing associations, meeting in 1939, approved a recommendation for a nation-wide program of licensing all who nurse for hire, and expressed an active interest in all aspects of such a licensing program. The nursing profession thus proved itself alert to the fact that its own carefully worked out course of action would be preferable to any which might be imposed by outside interests. Unfortunately, progress was interrupted by a growing possibility of participation in World War II. As a result, thought and energy were diverted to the task of providing a hitherto unheard-of number of nurses as quickly as possible, a task permitting no other expenditure of time or energy.

A CRITICAL SURVEY OF MEDICAL PRACTICE, 1927–1932

During the period of investigation of nursing by the Committee on the Grading of Nursing Schools, an extensive survey of medical practice was also going on in the United States of America. Public criticism of shortcomings in provision for medical care during illness had been growing louder and louder. The causes for complaint were many. On the one hand, scientific knowledge had increased to a phenomenal extent. Ancient plagues had been conquered. Infant and maternal mortality rates had been reduced. The practice of surgery had made marked advances. Potentially, it was possible to greatly reduce the incidence of illness and prolong life. On the other hand, with improved facilities had come higher costs, and opportunity to benefit by modern methods had been carried further and further away from the average person. For these and various other reasons, much newly acquired knowledge and skill were being unused by many people. At the same time, an ever-growing concept of the human right to possess and maintain health increased the general dissatisfaction.

In order to clarify the situation and meet the insistent clamor for more and better medical service, a *Committee on the Costs of Medical*

Care, composed of physicians, economists, and other specialists was established in 1927. A Research Staff was engaged and a five-year plan of fact-finding formulated. This developed into a nation-wide study of existing differences between the medical care needed and that being received by the people. The costs of such care, and its distribution, were also taken into consideration. On the other hand, statistics relating to annual incomes of physicians, dentists, and nurses were accumulated and shown to be unsatisfactory. Through the financial depression, many professional people were suffering from lack of employment while patients were suffering from lack of medical and nursing care.

Investigation of European provision for medical services revealed innovations. Many doctors in the countries studied were employed on a full-time salary basis, while others remained independent practitioners. The principle of *group insurance* had been put into effect, but patients so protected were still permitted the choice of a doctor. In a number of instances, persons earning less than a specified income were required, by one means or another, to carry medical insurance. In England, such expenses were divided among employee, employer, and the national government. In Germany, whose system antedates that of other countries, the benefits of insurance were extended to certain members of employees' families.

Conclusions reached by the Committee on the Costs of Medical Care aroused no little concern, both within and without the medical profession. It was more apparent than ever that citizens of the country as a whole were not receiving the full benefits of what medicine and related sciences had to offer. Medical and nursing services were unevenly distributed, with some areas left entirely without them. Unquestionably, opportunities for such benefits should be placed within reach of all, regardless of economic status. It was believed that if such a goal were to be attained, governmental bodies must assume considerable responsibility. By means of group insurance, adequate medical services could be provided by doctors, dentists, nurses, pharmacists, laboratory technicians, and others, with costs distributed over great numbers of people. It was further recommended that each community should be held responsible for coordination of effort of its hospitals, health centers, clinics, and laboratories, and for putting their services within the reach of all citizens. The question as to whether the carrying of medical insurance should be made compulsory or voluntary was regarded as controversial, and so it has remained in the United States up to the present time.

SOCIAL SECURITY ACT OF 1935

Satisfactory provision for care during illness is only one of many questions of a social nature as yet unanswered. Modern society is confronted with a complexity of problems, the solution of which involves development of methods never before employed in the history of the world. With an economic depression of global proportions, heralded by a spectacular crash of the stock market in 1929, vast throngs of people, regardless of personal abilities or years of service, were thrown out of employment with little or no hope of securing other positions. Those of proud and independent nature were forced to stand in bread lines with the less prideful, or to sell apples on street corners.

As poverty mounted, the incidence of illness as a cause of dependence increased with it. At the same time, more and more insistent grew the demand that society as a whole assume responsibility for the welfare of each of its citizens. Modern reasoning and application of the scientific method were bringing to light the errors of existing methods. With increasing awareness of the necessity for national planning to bring about alleviation of suffering, it was recognized that a comprehensive public welfare program must be forthcoming.

In a number of European countries, social laws which made easier the lot of the average man were put into effect about this time. In the United States, the Social Security Act of 1935 recognized a wide range of social needs, as indicated by the following statement:

"The act was devised to alleviate phases of economic distress such as are found even in normal times among the temporarily unemployed, dependent children, the aged, and the blind, and to strengthen maternal and child welfare, public health, and vocational rehabilitation services."[6]

The Social Security Act was amended in 1950 and 1954 to bring within range of its benefits, self-employed persons and employees of some religious, charitable and educational institutions which here-

[6] Informational Service Circular No. 1: A Brief Explanation of the Social Security Act, page 1.

tofore had been excluded. Many nurses engaged in private practice and institutional work thus became eligible. Monthly benefits to be received after the age of retirement were increased, the amount of which is based on the individual's average salary, up to a fixed maximum. A Federal fund for carrying on the project is maintained by means of taxes paid by employers, employees, and the self-employed.

IMPLEMENTING THE ACT

In order that benefits of the Social Security Act might reach all for whom they were intended, a nation-wide survey of existing health conditions was made by the United States Public Health Service soon after 1935. This revealed an uneven distribution of medical and nursing services, as well as an inadequacy of hospitals and other public institutions to meet health needs. That one-third of the population was receiving little or no medical attention and that an even larger proportion was suffering from economic burdens as the result of illness were among the alarming conclusions reached.

To meet the needs of rural areas, a large proportion of which lacked provision for care during illness, there followed a wide development of county health departments, and the greatest expansion of public health facilities in history. The best scientific knowledge and methods that modern medicine had to offer were afforded hitherto neglected places. The services of doctors and nurses with special preparation were secured, and through allotment of federal scholarships, provision was made for training others. Programs for maintaining maternal and child health received special consideration.

National Health Conference   In order to strengthen all aspects of the new program, a *National Health Conference* was summoned to Washington. Official representatives of the American Medical Association, of hospital and social service groups, and of the three major national nursing organizations attended. Annie W. Goodrich was the only speaker representing the nurses. Discussion centered in a *National Health Program*, with considerable emphasis on providing for better distribution of medical and nursing services. As a means of accomplishing desired ends, it was recommended that each community be held responsible for coordination of effort of its hospitals, health centers, clinics, and laboratories, and for putting them within reach of all of the people.

There was discussion also of the growing trend toward *socialized* or *state* medicine. If this were to come, conservation of health, like education, would become a function of the State. Plans developed for healthful living would reach into every activity of life, cover the needs of every community, be regulated from one central body, the National Government. The State would then become the employer of an army of laboratory and field workers necessary to give such health service, and be responsible for its distribution, equably, and according to the need of special functions that each profession has been prepared to offer. In this way, it might be possible to bring health to the family, to establish healthful working conditions, to reduce and ultimately, perhaps, to banish the waste of sickness.

A large group, however, did not accept the growing belief that the government owes complete medical services to the indigent and lower income groups. These expressed the opinion that instead of maintaining free medical services for those in need of them, the government should assure each man's opportunity to earn an income sufficient to cover his own and his family's health requirements.

SUMMARY, 1920–1939

By 1920 the aim of medical practice had reached the stage of teaching the principles of healthful living to all groups of people. Since the nurse was believed to be the person in the most advantageous position for effective teaching, the problem of health administrators was to supply expert nurse-teachers in sufficient numbers for the new program. There followed two critical surveys of nursing and nursing education.

The first survey, sponsored by the Rockefeller Foundation, covered the fields of private duty, public health, and twenty-three representative schools of nursing. In the private duty field, the influence of the nurse was found to be limited to one patient and his family, while in public health work, there was opportunity to teach many types of people. Findings in the hospital field disclosed many deficiencies in the conduct of nursing schools. Among recommendations made in the Winslow-Goldmark Report, emphasis was placed on making all schools of nursing financially independent of hospitals, raising nursing education to a college level, licensing subsidiary workers, and requiring preparation beyond the basic course for those holding administrative or teaching positions, or engaged in public health work.

An immediate answer to the recommendation that nursing schools be independent of hospitals and on a college level was the endowment of two university schools of nursing, one in connection with Yale University, New Haven, Connecticut, and the other with Western Reserve University, Cleveland, Ohio. With Annie W. Goodrich and Carolyn E. Gray as deans of these respective schools, the experiments proved both feasible and educationally sound.

A second and far-reaching result of the findings of the Rockefeller Survey was a critical examination of nursing schools, undertaken in 1925 under auspices of the National League of Nursing Education when May Ayres Burgess was named director of a Committee on the Grading of Nursing Schools. The general purpose of the Committee was defined as, "the study of ways and means for insuring an ample supply of nursing service, of whatever type and quality needed for adequate care of the patient, at a price within his reach."

As a result of the information disclosed, several hundred of the poorer schools closed their doors, and in many others educational standards were improved. In England and Canada, far-reaching results followed in the wake of similar surveys.

In order to provide for better distribution of nursing services, a *Joint Committee on the Distribution of Nursing Service* was appointed in 1928 by the three national nursing associations. It had the dual purpose of providing care for as many people as possible, and of ensuring needed employment for nurses during a major financial depression.

In an effort to strengthen the laws relating to nursing practice, a movement toward *licensing*, or legally permitting the qualified person to nurse, began about this time. With it arose the question of responsibility for the so-called "practical nurse." It was the opinion of many that she, too, should be required by law to complete an approved course of instruction before undertaking her work.

At the same time that nursing was undergoing a critical survey by the Committee on the Grading of Nursing Schools, a similar survey was being made of all phases of medical practice by a newly-appointed *Committee on the Costs of Medical Care*. Studies made of European methods revealed that, to a considerable extent, the principle of group insurance had been put into effect, with doctors, nurses, and other health workers employed on a full-time salary basis.

Among the conclusions reached by the Committee on the Costs of Medical Care was stressed the uneven distribution of medical services. Recommendations were made for the assumption by governmental bodies of responsibility for its provision for all citizens, regardless of financial ability. Through forms of group insurance, costs could be distributed over great numbers of people.

In line with public opinion that the Federal Government should assume responsibility for the economic and social welfare of each of its citizens, the Social Security Act of 1935 made its appearance. The greatest expansion of public health facilities in American history followed, with proportionate increase in demand for the services of doctors, nurses, and others having special preparation for the public health field.

TOPICS FOR DISCUSSION

1. Account for the fact that, with medicine's new aim of teaching personal hygiene to many people, the prevailing method of preparing nurses came under the fire of criticism.
2. What was the nursing situation at this time in regard to supply of workers for the public health field, and the number and type of students in the schools?
3. (a) What institution, closely associated with the public health movement, undertook a survey of the nursing field? (b) What committee was appointed, and who were its chairman and its secretary?
4. List important findings of the Committee, and some conclusions at which it arrived.
5. What two endowed university schools of nursing were founded in answer to one of the above conclusions?
6. (a) The appointment of what Committee was another and more far-reaching result of the Rockefeller Survey? (b) By whom was it sponsored? (c) Members of what organizations served on the Committee?
7. During its five year program, what three projects were undertaken by the Committee on Grading of Nursing Schools?

8. Why was a second survey made by the Grading Committee, and what were its findings?
9. What circumstances led to the appointment of a Joint Committee on the Distribution of Nursing Service?
10. What do you know of similar surveys of nursing education in other countries?
11. (*a*) In what project did organized nursing become interested after completion of the surveys by the Rockefeller Foundation and the Committee on the Grading of Nursing Schools? (*b*) What circumstances led to the new undertaking?
12. (*a*) What public criticisms led to an extensive survey of medical practice? (*b*) What Committee was appointed for this purpose? (*c*) Enumerate several conclusions reached.
13. (*a*) What changes in social outlook led to enactment of the Social Security Act of 1935? (*b*) What provisions were made for enforcement of the Act? (*c*) What field of nursing has it vitally affected?
14. Discuss the advantages and disadvantages of socialized or state medicine.

REFERENCES

Committee for the Study of Nursing Education: Nursing and Nursing Education in the United States. New York, The Macmillan Co., 1923.

Committee on the Grading of Nursing Schools: Nurses, Patients, and Pocketbooks, 1928.

———: Nursing Schools Today and Tomorrow, 1934.

Committee on Costs of Medical Care: Medical Care for the American People. Chicago, University of Chicago Press, 1932.

Curriculum Committee of Canadian Nurses' Association: A Proposed Curriculum for Schools of Nursing in Canada, 1936.

Curriculum Committee of National League of Nursing Education: Curriculum Guide for Schools of Nursing, 1938.

Falk, Rorem, and Ring: The Costs of Medical Care. Chicago, University of Chicago Press, 1933.

Goodrich, Annie W.: The Social and Ethical Significance of Nursing. New York, The Macmillan Co., 1932.

Johns and Pfefferkorn: An Activity Analysis of Nursing, 1934. Published by the Committee on the Grading of Nursing Schools.

Informational Service Circular No. 1: A Brief Explanation of the Social Security Act. The Social Security Board, Washington, D. C., 1938.

Nutting, Mary Adelaide: A Sound Economic Basis for Schools of Nursing. New York, G. P. Putnam's Sons, 1926.

Lancet Commission on Nursing: Final Report. The Lancet, Ltd., 7 Adam Street, Adelphi, London, W.C. 2.

Sigerist, Henry E.: American Medicine. New York, W. W. Norton & Co., Inc., 1934.

Stewart, Isabel M.: The Education of Nurses. New York, The Macmillan Co., 1943.

Weir, G. M.: Survey of Nursing Education in Canada. Toronto, Canada, University of Toronto Press, 1932.

XIII

World War II

By many observers, World War II is regarded as a continuation of the first World War, the twenty-one year period intervening representing merely an armistice which permitted the gathering of new strength for further hostilities. Credence is lent to this theory by the fact that the line-up of opposing powers was similar. The major shift in alignment was made by Italy and Japan, formerly in the Allied camp, but by 1939 in sympathy with Germany and willing partners in the so-called "Axis" which opposed the "United Nations." Provoked by the German attack on Poland, England declared war against Germany September 1, 1939. On December 8, 1941, the United States made a similar declaration against Japan. Two days later Germany and Italy retaliated by declaring war against the United States. The world was plunged into a new and terrifying form of conflict known as "total war," involving every man, woman, and child of belligerent countries.

In a relentless effort to break enemy morale, both sides sanctioned the bombing of cities and resultant destruction of civilian populations and property. What few rules of war mankind had built up to govern military campaigns were completely discarded, and the status of the noncombatant differed little from that of the front line soldier. The only answer to this total war must be total defense, with all civilians subjected to regimentation. Every able-bodied person had his station and his duties and was trained to carry out specific tasks in the event of bombing or invasion. The aged and the children were often evacuated in great numbers out of danger zones, taking noth-

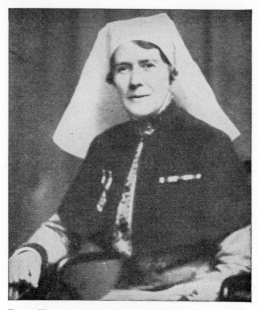

DAME KATHERINE H. JONES, D.B.E., R.R.C., S.R.N.
Matron-in-Chief Q.A.I.M.N.S. during World War II. (British Journal of Nursing, July, 1942.)

ing with them but what they could carry. Inevitably, anxiety neuroses and emotional instability accompanied such practices.

MEDICAL PROBLEMS

It was inevitable that the rapid massing of great numbers of troops in camps of the homeland would open up new channels for the spread of infection. Especially among men recruited from rural districts, the usual wartime outbreaks of children's diseases were frequent. With the transportation of troops to battle areas all over the globe, other varieties of disease put in their appearance. Lurking in pest-ridden African desert and South Pacific jungle, along with enemy snipers, were the organisms causing malaria, dysentery, and typhus.

Advances in Medical Treatment   As in previous conflicts, advances in medical treatment were great in some directions. The pre-

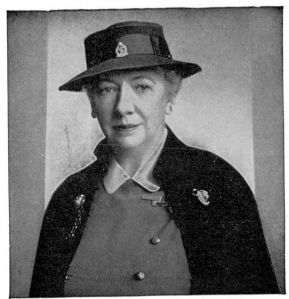

COLONEL ELIZABETH L. SMELLIE, C.B.E., R.R.C.
Matron-in-Chief Royal Canadian Army Medical Corps Nursing Service during
World War II.
(Courtesy of "The Canadian Nurse.")

vention and treatment of shock and infection showed marked improvement. Many a war veteran today owes his life to the effectiveness of blood plasma which could be transported to the battlefield and administered by a trained medical corpsman. The use of penicillin and the sulfonamides in relation to infection likewise was responsible for recovery of many of the wounded. When overseas sources of quinine were cut off by enemy action, synthetic preparations were perfected, giving promise of better results than the original. The new insecticide, dichloro-diphenyl-trichloroethane, better known as "DDT", was evolved and worked miracles in the elimination of insect-borne and rodent-borne diseases, notably malaria and typhus. Also among effective prophylactic measures introduced in World War II was the administration of tetanus toxoid and yellow fever vaccine to all members of the fighting forces.

PROCUREMENT OF NURSES

National Nursing Council for War Service In spite of revolutionary methods in treatment, a high incidence of disease and mounting casualties of war made it necessary that ever greater numbers of doctors, nurses, and related medical personnel be forthcoming. Recognizing the need for concerted action, the *National Nursing Council for War Service* was organized in July, 1940, to represent the nurses of the United States, and plans were formulated to (a) promote a national inventory of registered nurses, (b) expand facilities of existing accredited schools of nursing and (c) supply supplementary nursing services to hospitals and public health agencies.

The National Nursing Council for War Service soon proved effective as a coordinating link between organized nursing and the Federal program for supplying an adequate number of nurses to the armed forces. Launching an intensive campaign to attract candidates for nursing schools, it disseminated information that would be helpful in judging the relative merits of nursing schools, stated minimum entrance requirements, and outlined opportunities within the field of professional nursing. By magazine, poster, letter, and radio, the Nursing Council spread its message of need and opportunity. In addition, it served as a consultant to the *Procurement and Assignment Service for Physicians, Dentists, Veterinarians, Sanitary Engineers, and Nurses*, a Federal agency to which had been delegated responsibility for equable distribution of professional personnel in accordance with both military and civilian needs.

Red Cross Agencies The National Nursing Council for War Service was not alone in the struggle to secure adequate nursing personnel. Working side by side with it was the American Red Cross Nursing Service as it campaigned to enlarge the roll of reserve nurses who would be ready to augment the Army Nurse Corps and the Navy Nurse Corps as the need arose. Also, a *Red Cross Student Reserve* was set up in which senior student nurses were enrolled with the pledge to become active in war service upon graduation. At the same time, graduate nurses, with special preparation and holding responsible positions, were encouraged to remain at their posts. Unfortunately, however, this plea went unheeded by many.

In a determined effort to meet the desperate need of hospitals, first-aid stations, and similar organizations for trained assistants to

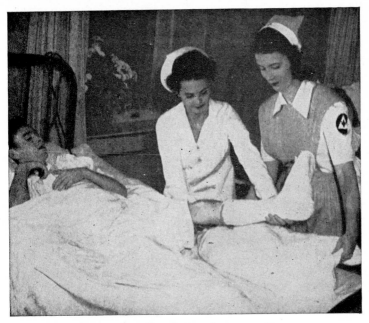

A Volunteer Nurse's Aide Assists the Nurse
(American Journal of Nursing, December, 1941.)

professional nurses, the *Red Cross Volunteer Nurses' Aide Corps* was organized by the American Red Cross. Composed of women between the ages of eighteen and fifty, many of them with homes and families, the Corps was trained by qualified nurse instructors in an eighty hour course, thirty-five hours of which were in the classroom, and forty-five in hospital wards. Their instructors were pleased by the efficient manner in which they took hold of simple nursing tasks for which housewifely experience provided a valuable background. They proved invaluable additions to professional staffs wherever institutions were fortunate enough to secure their services.

Additional help came from the American Red Cross in the employment of great numbers of nurse instructors to teach courses in *Red Cross Home Nursing* to housewives and mothers in order that they might take intelligent care of their families during minor illnesses, or periods of convalescence. Finally, the Red Cross greatly enlarged its personnel of instructors for teaching principles of *First Aid* to all types of people.

United States Public Health Service   Added to the efforts of the National Nursing Council for War Service, the American Red Cross, and the American Red Cross Nursing Service, were those of the *United States Public Health Service*. By conducting the National Survey of Registered Nurses, first promoted by the National Nursing Council for War Service, it was able to determine not only the total number of nurses throughout the nation, but also their preparation, experience, and availability. With its sanction and cooperation, Federal funds were granted to established schools of nursing of good standing, enabling them to increase their dormitory space and teaching facilities. In this way was made possible an increase in student enrollment, expansion of post-graduate courses, and institution of refresher courses for those who had been inactive in nursing.

United States Cadet Nurse Corps. So great was the need that, despite coordinated efforts of the organizations mentioned, there still remained an unfulfilled demand for military and civilian nurses. In one of the most effective steps taken to meet the emergency, Congress, in 1943, passed the Bolton Bill, so named because sponsored by Mrs. Frances Payne Bolton, congresswoman of Ohio whose endowment made possible the Frances Payne Bolton School of Nursing affiliated with Western Reserve University in Cleveland. Under provisions of the Bolton Act, the United States Public Health Service was authorized to establish the *United States Cadet Nurse Corps* through which young women desirous of entering schools of nursing would be extended financial aid, in effect, similar to a scholarship.

In a campaign to attract great numbers of recruits, it was widely advertised that students entering schools of nursing would be provided with books, indoor uniforms, all entrance and tuition fees, and paid a generous monthly allowance for personal expenses. In addition, an attractive gray outdoor uniform was designed featuring crimson epaulets, insignia of the United States Public Health Service, and a distinctive sleeve emblem patterned after the Maltese Cross, emblem of the Knights of St. John of Jerusalem, organized during the Crusades. In return, students pledged themselves to remain in some type of active nursing for the duration of the war.

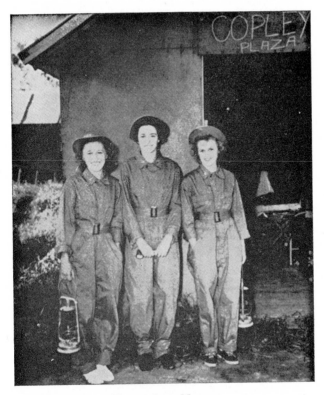

TRIO OF ARMY NURSES

(From Folder, "Enlist in a Proud Profession! Train as a Nurse!" Put out by the
U. S. Cadet Nurse Corps during the war.)

In order to be approved for receiving cadet students, accredited
schools of nursing were required to accelerate their curricula in order
that, during the last six months, senior cadets might be available for
service in military or other civilian hospitals where the need was
greater. In this way, cadet assistance was brought quickly to many
institutions, educational and dormitory facilities vacated by senior
cadets were made available for new recruits, and thousands of graduate nurses were released for military service without danger of collapse of nursing service at home. At the same time, nursing schools,
along with other educational institutions, grew more and more handi-

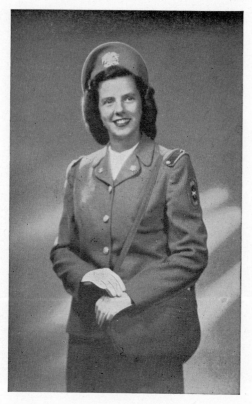

A MEMBER OF THE UNITED STATES CADET NURSE CORPS DURING WORLD WAR II

capped by a shortage of qualified teachers, as doctors and nurses continued to leave for war service.

Accepting the fact that a high percentage of their employees must be released, hospitals made heroic effort to ensure essential care for their patients. Part-time nurses and subsidiary workers were employed whenever possible. Refresher courses were instituted for retired nurses willing to return to duty, while the volunteer services of Red Cross Nurses' Aides for a few hours daily were gratefully accepted. At the same time an effort was made to discourage all types of "luxury nursing," and the employment of special nurses by pa-

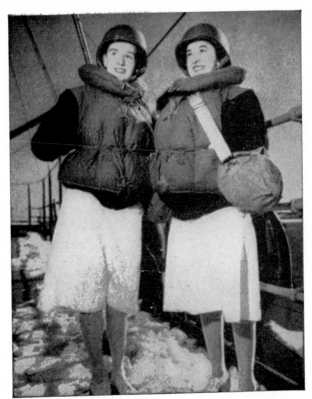

Two Navy Nurses on a Hospital Ship in the North Atlantic

(From Folder, "Enlist in a Proud Profession! Train as a Nurse!" put out by the U. S. Cadet Nurse Corps during the war.)

tients, or office nurses by doctors, was deemed contrary to the patriotic spirit.

Military Nursing And where, one may well ask, did all those nurses leaving for active service go? In the answer would be an almost complete tracing of geographical locations, for the nurse of World War II followed military operations, went with the fighting men. From Alaska to Australia, from England to Africa, from the Philippines to India, nurses of all warring countries carried on courageously, at times in face of enemy bomb, shell, and torpedo.

Assisting in underground operating rooms, evacuating patients from bombed positions, and salvaging equipment, nurses upheld the finest traditions of their calling. Some of their number were called upon to care for patients in the midst of tropical jungles, to part with all of their possessions as they evaded the trap of an enemy, to abandon sinking ships, to escape in submarines, to drift for days in life-boats. Others were taken prisoner, and some were killed in the line of duty.

Along with great advances in aviation prior to and during the war, it was not strange that the airplane should come to play an important role in transporting the sick and wounded, and neither was it strange that the nurse should have a place in the new method. With special training she might become a "flight nurse," caring for patients in air ambulances while in transit from battle fronts and emergency hospitals to institutions within zones of safety. A small group of selected nurses even learned parachute jumping at the Air Evacuation School set up at Bowman Field, Kentucky. A system providing rapid evacuation and the prompt, skilled services of doctors and nurses increased recovery rates perceptibly.

Industrial Nursing   While ever-increasing demands for nurses for the armed forces seriously depleted the civilian supply of graduates, another field of war effort was also draining off large numbers. With the production of hitherto unheard-of numbers of shells, ships, tanks, planes, and guns, *war industry* grew to vast proportions. To maintain this flood of equipment, calls for help were sent out everywhere to men, women, and children. By bus, train, and automobile they swarmed into manufacturing centers until scores of cities fairly bulged with the influx of workers. Also, in corn fields and deserts there grew like magic great industrial plants surrounded by their satellite areas of housing projects, overflowing with humanity. Only in what was considered a struggle for existence could such a transformation take place so rapidly.

As with the front line soldier, the health of the home front worker must be conserved if he was to remain at his post, turning out the materials of war. The great expansion in industrial nursing that followed proved a further drain upon available nurse power. At the same time, with the usual wartime increase in general wage levels, more and more workers participated in prepayment and group medical plans resulting in ever greater patient loads in hospitals. With

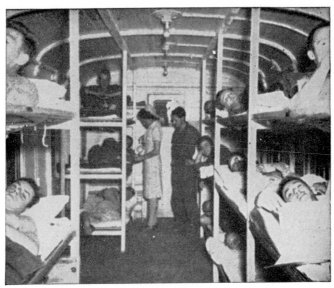

A HOSPITAL TRAIN

(From "Army Nursing"—a brochure published at Washington, D. C., August 7, 1947.)

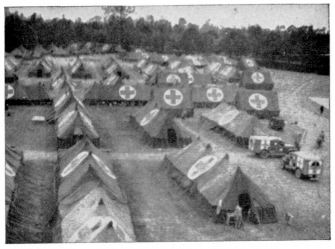

AN EVACUATION HOSPITAL NEAR A BATTLEFRONT

gathering speed the need for supplying doctors and nurses grew in all directions.

Like her sister in military uniform, the industrial nurse contributed her share to the war effort. Not only did she render nursing service under the direction of an industrial physician, but also she worked on safety education and accident prevention programs. Through her efforts loss of time due to occupational and nonoccupational illnesses and injuries was reduced to a minimum. In daily contact with the everyday worker and his family, she had opportunity to render assistance not only in relation to their physical ills, but many psychological and emotional problems as well. With a genuine liking for people and interest in health teaching, her influence penetrated through large groups of people.

The Nurse Draft Bill   In the closing months of the war, but before it was fully realized that the end was near, the President of the United States called upon Congress to prepare legislation permitting the government to draft nurses into military service. Although a large proportion of the active professional nurses of this country were in service, voluntary enlistments were not meeting anticipated needs. The American Nurses' Association went on record as approving such a move provided that it be made a part of Selective Service legislation to include all women.

In March, 1945, the House of Representatives designed and passed a Nurse Draft Bill and sent it to the Senate, but the subsequent train of events invalidated need for it. Realizing the urgency expressed in the president's words, additional nurses volunteered for war service, and a survey of cadet nurses showed that approximately nine tenths of them intended to enter the Army or Navy Nurse Corps upon graduation. Then the war in Europe came to an end on May 8, and need for a draft of nurses was over. The bill was dropped.

With final termination of hostilities in the Pacific, August 14, 1945, there came to a close the greatest nurse recruiting campaign in history.

REHABILITATION

Like other wars before it, World War II left in its wake an aftermath of hunger, fear, sorrow, and disease. This time, however, the loss of human life and human trust was greater. With these facts in

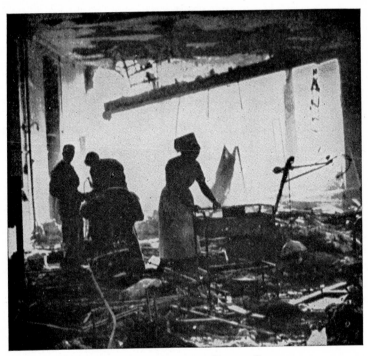

A British Hospital after Raiders Passed
(American Journal of Nursing, April, 1941.)

view, it is understandable that sociologists of today regard the elimination of war as the most urgent of man's problems, a practice of primitive man to be continued only at the risk of annihilating our entire civilization. Few who have seriously studied reports of the destruction of Hiroshima, Japan, in 1945 by the first atomic bomb used in warfare can discount this gloomy viewpoint. Then, too, as time goes on new scientific discoveries inevitably will lead to more and more terrible agents of destruction.

New weapons alone cannot serve as a measure of the horrors of war, for old destroyers sufficient to uproot social life as we know it, continue to accompany it. Moral deterioration and spread of social disease are concomitants of war, while poverty, broken homes and absence of parental guidance inevitably lead to an alarming increase in anxiety neuroses and juvenile delinquency. With such chaotic signposts as these to point the way, is it little wonder that at least a part of the world's people are striving to lead mankind out of old primitive pathways into a constructive era of peace and good will toward one's neighbors? However, the path leading to peace is a rocky one for it necessitates changes in long standing political and economic patterns. Nevertheless, there are reasons for encouragement.

UNITED NATIONS RELIEF AND REHABILITATION ADMINISTRATION

Active throughout the war in relieving suffering was the League of Red Cross Societies, and, late in 1943, forty-four countries banded together to bring into being the *United Nations Relief and Rehabilitation Administration*, a temporary organization to provide immediate assistance during a critical period. Surely there is cause for optimism concerning the future of civilization when it is realized that so many nations, in the midst of a war the outcome of which was as yet undetermined, instituted a program to provide food, shelter and clothing for millions of needy peoples. With the combined efforts of contributing nations were included the services of many doctors, nurses, dentists, social workers, and sanitary engineers. Through "UNRRA," as the organization was soon popularly called, stricken areas received not only essential primary assistance but also aid in the return to their homelands of prisoners-of-war and otherwise displaced persons, as well as help in the reestablishment of agricultural and industrial activities.

Some idea of the immensity of the task confronting UNRRA can be gathered from a study of Europe in the era immediately following total war. From France to western Russia and from the Baltic to the Mediterranean, an estimated twenty million human beings suffered from exposure, malnutrition, and disease, lived a pathetic day to day existence. With a complete lack of medical supplies, or even of that elementary adjunct to health, soap, it could be expected that disease and moral deterioration would run rampant. It was only natural, too, that tuberculosis would head the list of causes of death while scabies, influenza, and dysentery completed the incapacitation and decimation of millions of people.

Against this holocaust UNRRA threw its might, and the vast program was carried on in the face of crippling shortages of equipment and personnel. In addition to administering to the hungry, the homeless, and the sick, UNRRA was instrumental in determining the available medical and nurse supply in a given area, in establishing schools for nurses and nurses' aides, and in providing scholarships for graduate study.

Today the task of UNRRA is over. The size of that task may be measured by such statistical markers as the number of vaccines and serums administered, the tons of food dispensed, the quantity of clothing made available. Measure can never be made of the mental suffering alleviated by UNRRA's personnel, or of the message of hope that they brought to millions of hapless victims of war's ruthless desolation. While what has been described as "the most ambitious humanitarian effort ever undertaken by mankind" came to an end in December, 1946, its work to be taken over by numerous sr aller agents, the memory of its efforts will be lasting.

THE FOUR FREEDOMS

Before the entry of the United States into the conflict, but when gathering war clouds were making the future appear dark and gloomy, President Franklin D. Roosevelt in his message to Congress, January 6, 1941, gave hope to oppressed peoples through the following declaration:

"In the future days which we seek to make secure, we look forward to a world founded upon four essential human freedoms.

"The first is freedom of speech and expression everywhere in the world.

"The second is freedom of every person to worship God in his own way—everywhere in the world.

"The third is freedom from want—which, translated into world terms, means economic inderstandings which will secure to every nation a healthy peacetime life for its inhabitants—everywhere in the world.

"The fourth is freedom from fear—which, translated into world terms, means a world-wide reduction of armaments to such a point and in such a thorough fashion that no nation will be in a position to commit an act of physical aggression against any neighbor—anywhere in the world.

"That is no vision of a distant millennium. It is a definite basis for a kind of world attainable in our own time and generation."[1]

[2] Quoted in "An Adventure in World Order" by Philip C. Nash. The Beacon Press, Boston, 1944, pp. 129, 130.

THE ATLANTIC CHARTER

In August, 1941, Prime Minister Winston Churchill of Great Britain and President Franklin D. Roosevelt of the United States daringly met on shipboard in the Atlantic Ocean. At this time the fortunes of war appeared to be with the Axis powers; the oceans were infested with mines and submarines and every move of enemy officials was under rigid surveillance. On the fourteenth day of the month, what is known as the "Atlantic Charter" was drawn up to include the following:

"The President of the United States of America and the Prime Minister, Mr. Churchill, representing his Majesty's Government in the United Kingdom, being met together, deem it right to make known certain common principles in the national policies of their respective countries on which they base their hopes for a better future for the world.

"They desire to see no territorial changes that do not accord with the freely expressed wishes of the peoples concerned.

"They respect the right of all peoples to choose the form of government under which they will live; and they wish to see sovereign rights and self-government restored to those who have been forcibly deprived of them.

"They will endeavor, with due respect for their existing obligations, to further the enjoyment by all States, great or small, victor or vanquished, of access on equal terms to the trade and to the raw materials of the world which are needed for their economic prosperity.

"They believe that all of the nations of the world, for realistic as well as spiritual reasons, must come to the abandonment of the use of force. Since no future peace can be maintained if land, sea, or air armaments continue to be employed by nations which threaten, or may threaten, aggression outside of their frontiers, they believe, pending the establishment of a wider and permanent system of general security, that the disarmament of such nations is essential. They will likewise aid and encourage all other practicable measures which will lighten for peace-loving people the crushing burden of armaments."[2]

THE UNITED NATIONS

Recognizing the need for concerted effort in order to implement into action the spirit of the Four Freedoms and the Atlantic Charter, a group of representatives of the nations opposing the Axis met in San Francisco in February, 1945. Out of this gathering was born the "United Nations," a world organization designed to promote peace-time teamwork, and prevent future hostilities, which has been defined as follows:

[2] *Ibid.*, p. 130.

"The United Nations is an organization of sovereign states which have agreed to join their efforts in order to maintain international peace, to co-operate on the solution of economic, social, and cultural problems of international importance, and to promote human rights for all without distinction as to race, sex, language, or religion."[3]

The charter of the United Nations was signed by representatives of fifty-one nations, and came into force October 24, 1945, the anniversary of which is now observed as United Nations Day.

Despite the failure of its predecessor, the League of Nations, which slowly crumpled away as power after power abandoned it in pursuit of purely nationalistic ambitions, the United Nations was able to glean from the wreckage certain invaluable results of experience. In substance, it was recognized that the United Nations must have more power than had been allotted to the League of Nations. It must be upheld by the wealth, scientific resources, and armies of its member nations if it was to become an effective instrument for maintaining world peace. Upon its continuance and power to act in an emergency, the fate of civilization itself may depend.

The structure of the United Nations consists of six principal Organs: General Assembly, Security Council, International Court of Justice, Economic and Social Council, Trusteeship Council, and Secretariat.

General Assembly   At the base of the United Nations lies the *General Assembly*. Composed of all member nations, five delegates from each meeting annually, it has been compared to a sort of "town meeting of the world." Upon its shoulders rests responsibility for untangling perplexing problems arising between nations, and making recommendations in the interests of international peace and security. Its business is carried on according to parliamentary rule, and each member nation has one vote, whether large or small, rich or poor. The General Assembly is the only principal organ representing all members, and its decisions exert considerable moral influence over the great family of nations.

Security Council   With power to enforce international law, the *Security Council* is composed of five permanent members, England,

[3] Dolivet, Louis: The United Nations. New York, Farrar, Straus and Company, 1946, p. 15.

France, Russia, China, and the United States, as well as six non-permanent members to be elected for terms of two years each by the General Assembly. The Security Council is primarily responsible for effecting peaceful settlement of disputes that might otherwise lead to war. It has been empowered to settle such threats by diplomatic sanctions, by cutting off the offending nation from world trade, or, if necessary, by the use of armed force which will be placed at its disposal by member nations. Any nation, whether or not a member of the United Nations, may request action if it feels that it is being imposed upon by another nation, and the peace is being threatened. In the consideration of all disputes, world opinion exerts a powerful influence on the outcome.

International Court of Justice   With legal machinery to settle disputes, the *International Court of Justice* comprises fifteen judges from as many countries who have been elected by the General Assembly and the Security Council. It is permanently in session at the Hague, Holland, and the judges, on annual salary, are permitted no other occupation. The Court of Justice makes decisions which are in agreement with the principles of international law and the general legal principles recognized by civilized peoples.

Economic and Social Council   Composed of eighteen member nations elected by the General Assembly, the Economic and Social Council is of especial significance to doctors, nurses, social workers, and educators. As the name implies, it is concerned with matters affecting the economic and social life of all individuals. It is designed to promote conditions conducive to health, education, and higher standards of living throughout the world.

A number of *Specialized Intergovernmental Agencies* are associated with the Economic and Social Council, three of which are of interest to those in the field of health: The World Health Organization (WHO), the Food and Agricultural Organization (FAO), and the United Nations Educational, Scientific, and Cultural Organization (UNESCO).

Several *Specialized Commissions* also have been created, four of which are the Commission on Human Rights, the Commission on the Status of Women, the Commission on Narcotic Drugs, and the Social Commission. Under the heading of *Special Bodies* are the Permanent Central Opium Board, the International Children's

Emergency Fund (UNICEF), and the United Nations Appeal for Children (UNAC).

At the suggestion of Brazil and China, one of the first actions taken by the Economic and Social Council was the calling of a World Health Conference preliminary to drafting a constitution for a *World Health Organization,* in the preamble of which now appears:

"Health is a state of complete physical, mental, and social well-being and not merely the absence of disease or infirmity.

"The enjoyment of the highest attainable standard of health is one of the fundamental rights of every human being without distinction of race, religion, political belief, economic or social condition.

"The health of all peoples is fundamental to the attainment of peace and security and is dependent upon the fullest cooperation of individuals and States.."[4]

The World Health Organization has become the largest Specialized Agency of the United Nations, and now, once again, man's horizon in regard to a suitable viewpoint for health planning has assumed new proportions. The national health acts of various countries, considered radical measures when instituted, are now dwarfed by prospects of achievement by what might be compared to a great international public health service, the aim of which is to be mental, physical, and social health for each of the earth's inhabitants.

Among the first undertakings of the WHO were measures aimed at global control and ultimate eradication of malaria, tuberculosis, and the venereal diseases, and the development of maternal and child health services. To carry on its activities, a professional staff of more than five hundred is maintained which includes about thirty public health nurses and two nurse consultants.

In order to obtain a representative body of opinion on health subjects and ensure its constant support, a number of non-governmental organizations have been admitted to official relationship with the World Health Organization. In 1947, the International Council of Nurses became one of this group, and through such relationship, nurses are represented on the Expert Committees relating to nursing, and so enabled to act as advisers in regard to nursing education, nursing service, and other professional questions. It means that nurses are to have a prominent place in making special studies and collect-

4 Quoted in pamphlet issued by World Health Organization Interim Commission, 6306 Empire State Building, 350 Fifth Avenue, New York 1, New York.

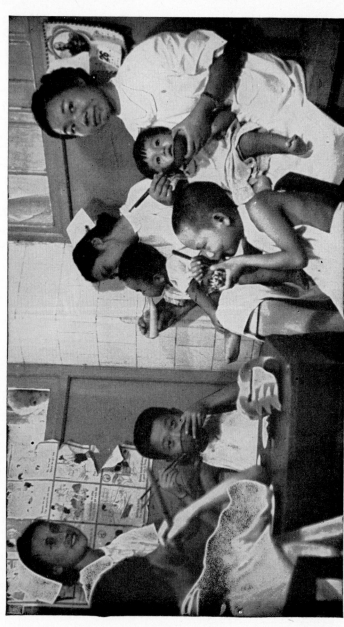

A WHO FIELD MISSION IN CHINA SUPERVISES RELIEF AND MEDICAL CARE PROVIDED FOR CHILDREN AT THE NANKING GENERAL HOSPITAL

(From American Journal of Nursing, January, 1948, by permission of American Journal of Nursing.)

ing information that will be of value in establishing nursing methods on a firm basis throughout the world.

The policies and programs of the WHO are determined by an annual World Health Assembly, made up of delegates from member countries. The new approach to world health which has been adopted is based upon the philosophy that by means of an unceasing, aggressive, world-wide attack upon disease with up-to-date methods, many of the scourges that have long troubled mankind can be either entirely eliminated or greatly reduced.

Closely associated with the aims and success of the World Health Organization is the *Food and Agricultural Organization* (FAO), pledged to improve the nutrition and general living standards of all peoples. So far in the world's history, at least two thirds of its inhabitants have been constantly hungry; but it is believed that with introduction of the best available farming methods into underdeveloped countries, they will be enabled to produce sufficient quantities of the right kind of food for all. With such increased production, greater employment opportunities and higher living standards can be expected to follow.

Another of the Specialized Agencies of the Economic and Social Council, the *United Nations Educational, Scientific, and Cultural Organization*, strives to promote the objectives of the common welfare of mankind and international peace by making universal the benefits that education, science, and culture have to offer.

UNESCO assists in the building of schools, universities, libraries, laboratories, and museums in war-torn and underdeveloped countries, and otherwise helps to promote education and combat illiteracy throughout the world. Since its ultimate purpose is to teach people to live in harmony with one another, it is making a special study of the various racial, religious, and social tensions that lead to war. Significantly, the Preamble to UNESCO's Constitution contains the following statement: "Since wars begin in the minds of men, it is in the minds of men that the defences of peace must be constructed."

Trusteeship Council   Faced with the responsibility of looking after those areas of the globe which are not self-administered, the United Nations provides for a *Trusteeship Council*. To it has been assigned the sacred trust of promoting the well-being and insuring the advancement of territories released from control by defeated powers of World Wars I and II, and also those voluntarily given over to it by the nations responsible for them.

Secretariat   Finally, the administrative body of the vast enterprise of the United Nations is the *Secretariat*, composed of a Secretary-General appointed for a period of five years, eight Assistant Secretary-Generals, and a staff of about three thousand citizens of many countries who have taken an oath of allegiance to the United Nations. Among the personnel of this permanent international civil service are many scientists, specialists in the fields of economics, social welfare, and health, as well as administrators, research workers, secretaries, and others. They are the first true international citizens, may be of either sex, and hold permanent positions with stipulated salaries.

What may well prove indicative of tomorrow's philosophy was expressed by Trygve Lie, the first Secretary-General, when, after taking the oath of office, he declared: "I no longer consider myself a Norwegian. I am a citizen of the world." The same thought was expressed more than two thousand years ago by Socrates when he said, "I am a citizen, not of Athens or of Greece, but of the world," and after World War I by Cale Young Rice, in the following poem:

THE NEW PATRIOT

"Within his heart, East shall be one with West,
And his effaceless thought shall be
That earth was made for all
Its driven millions sore distraught.
For he at last shall come to see
Through all the creeds about him hurled,
His nation is humanity,
His country, the world."

Even though civilization has been rendered chaotic by rapid social evolution, the assumption of new responsibilities and wide horizons by the United Nations indicates that there will be brought about a more even distribution of health, wealth, and happiness than has so far been experienced. Through international cooperation and scientific planning, its Constitution promises the peoples of the world a fair share of those factors which contribute to a good life for all. In the cost, however, must be reckoned the scrapping of many cherished traditions and such old loyalties as those which create a narrow nationalism. In return, the following advantages are to be gained: Security in place of instability, abolition of war, abundance instead of poverty, and opportunity to develop a finer culture than the world has yet known.

That the nurse plays a major role in the vast drama of struggle for peace and security throughout the world was made clear by the words of Katherine Densford, while President of the American Nurses' Association, as she reported to that organization following attendance at the first United Nations Conference in San Francisco:

"The nursing profession is one of the important groups in this country which must accept responsibility for helping to make an international organization work. Even as the nurse is the woman of the hour in time of war, she will play a vital role in the peace, and in the rehabilitation of the world of tomorrow. Obviously, a sound and healthful citizenry is essential to meet the tasks of peace no less than the emergencies of war. If we believe, as most of us do, that health is a fundamental in any international peace organization, we must accept the place of nurses as interpreters of health."[5]

It is evident that the nurse's contribution to world peace and security goes far beyond her individual knowledge and skill. It includes a half century's experience in international cooperation through the activities of the International Council of Nurses. Of vital importance to her country in time of war, she is no less so in the struggle for securing a workable and lasting peace.

POST-WAR DEVELOPMENTS

Now that the war was over, it was at first believed that in a short time conditions along all lines would assume a normal character. Soldiers, sailors, airmen, and nurses on foreign soil expressed eagerness to return to their homes immediately. Soon, however, it was realized that obstacles existed in many directions. A society that has been uprooted cannot return to old ground easily, if at all. Changes had taken place in homes and places of business, in those left behind as well as in those who served with the armed forces. Old patterns of life no longer fitted, and, in many instances, had lost their appeal. Restlessness and uncertainty on all sides became apparent.

Hospitals and other organizations looking to the nurse returning from active duty to relieve the emergency character of their work

[5] Quoted in Bulletin of California State Nurses' Association, May, 1945, p. 144.

were soon to be disappointed. Registries reported that many war-weary nurses were taking well-earned vacations; others found means of securing advanced education, or were determined to engage in new lines of endeavor offering more attractive hours or remuneration. Some, indeed, were incapacitated for further professional activity. At the same time, many married and retired nurses who had been giving valuable assistance suddenly left the field once more. Nursing staffs everywhere remained seriously depleted. As a final burden, termination of the benefits of the United States Cadet Nurse Corps, and the recruiting program associated with it, resulted in an alarming shortage of applicants for entrance to schools of nursing.

For a time, hospitals were left to their own resources for solution of their problems. Recognizing that a crisis was approaching, the National League of Nursing Education and the American Hospital Association devoted considerable time and energy to a study of the social implications of the situation, and soon engaged in a nation-wide recruitment program. It was not many months before the receding interest in nursing was once more showing signs of returning. Nevertheless, the task of rebuilding depleted nursing staffs remained difficult. Creation of new positions, increased hospital construction, prepayment hospital insurance, Federal social legislation, together with growing public interest in health education and early treatment, were constantly increasing the demand for nurses.

Recognizing the problem to be one involving the security of every citizen, the American Nurses' Association launched a publicity campaign of considerable magnitude. The purpose was to arouse the public to an understanding of its responsibility for correcting those factors contributing to a reluctance on the part of qualified young women to enter schools of nursing, and of graduates to remain in the profession. Moreover, it was believed that popular recognition of the fact that modern, complicated medical technics, involving the mind as well as the body, create a demand for nurses with a rich background of knowledge that will lead to the general establishment of nursing education in institutions of higher learning.

Practical Nurses   While effort was thus being directed toward providing satisfactory nursing care for all in need of it, the necessity for supplying great numbers of well-prepared practical or vocational nurses stood out with clearness. With their help, professional nurses would be relieved of many routine tasks, and so be free to assume greater responsibility in relation to teaching and treatment. To meet the demand, courses of about one year's duration began to appear in senior high schools, and to some extent in junior colleges. In order to give direction to the movement, and provide a consultant service to establish minimum standards for schools of practical nursing, the National Association for Practical Nurse Education was organized in 1940 by the American Nurses' Association. A definition of a practical nurse was formulated as follows:

"The practical nurse is a person trained to care for selected convalescent, subacute and chronically ill patients, and to assist the professional nurse in a team relationship, especially in the care of those more acutely ill. She provides nursing service in institutions, and in private homes where she is prepared to give household assistance when necessary. She may be employed by a private individual, a hospital, or a health agency. A practical nurse works only under the direct orders of a licensed physician or the supervision of a registered professional nurse."[6]

In the meantime, hospitals continued with brief courses of varying hours of instruction for nurses' aides, who practiced without any form of guarantee of their ability. There were indications, nevertheless, that adequate numbers of nursing service teams for institutional work eventually would emerge, the members of which would be professional nurses, practical nurses, and nurses' aides of stipulated preparation. Each would have knowledge of, and respect for, the ability and accomplishments of the others.

AMERICAN RED CROSS NURSING SERVICES

In the year 1947 changes were made in the method of enrolling Red Cross nurses. No longer was there need for providing a reserve for the Army Nurse Corps and the Navy Nurse Corps since these federal services were now doing their own recruiting. Need continued, however, for the maintenance of a roster of nurses who would go into immediate action in case of an epidemic or other local disaster. An earthquake, tornado, fire, flood, explosion, or train, bus, or plane wreck, or the bombing of a city would make it necessary to give first aid to, and evacuate from their homes, great

[6] "Practical Nurses in Nursing Services," a pamphlet prepared by the Joint Committee on Practical Nurses and Auxiliary Workers in Nursing Services. New York, American Nurses' Association, 1951, p. 11.

numbers of victims. Nurses would be needed to serve with the National Blood Program, to teach classes for Volunteer Nurse's Aides, and to give instruction in Home Nursing.

Public-spirited nurses, wishing to make their knowledge and skills available in case of emergency, or to assist with another of the Red Cross Services, now enroll through their local Red Cross Chapters. A badge and membership card, designating her as an American Red Cross Nurse, is awarded to each upon completion of such service. These symbols of a contribution to social welfare identify her with the humanitarian movement of the Red Cross, which knows no national boundaries.

THE RISE OF PSYCHIATRY

Two world wars, with their emphasis on mass destruction, inevitably focused medical attention on the care of patients with nervous and mental disorders. The revolution in the study of the human mind, which has followed, has restored many chronic invalids to health, and criminals and other social outcasts to their rightful places in society. Mental hygiene programs have come into being, child guidance clinics and psychiatric social work have been established in the large cities, all contributing to the peace and security that can be enjoyed by countless numbers of persons.

National mental health programs are in operation in many countries, and, in 1948, the *World Federation for Mental Health* came into being, the aims and purposes of which are defined as follows:

"To promote among all peoples and nations the highest possible standard of mental health, in its broadest biological, medical, educational, and social aspects.
"To work with the Economic and Social Council of the United Nations, UNESCO and the World Health Organization, with all of which the Federation has a consultant role."[7]

Membership of the World Federation for Mental Health is composed principally of societies "concerned to some degree with the establishment and maintenance of good Mental Health and better Human Relations in the home, the community, the state, and between nations."[7] Nurses can be justly proud of the fact that the

[7] Folder of the World Federation for Mental Health, 19 Manchester Street, London W. 1, England.

ANA and ICN are two of these societies. In 1950, the entire membership of societies and individual associate members represented about one million persons in thirty-three countries.

In the United States, passage of the National Mental Health Act in 1946 was followed by wide expansion of educational facilities to equip personnel for the practice of preventive Psychiatry in all its aspects. With the objective of eventual improvement of the services that all nurses will be prepared to offer, advanced courses in Mental Health and Psychiatric Nursing have been opened to qualified candidates. Scholarships to be used in preparation for positions as psychiatric nurses and mental health nurses have been made available.

Psychosomatic Medicine The practice of psychosomatic medicine has followed in the wake of Psychiatry. This science recognizes the body as a delicate instrument which, through the subconscious mind, responds to everything in its environment. It concerns itself with the whole pattern of everyday living of all patients and treats them as total organisms with mental and spiritual, as well as physical, requirements. Problems of life experiences, beginning in childhood, as well as disturbing social relationships encountered all through life, are now known to be the cause of many physical, as well as mental, illnesses. The degree of intelligence and understanding used in meeting such situations determines the outcome.

It has been demonstrated that, in overcoming their difficulties, many patients gain courage and substantial help through their particular interpretation of religion. The minister, priest, or rabbi then becomes an invaluable addition to the health team. In her contribution to its success, the capable nurse will have a sympathetic understanding of the healing power of all religions and be prepared to cooperate intelligently with prescribed forms of treatment, whether they be medical or surgical, psychological or spiritual, in character.

While peoples of the world are in disagreement upon many social and political issues, they are in complete agreement with the premise that mental and physical well-being is mankind's most valuable possession. This agreement led to establishment of the World Health Organization within the framework of the Economic and Social Council of the United Nations. It is now recognized that, in striving toward that millenium when the chief energies of man will be directed toward maintaining the highest possible standards of physical, men-

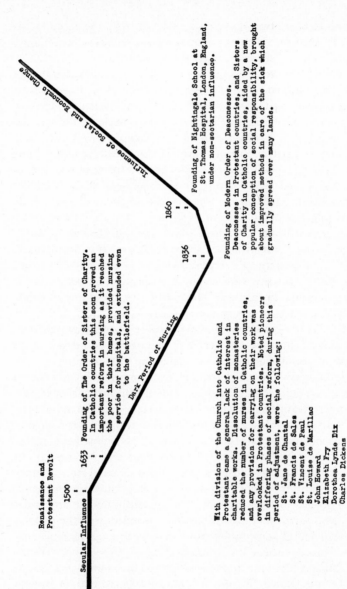

Renaissance and
Protestant Revolt

1500

Secular Influence :

1633   Founding of The Order of Sisters of Charity.
In Catholic countries this soon proved an
important reform in nursing as it reached
the poor in their homes, provided nursing
service for hospitals, and extended even
to the battlefield.

Dark Period of Nursing

1836

1860

Influence of Social and Economic Change

Founding of Nightingale School at
St. Thomas Hospital, London, England,
under non-sectarian influence.

Founding of Modern Order of Deaconesses.
Deaconesses in Protestant countries, and Sisters
of Charity in Catholic countries, aided by a new
popular conception of social responsibility, brought
about improved methods in care of the sick which
gradually spread over many lands.

With division of the Church into Catholic and
Protestant came a general lack of interest in
charitable works. Dissolution of monasteries
reduced the number of nurses in Catholic countries,
and any provision for carrying on their work was
overlooked in Protestant countries. Noted pioneers
in differing phases of social reform, during this
period of adjustment, were the following:
    St. Jane de Chantal
    St. Francis de Sales
    St. Vincent de Paul
    St. Louise de Marillac
    John Howard
    Elizabeth Fry
    Dorothea Lynde Dix
    Charles Dickens

NURSING OF THE MODERN ERA

1500—

tal, and spiritual well-being for all, a large share of responsibility must be assumed by doctors, nurses, ministers, dentists, public health experts, social workers, teachers, and others whose labors come within the field of health.

The trend of events indicates that the aim of nursing education is to be preparation for work in a complex social order, for human as well as individual well-being, for helping to provide a satisfying life for all. This will mean nurses who are experts in special fields and capable of guiding others to expertness. Knowledge of races and social history, psychology, sociology, economics, and international relationships will be a necessity. Thus, the work of doctors and nurses, and an army of other specialists will be brought into active cooperation, the aim of each to give to the public the best that their combined efforts have to offer.

SUMMARY, 1939–1945

With World War II came an unprecedented demand for doctors and nurses to serve with the army and navy, and for civilian defense as well. Responsibility for equable distribution of professional personnel to meet military and civilian needs was delegated to the *Procurement and Assignment Service for Physicians, Dentists, Veterinarians, Sanitary Engineers, and Nurses.* In order to provide an effective channel of communication and cooperation between the Federal Government and the three organizations representing the nurses of the United States, the *National Nursing Council for War Service* was created, and soon adopted a three-point course of action as follows:

(*a*) Making a National Inventory of Registered Nurses
(*b*) Expanding existing accredited schools of nursing
(*c*) Promoting supplementary nursing services for hospitals and public health agencies.

The United States Public Health Service gave its support to the program by conducting the proposed National Inventory of Registered Nurses. Through it also, Federal funds were granted to a limited number of nursing schools in order that they might increase their teaching facilities and admit larger classes. Its greatest contribution, however, was the expansion of great numbers of accredited schools through administration of the *U. S. Cadet Nurse Corps* authorized by Congress in June 1943. Funds were granted to cover costs of maintenance of cadet nurses, guarantee them a monthly allowance, and pay all expenses associated with the nursing course. Cooperating schools of nursing, in return, conducted accelerated programs of instruction that permitted senior cadets to finish their work in the home school in twenty-four to thirty months, and so be free to complete the three-year course in military establishments, or other civil institutions. Thus, while a new incentive attracted greater numbers of desirable applicants, a shortened course of instruction ensured space in dormitories and classrooms and made possible their acceptance.

The General Federation of Women's Clubs, the National Federation of Business and Professional Women's Clubs, the Women of the Moose, the United Daughters of the Confederacy, and other societies cooperated by assisting with the recruitment of students, and by raising funds to be used for educational purposes.

The American Red Cross Nursing Service gave assistance through a nation-wide campaign to enroll great numbers of nurses. It set up a Student Reserve composed of senior student nurses who promised to give needed service upon graduation, started a Red Cross Volunteer Nurses' Aide Corps to assist in hospitals, and employed greatly increased numbers of nurses to teach Red Cross Home Nursing to housewives and mothers.

The League of Red Cross Societies was active in bringing relief to distressed peoples throughout the war. The United Nations Relief and Rehabilitation Administration (UNRRA), organized while the war was still in progress, distributed enormous supplies of food, drugs, and clothing, aided in establishing schools for nurses and nurses' aides where none existed, and otherwise alleviated mental and physical suffering.

Nurses, serving with the army and the navy, cared for patients in many quarters of the globe, and under all sorts of circumstances. Nurses were stationed in air ambulances evacuating patients from combat areas to zones of safety. Nurses learned and practiced parachute jumping. On the home front, a new interest in industrial nursing developed when defense industries expanded to unprecedented proportions. Demands for nurses poured in from many sources which made it impossible to provide sufficient numbers in any direction. It was inevitable that the army and the navy, along with other services, should experience a serious shortage. A Nurse Draft Bill, representing an effort to remedy the situation, was passed by the House of Representatives and sent to the Senate in March, 1945, but the ending of hostilities on August 14th made further action unnecessary.

In 1941, President Franklin D. Roosevelt outlined the four essential freedoms for the human race, as freedom of speech, freedom of religion, freedom from want, and freedom from fear. Later in the same year, Prime Minister Winston Churchill of Great Britain and President Roosevelt brought forth the Atlantic Charter. For the purpose of bringing into actuality the spirit of the Four Freedoms and the Atlantic Charter, the United Nations was born in 1945.

Of the six principal organs of the United Nations, the Economic and Social Council is of greatest significance to doctors and nurses. Its specialized agencies, the World Health Organization (WHO) and the United Nations Educational, Scientific and Cultural Organization (UNESCO) are designed to promote health, education, science, culture, and, finally, peace for all peoples.

The close of World War II by no means put an end to the need for nurses. While they were no longer recruited for the armed forces, requests poured in from other sources, and the staffs of civilian hospitals and public health agencies remained critically depleted. Nurses returning from front-line duty took extended vacations, found means of securing advanced education, or even engaged in other occupations, while married and retired nurses who had given service left the field once more.

As in previous wars, noteworthy advances were made in medical science. Among these were improved methods for preventing shock and infection and for dealing with patients suffering from nervous and mental disorders. A new emphasis on the study and practice of psychology, psychiatry, and psychosomatic medicine followed. In 1946, the National Mental Health Act came into being in the United States, and similar acts were introduced in other countries. In 1948, the *World Federation for Mental Health* was founded, its membership made up of organizations concerned with the maintenance of mental health and improved human relationships. In this group are to be found the International Council of Nurses and the American Nurses' Association.

TOPICS FOR DISCUSSION

1. How did the conduct of World War II differ from previous wars, and with what effect on the civilian population?
2. What diseases were prevalent, and what advances made in treatment of these and other conditions
3. In making plans to provide nurses for war service, what coordinating link was developed between organized nursing and the Federal government?
4. Through what agencies and by what ways and means were ever increasing numbers of nurses made available for war service and civilian needs?
5. Tell what you know of industrial nursing, and the effect of the war upon it.
6. What great relief agency was organized during the war to provide immediate assistance to destitute peoples?
7. Give your estimate of the principles set forth in the Four Freedoms and the Atlantic Charter.
8. Make an outline of the structure of the United Nations, its principal organs and specialized agencies, putting emphasis on those with which medicine and nursing are closely associated.
9. Give reasons for the fact that termination of hostilities did not put an end to the demand for greater numbers of nurses.
10. What advances in medical science were achieved during World War II, with impetus given to what branches of study?
11. What do you know of the National Mental Health Act of the United States, and of the World Federation for Mental Health?
12. Ownership of a membership card and the badge of the American Red Cross Nursing Services signifies what today?

REFERENCES

American Journal of Nursing. 2 Park Ave., New York.
American Journal of Sociology, University of Chicago Press.
Journal of the American Medical Association. 535 N. Dearborn St., Chicago.
Pamphlets on International Conciliation. Carnegie Endowment for International Peace, 405 West 117th Street, New York 27, New York.

United Nations News. Woodrow Wilson Foundation, 45 East 65th Street, New York 21. In cooperation with Carnegie Endowment for International Peace.

Committee on Medicine and the Changing Order of the New York Academy of Medicine: Medicine in the Changing Order. New York, The Commonwealth Fund, 1947.

Arne, Sigrid: United Nations Primer. New York, Rinehart and Company, Inc., 1945.

Charter of the United Nations. Department of State Publication 2353, Conference Series 74.

Dolivet, Louis: The United Nations. New York, Farrar, Straus, and Co., 1946.

Department of State Publication 3624: The United Nations—Four Years of Achievement. Washington, D. C., U. S. Government Printing Office, 1949. (A pamphlet)

General Assembly of the United Nations: Universal Declaration of Human Rights. Lake Success, New York, United Nations Department of Public Information, 1950. (A pamphlet)

Hume, Edward H.: Doctors Courageous. New York, Harper and Brothers, 1950.

Public Health Service Publication No. 38: The United States Cadet Nurse Corps. Federal Security Agency, Washington, D. C., 1950.

United Nations Department of Public Information: Everyman's United Nations. New York, Funk and Wagnalls in association with United Nations World. (Introduction by Trygve Lie)

Modern Trends in Nursing

Today we find ourselves in the midst of the greatest and most rapid transition phase in the evolution of human society that the world has yet experienced. Along with fast-moving developments many ideological and spiritual conflicts have come to the foreground. A new concept of the rights of peoples of all races, religions, and levels of society to personal liberty and a fair share of the essentials to ensure health and happiness has become a principal issue. Speed in transportation, ease of communication, mixing of populations during large-scale wars, the work of the United Nations, all are contributing to an awakening to the possibilities of a peaceful world in which every human being will benefit from the goods and services that it can be prepared to offer. Despite many such encouraging signs, the threat of an atomic war casts a shadow at our gates and puts the fate of each and every person in peril. Only through the colossal effort of an informed and socially minded citizenry can such a cataclysm be averted.

NURSING RESEARCH

Nursing, now recognized as one of the great social services, is of necessity assuming a new importance. In order that it may be prepared to give what is expected of it, various studies and research projects relating to all phases of nursing service and nursing education are being undertaken. By this means a scientific approach to the varied issues confronting the profession will be provided and conclusions reached upon which satisfactory and stable policies can be based. Some of these studies are being carried on by educational institutions and others by state, national, and international organizations associated with nursing. The following definition makes clear their value:

"Research is the orderly, systematic collection of facts, and the classification, analysis, and interpretation of those facts in relation to a specific problem. It is free from prejudice and is carried on with an open mind. . . . Research, as a state of mind, seeks change rather than 'letting well enough alone,' and looks for solutions to problems arising from social changes."[1]

RESEARCH AND STATISTICS UNIT OF THE A.N.A.

The Research and Statistics Unit of the American Nurses' Association was developed for the purpose of initiating studies and interpreting and reporting their findings. It also aids in implementation of the recommendations made and acts as a clearing house for the dissemination of information. Since all research projects involve the expenditure of considerable sums of money, procedure can take place only as necessary funds become available.

Socio-Economic Study A research project of considerable size was undertaken in 1947 when the National Nursing Council[2] cooperated with the Bureau of Labor Statistics of the United States Department of Labor in conducting a socio-economic study of nursing for the purpose of comparing the working and living conditions of nurses with those of women in the other professions. The facts elicited from replies to questionnaires sent to individual nurses and other sources of information were published in the pamphlet, "The Economic Status of Registered Professional Nurses 1946–47," prepared by the Bureau of Labor Statistics. Statistics contained therein indicate, among other things, that while salaries of teachers in city schools were higher at that time than those of nurses, the average for city and rural teachers combined was about the same.

A.N.A. Economic Security Program On the basis of information provided by the report of the Socio-Economic Study, a subsequent *Economic Security Program for Nurses* was set up by the American Nurses' Association and implemented through its Economic Security Unit and the state nurses associations. Social security for nurses, group plans for sickness and accident insurance, and wage stabilization were promoted. The program was based upon the

---

1 American Journal of Nursing, December, 1950, p. 767.
2 Successor to the National Nursing Council for War Service.

use of collective bargaining in securing improved working conditions, with the state nurses' associations acting as bargaining agents, a principle which previously had been given an approval vote by nurses. Improvement in employment conditions was brought about in many states, with a greater stability in nursing staffs and a corresponding improvement in nursing service.

Study of Nursing Functions   Since it is the responsibility of a profession to determine its own activities, the American Nurses' Association was requested by the state associations and some other groups to initiate a program for the study of nursing functions. Such a program, which is expected to cover a period of five years, is now under way. The purpose is to determine the functions and relationships of professional nurses, practical nurses, and auxiliary workers in institutions, and the proportion of nursing time which should be provided by each group under varying circumstances. In this way, a national viewpoint can be reached which may be applied to plans for providing nursing service in all types of hospitals. Institutions were chosen for this study because the greater number of professional nurses are employed by them.

Necessary funds are being provided by nurses through their state associations. Grants are then made by the A.N.A. to the state associations, a few hospitals, and other groups, each of which will carry on that part of the total program in which it has expressed a special interest. One of the most extensive studies was carried on by the state of California. Beginning with a pilot study in one hospital, for the purpose of developing forms and procedures, it was extended to eight other institutions, and finally to forty-two representative California hospitals.

At the same time, the Division of Nursing Education at Teachers College, Columbia University, is making its own study which began with appointment of a *Committee on the Function of Nursing* in 1947. Other universities and philanthropic foundations are expressing interest in the study of this phase of national welfare by contributing toward its success in numerous ways.

National Inventory   Another research project of the American Nurses' Association, which is to be repeated at regular intervals, was that of making national inventories of all professional registered nurses of the country in 1948 and 1951. In this way, the number of active nurses, their location, and type of work engaged in, was determined. Information in regard to inactive nurses, also obtained, would prove of value in the event of a national emergency.

Other research projects, which have been undertaken or are being contemplated, all aiming at providing better nursing care for a greater number of people, are as follows

Causes of the nursing shortage

The nursing needs of expanding health programs on local, national, and international levels

The type of education for all nursing personnel that will meet future needs

Nursing care of hospital patients, with emphasis on those with psychiatric and chronic illnesses

Functions that can be assumed legally by professional nurses of all types

Methods to improve inter-group relations and skill in handling personality problems

Research in Regard to the Nursing Shortage   In an effort to ensure adequate numbers of nursing personnel to meet present and future needs, a study of causes of the existing shortage was undertaken as a major responsibility by the national nursing organizations of a number of countries, by the International Council of Nurses, and by the World Health Organization. It was brought to light that while there are more nurses in active work than at any previous time in history, an unprecedented development of public health programs on local, national, and international levels, wide expansion of federal army, navy, and air services, new group hospital insurance plans, expansion of the bed capacity of hospitals, greater life expectancy with an increase in the number of chronic diseases, and the introduction of complicated technics in the treatment of patients, inevitably has been accompanied by a world-wide scarcity of health workers of all types. This circumstance is most keenly felt in nursing, especially in the fields of mental health, psychiatry, and public health.

The facts elicited make it clear that in order to rectify the condition, a greater proportion than ever before of both young men and young women, with no distinction as to race or creed, must be

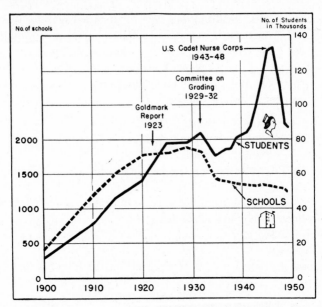

FEWER SCHOOLS OF NURSING BUT MORE STUDENTS

(From Nursing Schools at Mid-Century, published by the National Committee for the Improvement of Nursing Services, New York.)

attracted into the profession. At the same time, it is gratifying to note that while the trend is toward the establishment of fewer and better schools of nursing, those now in existence are prepared to accommodate greater numbers of students than formerly, and the proportion of young people in them has been increasing appreciably. However, professional schools alone cannot produce sufficient numbers of nurses to meet the demand.

CARNEGIE STUDY OF NURSING SCHOOLS

Progress toward the goal of ensuring to society a type of nursing service that is satisfactory in quality has been aided by extensive surveys of educational method as it applies to nursing schools. Such surveys have been carried on in the United States, England, Canada, and some other countries since the close of the second world war. In the United States, two previous surveys of schools had been made, each of which proved instrumental in bringing about better preparation of nurses. Good schools were encouraged to improve their programs of education, and some of the poorer ones were discouraged to the extent of closing. Helpful indications of the general direction in which all of the health services were moving also were brought to light.

It will be remembered that the *first study* of considerable magnitude in the United States was completed in 1923 by the *Committee for the Study of Nursing Education*, financed by the Rockefeller Foundation with Josephine Goldmark, expert in social research, in charge of the investigation. Three years later a *second study*, sponsored by the national nursing organizations, was begun by the *Committee on the Grading of Nursing Schools* with May Ayres Burgess, statistician, acting as director. This extended over a period of eight years and cost more than a quarter of a million dollars.

The *third study* was financed by the Carnegie Foundation and carried on as a final project of the *National Nursing Council* before its dissolution, for "examination of the question of who should organize, administer, and finance professional schools of nursing."[3] Esther Lucile Brown, expert in the field of social research, working with both a professional and a lay advisory committee, served as director. An early decision of the group to "view nursing service and nursing education in terms of what is best for society—not what is best for the profession of nursing as a possibly 'vested interest',"[4] indicates the objective nature of their work.

Brown Report   Dr. Brown visited about fifty selected schools conducted by voluntary and public hospitals over a cross-section of the country. Findings were evaluated which she described as "both better and worse than expected."[5] In addition, individual interviews were carried on with those responsible for nursing education and members of other health services and university faculties. Three regional conferences were conducted to which the director and one other member of each nursing school were invited. The conclusions reached, with recommendations for improvement, were published in 1948 in the volume, *Nursing for the Future*, by Esther Lucile Brown.

[3] Brown, Esther Lucile: Nursing for the Future. New York, Russell Sage Foundation, 1948, p. 10.
[4] *Ibid.*, p. 11.
[5] *Ibid.*, p. 18.

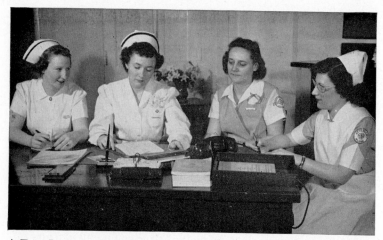

A TEAM LEADER AND HER NURSING TEAM CLARIFY THEIR ASSIGNMENTS BEFORE
STARTING THE DAY'S WORK.
(Reproduced by permission from the American Journal of Nursing, February,
1952.)

In this volume, prevailing methods in relation to nursing education
and nursing service were reviewed. In answer to the chief question
under consideration it was recommended "that effort be directed to
building basic schools of nursing in universities and colleges, comparable in number to existing medical schools, that are sound in
organizational and financial structure, adequate in facilities and
faculty, and well distributed to serve the needs of the entire country."[6] It was pointed out that federal assistance with financing
would be necessary. The feasibility of a combined general and professional university course shortened to four years was set forth,
but, at the same time, the necessity for continuing hospital schools
far into the future was acknowledged.

Recommendations of the Brown Report for providing adequate
numbers of well-qualified nursing personnel included the following:

1. *Building integrated service teams for care of patients in institutions.* These would consist of professional nurses, trained practical
nurses, and, possibly, an intermediate level of "graduate bedside
nurses," each group of stipulated preparation defined by law, and

[6] *Ibid.*, p. 178.

licensed to practice. Professional nurses would then be relieved of many routine duties and free to exercise their especial knowledge and skills.

2. *Recruiting large numbers of men into schools of nursing.* The advisability of this move was expressed in the following statement:

"There is a general agreement that men are much needed both as graduate and as trained practical nurses. The number that could be utilized immediately in positions of all kinds on men's wards both of psychiatric and general hospitals, as well as in the field of private duty, is large. Because so few are available, women graduate nurses and orderlies divide the nursing care of men patients. It could probably be better performed by men graduate and trained practical nurses, besides freeing women nurses for other duties."[7]

3. *Recruiting "minority groups" into schools of nursing.* A growing concern over restriction from nursing schools of members of some ethnic and cultural groups who are personally qualified to enter the field of nursing was indicated in the following:

"It is a problem of our national life about which conscientious persons are profoundly uneasy, because they realize that it is not in keeping with what they understand the tenets both of democracy and Christianity to be."[8]

4. *Preparation of nurse specialists.* It was pointed out that while there is a dearth of nurses with preparation for administrative, supervisory, teaching, and public health work, there is demand also for specialists in certain areas of clinical nursing, such as the care of patients with tuberculosis, heart disease, cancer, orthopedic conditions, and mental illnesses. Nurse specialists are needed in homes, hospitals, schools, industrial plants, public health services, and in the army, navy, and air force nursing services. It was disclosed, too, that the public looks for certain personal qualifications in its nurses. It seeks those having a calm, kindly, understanding manner and moderated voice, who will impart an inner sense of security and well-being.

OTHER POSTWAR STUDIES OF NURSING

Simultaneously with the Carnegie study to determine ways and means to meet the constantly growing demand for more and better nursing care, two other authorized groups were making similar

[7] Brown, Esther Lucile: Nursing for the Future, p. 188.
[8] *Ibid.*, p. 193.

studies and submitting findings and recommendations. One was sponsored by the Division of Nursing Education, Teachers College, Columbia University; the other by the American Medical Association.

Ginzberg Report   Through the efforts of Professor R. Louise McManus, Director, Division of Nursing Education, Teachers College, the *Committee on the Function of Nursing* was formed in 1947. Composed of representatives of the nursing profession and experts in the fields of medical and social science, the Committee reviewed "a selected group of problems centering around the current and prospective shortages of nursing personnel."[9] Eli Ginzberg, Associate Professor of Economics, Columbia University, acted as chairman and Dr. Thomas P. Murdock of the American Medical Association served on the Committee.

Conclusions and recommendations of the Committee on the Functions of Nursing were similar to those set forth by the Brown Report. To meet the critical nurse shortage, it was recommended that nursing teams be developed which would consist of four-year professional nurses, two-year registered nurses, and one-year practical nurses. It was anticipated that, eventually, the majority of registered nurses would prepare for full professional status, leaving but two groups to practice.

Murdock Report   A *Committee to Study the Nursing Problem in the United States* was appointed in 1947 by the American Medical Association. Composed of five doctors with Dr. Thomas P. Murdock acting as chairman, it held conferences with representatives of the American Hospital Association, the American College of Physicians, the American College of Surgeons, the American Nurses' Association, and others. Conclusions and recommendations were published in the *Journal of the American Medical Association* for July 3, 1948 and the *American Journal of Nursing*, July, 1949.

Recommendations for immediate relief of the nursing shortage emphasized the need for assigning auxiliary personnel to housekeeping and other non-nursing duties in institutions. To meet future needs, three groups of nurses were proposed: nurse educators, clinical nurses, and trained practical nurses. Nurse educators would

[9] Committee on the Function of Nursing: A Program for the Nursing Professions, p. IX.

have college preparation. Clinical nurses would have a hospital course shortened to two years and care for general duty and private duty patients. Trained practical nurses would have uniform standards of training throughout the country.

It was further recommended that nurses be made eligible for the benefits of social security and retirement plans in effect for those in corresponding professions, and that the cost of special nursing care to the patient be covered by prepayment nursing plans or be included in prepayment hospital and medical plans.

Following this study, a permanent *Joint Commission for the Improvement of the Care of the Patient* was set up. Composed of representatives of the American Nurses' Association, the National League for Nursing, the American Hospital Association, and the American Medical Association, its function is the continued study and solution of problems common to all groups.

NURSING TECHNICIANS

A more recent proposal than those offered by the Brown, Ginzberg, or Murdock Reports for providing sufficient numbers of nursing personnel has come from the Division of Nursing Education, Teachers College, Columbia University. This calls for the preparation of nursing teams composed of aides with on-the-job training, professional nurses, and an intermediate group of "nursing technicians" with two years of preparation.

Plans are now under way to test the workability of this latest proposal by assisting a group of local junior and community colleges to "organize training programs comparable to the semi-professional education available for medical, dental, and engineering technicians."[10] Their graduates are being prepared for the registered nurse examination. The feasibility of later adaptation of the program to hospital schools is under consideration.

Whether or not implementation of any one of the recommendations so far offered will prove satisfactory in providing nursing service, adequate both in quality and quantity, without considerable alteration and adaptation can be determined only through time and experience. In the meantime, a number of colleges are instituting four or four and one-half year combined general and nursing educa-

[10] American Journal of Nursing, March, 1952, p. 344.

tion courses, and more and more junior colleges and high schools are offering programs for the training of practical nurses. The United States Army, too, is conducting a course for practical nurses who are designated in its nomenclature as "medical technicians." However, it is the opinion of many that the three-year hospital school will continue to be the mainstay of American nursing.

THE SCHOOL DATA SURVEY OF 1949

In order to implement into action what were judged most urgent of the recommendations set forth in the Brown Report and elsewhere, the Joint Board of Directors of the national nursing organizations appointed, concurrently with its publication, a *National Committee for the Improvement of Nursing Services*. This was made up of representatives of the nursing organizations, the fields of general education, hospital administration, public health, and the American Medical Association.

The newly appointed Committee soon decided that up-to-date information on the administration of all schools of nursing was essential, and their first undertaking would be to make a *School Data Survey*. Information gathered by means of questionnaires would be used as a basis for determining the major problem areas of nursing education and nursing service and making recommendations for improvement. That the schools themselves welcomed this opportunity for evaluation of their policies is indicated by the following statement:

"Questionnaires were sent to every state-approved school of nursing in the United States, Puerto Rico, and Hawaii during March, 1949. Participation in the survey was voluntary, but the extraordinary return of 97% of the questionnaires demonstrated the cooperative spirit of the nursing school directors and the state and local nursing organizations, whose united efforts made this high percentage of returns possible."[11]

Interim Classification   The data received were analyzed and the schools classified in three groups according to findings. This *Interim Classification of Schools of Nursing Offering Basic Programs*, which appeared in November, 1949, in the American Journal of Nursing, "was the first critical listing of schools of nursing on a national basis

[11] Annual Report of the National League of Nursing Education, 1950, p. 202.

which had ever been published by the profession."[12] It was published again in 1950, with an analysis of all data received, in a paperbound volume entitled, *Nursing Schools at the Mid-Century*, compiled by the National Committee for the Improvement of Nursing Services. Opportunity was thus provided for those administering schools of nursing to evaluate their practices in relation to those in vogue in all other schools of the country.

NATIONAL ACCREDITATION OF NURSING SCHOOLS

After publication of the Interim Classification in 1949, responsibility for a second survey and reclassification was turned over to a new Accrediting Service, now known as the *National League for Nursing Accrediting Service*. Since 1939, the National League of Nursing Education had been carrying on the work of accreditation, which was now taken over by the newly established Service. Necessary funds to carry on the proposed project were solicited and received from the following:

Commonwealth Foundation, $75,000
National Foundation for Infantile Paralysis, $61,250
Rockefeller Foundation, $65,000

Temporary Accreditation   A program of action was then set into operation during the first part of which, data in addition to that supplied by the School Data Survey were gathered from each participating school. Information returned on questionnaires was supplemented by a one-day visit of a representative of the nursing organizations. Lists of schools to which *Temporary Accreditation* was then granted were published in the *American Journal of Nursing and Nursing Outlook*.

Full Accreditation   A series of individual and regional conferences was then conducted for the purpose of assisting those schools on the temporary list to meet requirements for *Full Accreditation*. By June 1945, two hundred and forty-five schools had reached this goal, 192 of which were diploma schools and 53 were basic collegiate programs.

[12] National Committee for the Improvement of Nursing Services: Nursing Schools at the Mid-Century, p. 6.

CHANGES IN STRUCTURE OF ORGANIZED NURSING

In order to guide emerging patterns of nursing into forms best suited to changing times, a trend toward alteration in structure of their national nursing organizations is taking place in a number of countries. Such structure changes, aimed at providing greater efficiency in serving the many and varied interests and responsibilities of nurses and nursing, are preceded by exhaustive studies of the existing structure and of possibilities for improvement. In the United States, such a study was sponsored by the national nursing organizations and originally conducted by the Raymond Rich Associates, "a research organization experienced in the study of organizations (especially nonprofit ones), their structure and functions, and their relationship to each other and to the public."[13] A report of this study was presented to the nurses at the 1946 Biennial Convention. Extensive studies and discussions then were carried on by nurses themselves through their district, state, and national associations until a decision could be arrived at which would be in accordance with the judgment of a majority of the membership.

There were by this time the following six national nursing organizations, each working within a field limited by the provisions of its constitution or articles of incorporation and without authority to enter another:

Three major organizations (see page 411):
American Nurses' Association (A.N.A.), organized in 1896 and re-organized in 1911
National League of Nursing Education (NLNE), organized in 1893 and re-organized in 1912
National Organization for Public Health Nursing (NOPHN), organized in 1912

Three organizations representing special groups:
National Association of Colored Graduate Nurses (NACGN), organized in 1908
Association of Collegiate Schools of Nursing (ACSN), organized in 1933
American Association of Industrial Nurses (AAIN), organized in 1942

[13] American Journal of Nursing, July, 1946, p. 442.

At the Biennial Convention of 1950, held in San Francisco, an approval vote was cast for a general plan to change the structure and reduce the number from six to two organizations. It was destined to require two more years, nevertheless, before the change could be complete. After months of discussion and deliberation, two companion organizations emerged, the *American Nurses' Association* and the *National League for Nursing*, with "a common overall purpose—to further the development of the best possible nursing service for the people of the United States of America."[14] The Constitution and By-laws of the American Nurses' Association were made the nucleus for the reconstructed association, and the structure of the National League of Nursing Education became the nucleus for the new National League for Nursing.

Each of the six national nursing organizations voted separately on the question of whether or not to change its structure and be absorbed by one of the emerging organizations. All voted in the affirmative with the exception of the American Association of Industrial Nurses which expressed itself as desiring to retain independent status but to continue to work in close cooperation with the other two associations. First to disband was the National Association of Colored Graduate Nurses which was absorbed by the American Nurses' Association in January, 1951, leaving a notable record of forty-three years of achievement. At a banquet in New York City to mark the occasion, an address by Judge William H. Hastie contained the following statements:

"It is a grand thing that there is no longer need for a separate organization of Negro nurses. It is also a grand thing that these ladies have recognized that fact and have cheerfully embraced the opportunity to give up an organization of which they deservedly are very proud.

"To me the meaning of this far transcends the nursing profession, its organization, and its internal policies. It points up a change of great consequence which is coming about in the patterns of American life and the reaction of the Negro to this change as well.

"The pattern of racial segregation in American life is breaking up. . . . As this process goes on and its pace accelerates, I can think of no incident which symbolizes the dynamics of constructive social evolution at its best more effectively or more dramatically than this gathering and its occasion."[15]

While the NACGN was thus acknowledged to have achieved its

---

[14] *American Journal of Nursing*, May, 1951, p. 288.
[15] *American Journal of Nursing*, March, 1951, p. 154.

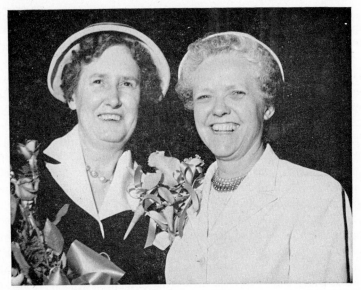

ELIZABETH K. PORTER   RUTH SLEEPER

First presidents of the reconstructed A.N.A. and the new N.L.N. (Reproduced from the American Journal of Nursing, August 1952. By permission of the American Journal of Nursing.)

purpose and consigned to the pages of history, various committees were forging ahead with plans for completion of details for the structure of the two major organizations. Decisions arrived at were subjected to the vote of all the membership at the Biennial Convention of 1952, held in Atlantic City, New Jersey. At this time, the National Organization for Public Health Nursing and the Association of Collegiate Schools of Nursing formally merged with the National League for Nursing, thus finally reducing the number to the following three organizations:

Two major organizations
    American Nurses' Association
    National League for Nursing
One organization representing a special group
    American Association of Industrial Nurses

Responsibility for *nursing practice* was assumed by the reconstructed American Nurses' Association. The objectives of this organization, composed exclusively of professional nurses, were well expressed in the following statement in regard to its necessity:

"Nurses as members of a profession must establish professional standards of practice for the individual practitioner, must promote effective counseling and placement for her, must define her functions and qualifications, must have a strong voice in legislation affecting her practice, must look after her economic interests, and represent her in the International Council of Nurses."[16]

The interests of nurses, grouped according to occupational status, are represented by the following A.N.A. *sections:*

1. Educational Administrators, Consultants, and Teachers Section
2. General Duty Nurses Section
3. Industrial Nurses Section
4. Institutional Nursing Service Administrators Section
5. Private Duty Section
6. Public Health Nurses Section
7. Special Groups Section, including such persons as registrars, office nurses, executive secretaries, counselors, and others not eligible for any other section.

Responsibility for *nursing services* and *nursing education* was assumed by the new National League for Nursing. Membership in this organization is open to such special groups as nursing service agencies, schools of nursing, interested non-nurse citizens, as well as professional nurses and qualified practical nurses. The need for this type of organization was expressed as follows:

"The determination of community and institutional patterns and standards for *nursing service* and *nursing education* and their promotion, organization, and distribution, and financing are the responsibility, not only of nurses but of the people themselves as supporters and consumers, and of other professional and allied groups. To carry out this responsibility, nurses in all fields and in all types of community agencies concerned with nursing, the medical and other health professions, legislators, employers, educators, and users of nursing service should work together."[16]

The interests of members of the National League for Nursing are represented by two main divisions, subdivided into departments, as follows:

16 American Journal of Nursing, February, 1951, p. 80.

I. Division of Nursing Services
    1. Department of Hospital Nursing
    2. Department of Public Health Nursing
II. Division of Nursing Education
    1. Department of Diploma and Associate Degree Programs
    2. Department of Baccalaureate and Higher Degree Programs

Membership of the American Nurses' Association includes all the members of its fifty-four constituent units: associations of the forty-eight states, District of Columbia, Alaska, Panama Canal Zone, Hawaii, Puerto Rico and the Virgin Islands. Each state association is made up of the members of its district associations. By joining her district association, the nurse becomes, automatically, a member of her state association and of the American Nurses' Association as well. Similarly, the National League for Nursing includes all state and local Leagues, and the nurse becomes a member of all three by joining her local League.

National Student Nurse Association   More than one thousand nursing students attended the Biennial Convention of 1952, representing Student Councils from forty-three states and two territories. The group was presented with several choices in regard to the place of their organization in the new structure. They voted in favor of the plan which provided for a *National Student Nurse Association* under sponsorship of the Coordinating Council of the American Nurses' Association and the National League for Nursing.

Membership of the National Student Nurse Association is composed of the membership of state student nurse associations, each of which, in turn, is made up of district associations. Each district association is composed of a group of local schools of nursing, not individual students.

A.N.A. Professional Counseling and Placement Service   An undertaking of the American Nurses' Association, which extends over a wide area and is proving of value to many nurses, is that of maintaining a *Professional Counseling and Placement Service* at headquarters in New York City, with a branch office in Chicago. These cooperate with, and act as clearing houses for, similar offices maintained by the state nurses associations. State offices, in turn, cooper-

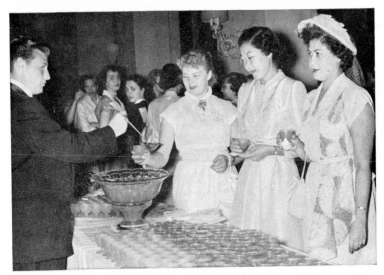

STUDENT NURSES ATTENDING THE BIENNIAL CONVENTION OF 1952 AT A PARTY
GIVEN BY THE NEW JERSEY STATE STUDENT ORGANIZATION

(Reproduced from the American Journal of Nursing, July 1952. By permission
of the American Journal of Nursing.)

ate with the same type of district offices. A district office is often
shared by a registry for nurses which has been approved by the state
nurses' association. All PC and PS offices are staffed with counselors
who are specially prepared to guide the individual nurse toward a
type of work for which she is suited, and to assist with educational
plans or employment problems. With the objective of providing well
qualified candidates for available positions, they are able to supply
information on state, national, and international levels.

Professional Nursing Journals   There are now three professional
journals published in the United States by and for nurses. The *American Journal of Nursing*, first published in October, 1900, continues
to be the mouthpiece of the American Nurses' Association. *Nursing
Research*, sponsored by the N.L.N. and first published in June, 1952,
provides current comprehensive information on research activities.
The *Nursing Outlook*, with which is combined the former magazine,
"Public Health Nursing," was first published in January, 1953, and
is the official organ of the National League for Nursing.

REVISION OF NURSING PRACTICE ACTS

Interest continues to be manifested in revision of nursing practice acts. Since need for such revision was recognized officially by the national nursing organizations in 1939, one by one the state nurses associations have been promoting new nursing practice legislation. In some states, effort is directed toward obtaining acts which will provide for mandatory licensing, or granting of legal permission to practice, of professional nurses only. Nurses of other states are working toward securing licensing of both professional and practical nurses on either a permissive or mandatory basis. Still others are working for licensing of practical nurses only.

If the law of a state relating to the practice of nursing is *mandatory*, it will be illegal for a nurse to practice for compensation in that state without first being licensed. If the law is *permissive*, she will be permitted to practice without a license, but it will be illegal for her to claim in any way to be a registered or licensed nurse. In any case, opportunities for employment are reduced to a minimum for the nurse without a license.

Practical Nurses   A minimum program of one year for schools of practical nursing is recommended by the National Association for Practical Nurse Education. Upon graduation from a state accredited school and passing a state board examination, a practical nurse becomes legally entitled to affix to her business signature the letters, "L.P.N.," or "L.V.N.," depending upon whether the law recognizes her as a practical or vocational nurse. As in the case of a professional nurse, the state law may be either mandatory or permissive.

Interstate Licensure   The nurse who wishes to practice in a state other than the one in which she originally obtained her license, continues to meet with the problem of *interstate licensure*. Since passage of the first registration act in North Carolina in 1903, it has been more or less difficult for a nurse registered in one state and desiring to practice in another, to show evidence of meeting in every detail its personal and educational requirements. Only by development of national minimum standards for the accreditation of nursing schools, the use of a national licensing examination throughout the country, and agreement upon a passing grade, will it be possible to eliminate this difficulty. Even then differences in preliminary educational requirements and their evaluation may present further obstacles.

In recent years, two steps have been taken which may prove to be in the direction of the long-hoped-for goal of national recognition. The first was provision for a *state board test pool* to be used in licensing examinations. This has been adopted by all of the states, although they continue to differ in regard to passing scores and grades. The next step was assumption of responsibility for accreditation of nursing schools on a national basis by the national nursing organizations, and carried on by the N.L.N. Accrediting Service. Ii it is possible to overcome other variations after national accreditation has been completed, a nurse who has passed a state board examination will be eligible for licensing in any state.

The board of nurse examiners of each state is the licensing agency for professional nurses who practice within its borders, and there is a corresponding board for practical nurses. Therefore, before a move to another state is made, either the professional or the practical nurse should apply for a license by writing to the Examining Board of the desired location. The professional nurse will find this listed in the Official Directory of the American Journal of Nursing. It may be that she can be licensed without difficulty. On the other hand, it may be that, even though a graduate of an excellent school, she will be required to pass another state board examination, complete additional class work or acquire clinical experience and pass another examination, or even that she is entirely ineligible for licensing.

A NEW STATUS FOR WOMEN

Although manifold problems present themselves for solution, there are encouraging indications of public awakening to the capabilities of nurses, and, indeed, of all women, in their special fields and in public affairs as well. One evidence of this is the gradual assumption of responsibility for nursing education by established educational institutions. Another evidence is the granting of financial aid to nursing schools, and scholarships to nursing students, both professional and practical, by some state legislatures. The employment of women in industry indicates a trend toward freedom which was accelerated during World Wars I and II. These two great struggles for human justice and human freedom embraced the rights of women, which were officially recognized in 1948 in the Preamble of the *Universal Declaration of Human Rights*, proclaimed by the General Assembly of the United Nations.

Labor saving devices in the home permit time for outside interests for the housewife. She is enabled to contribute the benefits of her intelligence and her character not only to business and industry and the professions, but to politics and education and religion as well. Her active participation in public affairs and the promotion of social progress has been accompanied by the removal of emphasis on old customs. Fashions in dress now conform to requirements for freedom of movement. In India and Pakistan and some other sections of the Middle East, veils have been discarded in the interests of efficiency. With them, the old ideal of submissiveness to male authority has been discarded too. Is the day awaiting woman's spiritual influence when war, with all of its present possibilities for wholesale destruction, will be banished from the earth?

Even though peoples of the earth find themselves in the grip of revolutionary ideologies relating to principles of freedom and equality and justice, the dawning of an era expressing the humanitarian ideals of Christianity and offering new hope to the destitute and sick of every land is already discernible. Possibilities for the peace-time application of atomic power to medical and agricultural purposes foreshadow an unprecedented increase in health facilities, in foodstuffs made available to gigantic populations now continually ill-fed and miserable with sickness. A growing acceptance of the mental and emotional causes of disease is opening new avenues of diagnosis and treatment. An enormous increase in respect for the individual which reaches out to the weak, superstitious, and fear-ridden peoples of backward races is being accompanied by a new and strong conviction that, to an amazing extent, man is equipped with the power to make this a satisfactory world in which to live.

SUMMARY

Numerous *research projects* are being undertaken by nurses, through the medium of their professional organizations, for the purpose of providing a solid foundation for long-term planning toward the adjustment of nursing to the needs of a changing society. All established methods of providing nursing services and nursing education are being questioned, and information sought of a scientific and objective nature.

A *Socio-economic Study of Nursing* was launched in 1947 by the National Nursing Council in cooperation with the United States Department of Labor. *National inventories of all professional nurses* of the country were made in 1948 and 1951 and others are to follow. *Studies of the causes of, and remedies for, the world-wide shortage of nurses* were made by the national nursing organizations of a number of countries and by the International Council of Nurses and the World Health Organization. A *Study of Nursing Functions* is now under way.

Comprehensive studies of nursing service and educational method have been undertaken by the nurses of several countries. In the United States, two previous studies of this kind were known respectively as the "Rockefeller Survey" and the "Grading of Nursing Schools." The third study, sponsored by the National Nursing Council, financed by the Carnegie Foundation, and directed by Esther Lucile Brown, arrived at conclusions and recommendations which were published in 1948, in the volume, *Nursing for the Future*, popularly termed, "The Brown Report."

To aid in implementation of what appeared most urgent of the recommendations of the Brown Report, a *National Committee for the Improvement of Nursing Services* was appointed. This committee soon discovered that first-hand information was needed on the methods in vogue in all nursing schools of the country, and a *School Data Survey* was launched. Through information elicited by means of detailed questionnaires, all participating schools were classified in three groups in what is known as the *Interim Classification of Schools of Nursing Offering Basic Programs*.

Responsibility for completing the survey was turned over to the *N.L.N. Accrediting Service* which set into action a program for granting *Temporary Accreditation*, and, finally, *Full Accreditation* to those schools which would improve their methods sufficiently to meet requirements.

Two other studies of nursing service and educational method, in addition to the Carnegie Study, were made at this time and followed by reports published in 1948. The *Ginsberg Report* sets forth the findings and recommendations of the Committee on the Function of Nursing of Teachers College, Columbia University. The *Murdock Report* gives corresponding information propounded by the Committee on the Nursing Problem of the American Medical Association. There were, therefore, three major reports on nursing published in the year 1948.

The national nursing organizations in this and some other countries have undergone changes in their structure. In the United States, after exhaustive studies and some preliminary voting, the number of organizations was reduced from six to the following:

Two major organizations
American Nurses' Association
National League for Nursing
One organization representing a special group
American Association of Industrial Nurses

The National Association of Colored Graduate Nurses was absorbed, voluntarily, by the American Nurses' Association. The National Organization for Public Health Nursing and the Association of Collegiate Schools of Nursing merged with the National League of Nursing Education to form the new National League for Nursing. The American Association of Industrial Nurses retained independent status. A new *National Student Nurse Association* also was formed at the 1952 Biennial Convention in Atlantic City which will function under the sponsorship of the Coordinating Council of the American Nurses' Association and the National League for Nursing.

Membership of the A.N.A. is composed exclusively of professional nurses, while that of the N.L.N. is open to interested special groups and lay people as well as professional nurses and qualified practical nurses. Schools of nursing make up the membership of the *National Student Nurse Association*. For the purpose of keeping all nurses and the public informed of the activities of their associations, three journals are owned and published by nurses, namely, the *American Journal of Nursing*, the *Nursing Outlook* with which is combined "Public Health Nursing" and *Nursing Research.*

Practical nurses, in addition to being eligible for membership in the National League for Nursing, have exclusive membership in their own organization, the *National Federation of Licensed Practical Nurses*, which corresponds to the A.N.A. for professional nurses.

Revision of Nursing Practice Acts is taking place in many states with passage of new laws providing for licensing of either or both professional and practical nurses. The greater number of these laws are *permissive* rather than *mandatory*. The problem of *Interstate Licensure* continues to elude a satisfactory solution.

Women of the world are experiencing a new freedom. With achievement of woman suffrage by more and more countries and participation in business and politics, woman's spiritual and humane influence has become an appreciable factor in world affairs.

TOPICS FOR DISCUSSION

1. Name several modern trends in nursing.
2. What do you understand by the term, *research*, and what do you know of its value?
3. Name several research projects that have been undertaken by nurses.
4. Outline the steps toward improving the quality of nursing services which began with the Carnegie Study of Schools of Nursing.
5. Give your estimate of the recommendations of the Brown, Ginzberg, and Murdock reports for overcoming the nursing shortage.
6. Define: Interim Classification. Temporary Accreditation. Full Accreditation.
7. Make an outline of the national nursing organizations of the United States, their membership, and objectives.
8. (*a*) What is the name of the national organization of nursing students? (*b*) By what group of professional nurses is it sponsored? (*c*) Of what is its membership composed?
9. What journals, owned and published by nurses, report the activities of their national associations?
10. (a) What organization restricts its membership to professional nurses? (b) practical nurses?
11. Differentiate between *permissive* and *mandatory* nursing practice acts.
12. Discuss the subject of *interstate licensure.*
13. Through what service of the A.N.A. may the young graduate seek counseling and guidance in regard to obtaining the type of nursing in which she will be most happy and successful?

14. (a) Make a list of the Units of the A.N.A. as you find them in the official directory of the American Journal of Nursing. (b) Which of these is sponsoring research programs? (c) Which is sponsoring economic security for nurses?
15. Enumerate reasons for optimism in regard to the direction in which all of the health services are moving.
16. Referring to the charts on pages 108, 200, and 484, make one large and improved chart of similar type.
17. It is suggested that one member of the class write to the national headquarters of the A.N.A. for a copy of its Constitution and By-laws and other literature concerning its activities; and another member write to the N.L.N. for similar information.

REFERENCES

Brown, Esther Lucile: Nursing for the Future (Brown Report). New York, Russell Sage Foundation, 1948.

Bureau of Labor Statistics: The Economic Status of Registered Professional Nurses 1946–47. Bulletin No. 931. Superintendent of Documents, U. S. Government Printing Office, Washington 25, D. C.

California State Nurses' Association: Nursing Practice in California Hospitals. California State Nurses Association, 185 Post Street, San Francisco 8, 1954.

Commission on Hospital Care: Hospital Care in the United States. New York, Commonwealth Fund, 1947.

Committee on the Function of Nursing: A Program for the Nursing Profession. (Ginzberg Report) New York, The Macmillan Company, 1948.

Committee on the Nursing Problem: The Murdock Report. Journal of the A.M.A., July 3, 1948, pp. 878–879.

Deming, Dorothy: The Practical Nurse. New York, The Commonwealth Fund, 1947.

General Assembly of the United Nations: Universal Declaration of Human Rights. U. N. Department of Public Information, Lake Success, N. Y.

Montag, Mildred L.: The Education of Nursing Technicians. New York, G. P. Putnam's Sons, 1951.

Murdock, T. P.: A Physician's Viewpoint. (Murdock Report) American Journal of Nursing, July, 1949, p. 439.

Newell, Hope: The History of the National Nursing Council. National Organization for Public Health Nursing, 2 Park Ave., New York, 1951.

West and Hawkins: Nursing Schools at the Mid-Century. National Committee for the Improvement of Nursing Services, 2 Park Ave., New York, 1950.

International Relationships

In spite of drawbacks, there is evidence that the world is moving toward achievement of international understanding and an international conscience as well. Slowly it is learning that circumstances surrounding the most backward and lowly of its inhabitants influence other peoples living in every quarter of the globe; that those who are mentally or physically handicapped inevitably become a menace to all members of society. Such understanding has been demonstrated in the World Health Organization, where there exists a greater degree of cooperation than in any other department of the United Nations.

The International Council of Nurses, through official relationship with the WHO, is active in promoting its objectives by encouraging the development of nursing throughout the world. By 1950, nurses filled thirty of more than five hundred full-time positions of the Secretariat of the WHO. Nurses of many nationalities express modern viewpoints as they work together on the *World Health Expert Committee on Nursing*. To this group, *Lucile Petry Leone*, Assistant Surgeon General of the United States Public Health Service, was appointed. Two nurse consultants, *Olive Baggally* of England and *Lyle Creelman* of Canada, have offices in the Palais des Nations in Geneva, Switzerland, one time home of the League of Nations and now the permanent headquarters of the WHO. Miss Baggally was formerly executive secretary of the Florence Nightingale International Foundation, and, therefore, is acquainted with nursing conditions throughout the world; and Miss Creelman is especially qualified in the field of child welfare.

A nurse is stationed in each of the regional offices of the WHO, six of which had been established by 1951 for the purpose of conforming to the health needs of specific areas. In many parts of the world, public health nurses are at work with WHO demonstration teams, usually made up of a doctor, a nurse, and a sanitary engineer. In order to ensure adequate nursing personnel to carry on its many activities, the WHO grants a limited number of fellowships for observation and study in the fields of malaria, tuberculosis, venereal diseases, maternal and child health, mental health, nutrition, sanitation, and public health administration. Applicants are chosen from among those engaged in some type of public health service.

Other opportunities for participation in promotion of world health are open to nurses in addition to those provided by official relationship of the ICN with the *World Health Organization*. The ICN is a member of the *International Hospital Federation*, a trans-national member of the *World Federation for Mental Health*, and is on the Consultative Register of the *Economic and Social Council of the United Nations*. Representatives of the ICN attend the Nursing Advisory Committee of the *League of Red Cross Societies*, and they have been present at the last few meetings of the Committee on the *United Nations International Children's Emergency Fund* (UNICEF). Representatives are sent, by invitation, to the Annual Congresses of the *World Medical Association*, the Congresses of the *International Dental Federation*, the *World Confederation for Physiotherapy*, and some other international organizations.[1] In the final analysis, however, it will be the sum of the abilities and the character of all individual nurses that will weigh in the balance toward the success or failure of the purposes of these organizations.

Exchange of Nurses   Another trend toward widened horizons and greater responsibility that is gaining momentum is the exchange of nurses by one country with another, for appointment to positions for a stipulated period, or for study. The ICN maintains a clearing house through which such exchanges are arranged, and policies relating to them defined. Some national nursing organizations also have assumed responsibility for exchange of their nurses. A working permit for each applicant and membership in her national nursing organization are always necessary. Knowledge of the language of the country to which assignment is to be made is usually a requirement.

A satisfactory exchange of nurses has been carried on since 1938

[1] Above information supplied by Daisy C. Bridges, executive secretary, ICN.

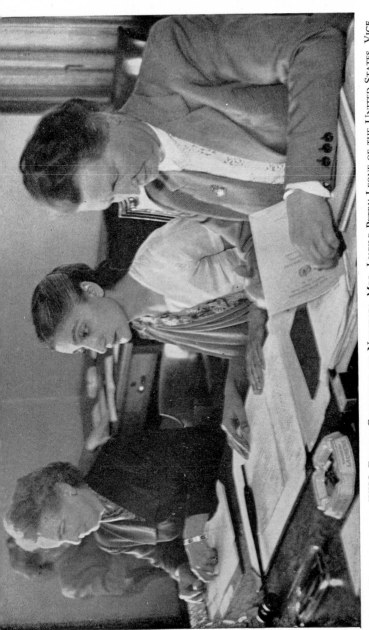

AT A MEETING OF THE WHO EXPERT COMMITTEE ON NURSING: MRS. LUCILE PETRY LEONE OF THE UNITED STATES, VICE CHAIRMAN, MISS T. K. ADRANVALA OF INDIA, CHAIRMAN, AND MISS OLIVE BAGGALLY OF ENGLAND, SECRETARY TO THE COMMITTEE AND CHIEF OF THE WHO NURSING SECTION

(From International Nursing Bulletin, Winter Issue, 1951.)

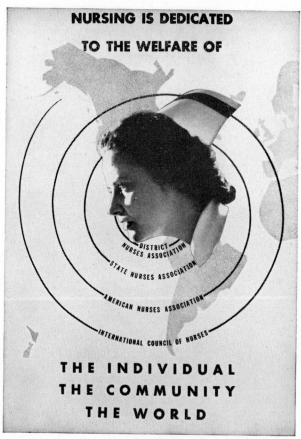

NURSING IS DEDICATED
(From A.N.A. Poster, American Nurses' Association.)

by the countries of northern Europe, and, between the years 1945 and 1948, foreign nurses are known to have been employed in fourteen countries. The educational institutions of Canada, England, New Zealand, northern and western European countries, and the United States provide study opportunities for foreign nurses. Mastery of the language is always a requirement.

Regional Associations   The successful exchange of nurses is facilitated by *Regional Federations* of nurses. The *Association of*

Northern European Nurses is such an association which is made up of the national associations of Norway, Sweden, Denmark, Finland, and Iceland. A more recent federation of nurses, known as the *Western European Group*, is composed of the national associations of France, Belgium, the Netherlands, Luxembourg, Switzerland, and the National Council of Nurses of Great Britain and Northern Ireland. A Regional Federation of Nurses of North and South America has been proposed and is under consideration.

Regional planning on a smaller scale is proving to be advantageous. It may be several states, several sections of one state, or any other divisions of territory that discover that they have common purposes and common problems, and can derive mutual benefit by working and planning together. The maintenance of central schools of nursing and of affiliations for nursing students express regional cooperation. District and state organizations of nurses are regional associations that long ago demonstrated their value through the exchange of ideas at their gatherings.

Another means by which nurses are attaining an enlarged viewpoint is assignment with the nursing services of the army, navy, air force, and other federal services of their respective countries. If they arrive on foreign soil with a knowledge of its general and nursing history, their accomplishments usually prove to be greater. A glimpse into the history of a number of countries which is here provided reveals the religious motive as the common factor in the inception of all nursing. It reveals also that the major trends of nursing development in one country usually parallel those of other lands.

FRANCE

In Catholic France, through the Middle Ages and up to the present time, religious orders have carried the chief burden of nursing. A daring movement of the sixth and seventh centuries was the building of the Hôtels Dieu of Lyons and of Paris outside the protecting walls of their monasteries. Of the loyal and selfless service of the Augustinian nuns at the Hôtel Dieu of Paris, we have already learned. The next event of great significance in French nursing history was the organization of the Sisters of Charity by St. Vincent de Paul and St. Louise de Marillac in 1633. This proved to be a reform movement which was to grow to international proportions.

Important changes in nursing method came about in the nineteenth century as a result of discoveries by the Frenchman, Louis Pasteur, who, in 1865, began a series of experiments which were to revolutionize the practice of medicine and surgery. Necessary adjustments, however, did not come as quickly as might be expected. A few enlightened leaders recognized the need for changes in accord with new understanding of the transmission of infection, yet reform in nursing was gradual throughout Europe, and especially so in France, birthplace of the new knowledge.

As in other European countries, some improvement in nursing practice came with establishment of Red Cross hospitals where nurses were trained for work in the home and for service during wartime. In the beginning, little was accomplished because the courses covered a period of not more than six months and offered little in the way of instruction. As a means of guiding the lives and work of their graduates, the motherhouse system of monasteries and deaconess institutions was adopted and so became common practice throughout Europe.

Founding of Nursing Schools   It was the privilege of a young woman physician to introduce into France reforms based on Nightingale principles. Possessed of high ethical principles, *Dr. Anna Hamilton*, as a medical student, had observed a crudeness and inefficiency in the care of hospital patients that was shocking to her. Upon graduation in 1900, her thesis, "Considérations sur des Infirmières Hôpitaux," not only exposed poor nursing methods but suggested reforms similar to those effected at the Nightingale School in London. Among her suggestions, chief emphasis was placed upon having a trained nurse, rather than a physician or a layman, in charge of each nursing school. The following year, when Dr. Hamilton became head of the Protestant Hospital at Bordeaux, she was able to put her ideas into practice. It was here that she founded the Ecole Florence Nightingale and placed responsibility for conducting it in the hands of a young graduate of the London Hospital.

Because it established a precedent, Dr. Hamilton's move was helpful, although years were to elapse before existing prejudices could be displaced and up-to-date nursing methods become popular in France. About this time, some contribution to progress was made by the appearance of two private nursing schools designed to train

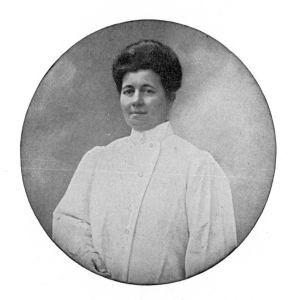

DR. ANNA HAMILTON

young women of good families, a development paralleling that of England's "lady nurses." The *School of the Rue Amyot* was established in Paris by a group of philanthropists acting upon the advice of the principal of a girl's high school who desired to provide for her graduates an opportunity other than teaching. Probably the greatest obstacle to the success of this school was the fact that the gentlewoman placed in charge of it was neither trained in, nor even familiar with, the art of nursing.

The *Rue Vercingetorix Private School for Nurses*, also in Paris, was founded and put under the direction of *Mlle Chaptal*, a woman whose girlhood attraction to social work had prompted her to give voluntary service on a number of occasions. She had assisted with a national campaign against tuberculosis, earned a diploma for work with the French Red Cross, graduated from the training school of the hospital La Pitié of Paris in 1903, and rounded out her experience by visiting hospitals in London. Revealing as to the conditions to which nurses of that time were subjected is a description of the dormitory in which Mlle Chaptal lived while in training at the

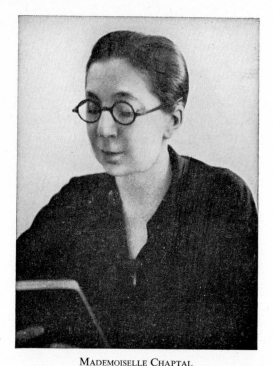

MADEMOISELLE CHAPTAL
(From "Mademoiselle Chaptal," by Marguerite Peltier, Editions Spes, Paris,
France.)

hospital La Pitié. Located in the attic of the oldest building on the
grounds, it was rat-infested, and so crowded with beds that the feet
of one nurse would touch the pillow of her neighbor.

For many years Mlle Chaptal remained as directress of the Rue
Vercingetorix Private School for Nurses. In the beginning there was
inadequacy of equipment, but eventually organization and instruction came to be superior to those of the large municipal hospitals.

Progress continued to be won by slow moves in France until sud-
den changes were precipitated by the outbreak of the first World
War. Working together in a common cause, nurses of Great Britain,
America, and France succeeded in breaking down some of the usual
French indifference to foreign ideas, and in fostering interest in im-
provement. Again, Mlle Chaptal became a leader in the revitalized

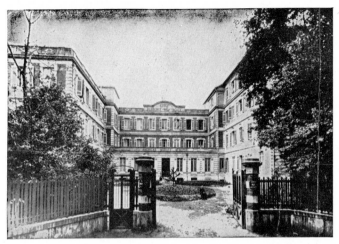

THE AMERICAN NURSES' MEMORIAL, BORDEAUX, FRANCE, AS IT LOOKED BEFORE
WORLD WAR II
(From American Journal of Nursing, May, 1946, by permission of American
Journal of Nursing.)

movement to raise the level of nursing practice, and it was through
her influence that state registration of nurses became effective in
1922. This progressive move was followed by an increase in the
number of nursing schools, all conforming to a requirement for a
two year period of instruction which was to be increased to three if
Public Health nursing were included in the curriculum. In 1923 the
National Association of Graduate Nurses of France was organized
with Mlle Chaptal as first president. More recently, as a result of
organization, registration, and progressive thinking, the profession
has been making many noteworthy advances. Until her death in
1937, Mlle Chaptal continued to be a prominent figure in French
nursing history, and, indeed, international history, for she was
elected president of the International Council of Nurses at the Congress held in Montreal in 1929.

American Nurses' Memorial. For American nurses, the Ecole
Florence Nightingale of Bordeaux has come to hold a unique interest, for it is here that their individual contributions were used to
erect the stately structure that provides classrooms and residence for
student nurses. As a tribute to the two hundred and ninety-six of

their sisters who died in service during World War I, about one third of whom are buried in France, it bears, engraved in stone over the main entrance, the inscription: "American Nurses' Memorial." Within, on one side of the fireplace in French and on the other in English, is the following dedication:

"To the Florence Nightingale School in memory of our comrades who died in service in the Great War, we, the nurses of America, dedicate this memorial to the higher education of nurses."

The rooms of this residence for students of the Florence Nightingale School include a large assembly hall, libraries, a lecture hall, and a demonstration room. The bedrooms, all of which are single, have been made individual in one wing by the name of a flower, and in the other by the name of a state of the United States of America.

The decision to erect this type of memorial was the outcome of a visit to the United States by Dr. Anna Hamilton soon after the close of the war when seeking financial assistance for the erection of new buildings to replace the dilapidated and inadequate hospital. Having already contemplated some suitable tribute to their comrades, the American Nurses' Association readily gave approval to a proposal by one of its members that it provide for the Florence Nightingale School a suitable building where a modern school of nursing might be maintained.

A fine old estate known as "Bagatelle" had come into the possession of the hospital. Here the memorial was erected amid the gardens and trees of a French countryside. The main structure and one wing were completed and opened in 1922, but insufficient funds prevented going ahead with the entire project. Finally, in 1931, the memorial was finished and formally dedicated, and a golden key turned over to the headquarters of the American Nurses' Association in New York City. The completed building stands as a memorial, not only to the American nurses who gave their lives in a great humanitarian struggle, but also to the life work of a woman engaged in a similar but less spectacular undertaking. Under Dr. Hamilton's guidance, the care of patients at the hospital at Bordeaux gradually emerged from that provided by disinterested, untrained men and women, to the understanding and skillful ministrations of young ladies from the best French families.

Unfortunately, the Protestant Hospital of Bordeaux did not emerge from World War II unscathed, for Bordeaux was invaded and the hospital taken over for military purposes. Partitions were knocked out and erected in new places; furnishings were removed and only a few beds left for patients. Funds for restoration were raised in the United States through the efforts of the Board of Directors of the American Nurses' Association.

Great numbers of new graduates are needed throughout France during the present period of reconstruction; a fact made evident by the existing shortage of nurses in all types of positions. As in other countries laid waste by the ravages of war, it is for the services of nurses with knowledge of public health and social work that the demand is greatest. New schools are being established which are independent of hospitals but may be associated with several. Students often live apart from both and arrive daily for classes and clinical experience. The French Red Cross continues to develop and maintain a large number of schools. Doctors always provide most of the instruction and give all of the state board examinations.

GERMANY

The foundation for nursing in Protestant Germany was laid during the early Christian period by the ancient order of deaconesses. Deaconesses were succeeded by monks and nuns as the monasteries grew, and, in order to meet the war-time call for nurses who would assuage the sufferings of sick and wounded soldiers, there appeared during the Crusades that unique combination of knight and monk known as the Military Nursing Orders, or Knights Hospitallers. Most famous of this singular development were the Knights Hospitallers of St. John of Jerusalem, the Teutonic Knights, and those willing to minister to lepers, the Knights of St. Lazarus.

In the late Middle Ages, as need for a less restricted service was recognized, secular orders of nurses flourished. Well known among these groups were the Beguines, a group composed entirely of women. Inaugurated at Ghent and Bruges in Flanders, the order soon spread through the larger cities of thirteenth century Germany.

The Kaiserswerth institution, founded in 1836, introduced into Germany principles similar in many respects to those of present-day schools of nursing. Thereafter, though Catholic nursing orders never disappeared completely from Germany, Protestant deaconesses carried the chief burden of nursing, and were transplanted far afield, even across the seas to America.

Soon after 1864 when national Red Cross societies were springing into being, thirty or forty Red Cross hospitals were set up in Germany within a brief period of time. In a remarkably rapid expansion these hospitals soon added to their staffs more than three thousand graduates of their short courses in nursing. Finally, the Nightingale System made its appearance, but not before revolt and leadership had led the way.

The motherhouse system, patterned after the custom of monasteries, had been spread throughout Germany by both deaconess and Red Cross hospitals. Under this arrangement, which supposedly operated to the advantage of all concerned, nurses, graduating from schools, remained associated with them and governed by them for the remainder of their lives. While permitted no voice in matters pertaining to conditions under which they lived and worked, more and more came to be demanded of them, and less and less given in return. A working day of from fourteen to seventeen hours with responsibility for the care of as many as twenty patients, and meager remuneration, inevitably led to mental depression, invalidism, and poverty.

An appalling sequence of tuberculosis, alcoholism, and drug addiction, together with an alarming number of suicides, failed to elicit any tendency toward reform in institutions where lived the deep-rooted conviction that the established order of things must be right. That nursing could exist apart from the control of motherhouses was regarded as utterly impossible.

Organization of German Nurses' Association   First to display open dissatisfaction and daring by breaking away from traditional patterns was a group of nurses who soon came to be known as the "Free Sisters" or "Wild Sisters" of Germany. In the attempt to earn their living, these free lancers were forced to compete with the nursing service of institutions partly supported by charity or endowment and hence able to undercharge. Unorganized, the rebels suffered many hardships. In banding together lay their only hope for success, and in *Sister Agnes Karll* they found an able leader. Through the cooperative effort of this group the German Nurses' Association was organized in 1903 with Sister Agnes Karll as first president.

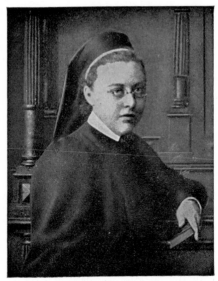

SISTER AGNES KARLL
(Courtesy of Lakeside Publishing Co.)

Encouraged by the unexpected interest and understanding of the International Council of Women, meeting in Berlin in 1904, the new organization formulated plans for its own protection, and, in addition, for the promotion of a three year course with more adequate instruction for student nurses. Possessed of an interest in statistical procedure anticipating that of her associates, one of the many accomplishments of Sister Agnes Karll was use of the questionnaire method to compile a health census. In this way the shocking health conditions existing among German nurses were revealed and some badly needed reforms brought about. In 1905, also through the efforts of the organization, the German Registration Act came into being. Finally, by the time of the third Reich, dominated by Adolf Hitler, there were four well-organized groups of German nurses:

(a) Catholic Nursing Sisterhoods
(b) Protestant Deaconess Sisterhoods
(c) Red Cross Nursing Sisterhood
(d) German Free Nurses, represented by the German Nurses' Association.

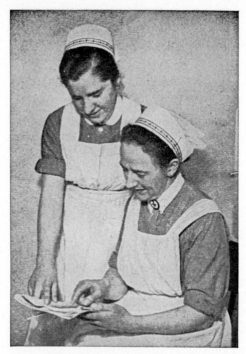

GERMAN RED CROSS NURSE IN WORKING UNIFORM

(Photograph furnished by the German Red Cross.) (From League of Red Cross
Societies Bulletin.)

Educational Program of Nursing Schools   In 1938, control of
the educational programs of all nursing schools was turned over to
the Nursing Division of the German Red Cross. As a result, uniform
standards were established.

In the position of director of each nursing school was placed a
licensed physician, with a licensed nurse acting as his deputy. The
class work offered covered two hundred hours of instruction, one
half of which was provided by physicians. The main emphasis, however, was to be upon ward practice. While schools were maintained
separately from hospitals, they might affiliate with more than one
institution. If adequate funds for operation were lacking, state sub-
sidies were granted. Graduate nurses were *licensed* to practice, and

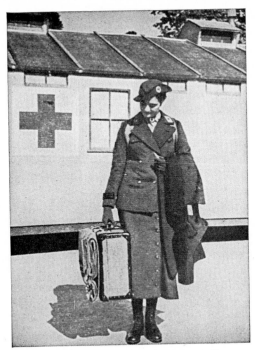

A GERMAN RED CROSS NURSE READY FOR SERVICE

The suit-case and rucksack contain, in addition to her uniform, everything the nurse is likely to need during what may be a prolonged stay at the Front. (From League of Red Cross Societies Bulletin.)

only they and the Catholic nuns were permitted to use the title, "Sister." Graduates serving with the armed forces were accorded the rank of officer.

Since the close of World War II, many new schools of nursing have been opened in Germany, to operate according to the principles in vogue in the nation controlling each zone of occupation. Because of overcrowding in hospitals and other unfavorable working conditions, the average health level of German nurses remains low. With the exception of members of the German Nurses' Association, they continue to find some measure of security in the motherhouse system.

BELGIUM

Sandwiched in-between France and Germany and sensitive to happenings in both, is the little country of *Belgium*, the most densely populated of Europe. Its people are adherents of the Catholic religion, and have for their official languages both French and Flemish. As in France, nursing has been carried on chiefly by nuns with the assistance of untrained and uncultured helpers of a position so low in society as to be looked down upon by higher grade servants.

School of the Rue de la Culture   Edith Cavell, martyred English nurse of World War I, introduced up-to-date educational methods for lay nurses at the *Ecole Belge d'Infirmières Diplomées*, popularly known as the "School of the Rue de la Culture," in Brussels. Opened in 1907, the school was fostered by Miss Cavell in the capacity of matron, and by Dr. Antoine Depage and his wife, Marie Depage, its founders. Steady progress was made until a solid foundation had been laid in time for its nurses to render skilled service to men of the French, Belgian, and German armies of the first World War.

After several important battles had been fought on Belgian soil in which Germany was victorious, hundreds of Allied soldiers were left separated from their regiments. In order to avoid capture and possible death, these unfortunate men were compelled to seek shelter in nearby woods and villages. With the avowed purpose of assisting them to escape into neutral Holland, a secret organization of considerable size was formed to which Edith Cavell and Marie Depage gave their support. German forms and stamps were secured, and passes forged. Personal guides were provided, and Philippe Baucq, a Belgian lawyer and father, was among these daring men.

As time went on, one after another of the group came under suspicion of the German secret police until thirty-five of their number, including Edith Cavell and Philippe Baucq, were apprehended and placed within the walls of St. Gilles prison. At the ensuing trial, two months later, all were found guilty of giving aid to the enemy by assisting in the escape of able-bodied men. The death sentence, "Todesstrafe," for five of the prisoners rang through the somber halls of the jail.

For a reason that has never been clearly understood, Edith Cavell and Philippe Baucq were singled out for immediate execution. At dawn on the following day, October 15, 1915, they died before a gray-clad firing squad. The following words of Miss Cavell, uttered to a clergyman as she was leaving her prison cell, are expressive in many ways:

"I have nothing to regret. If I had it to do over again, I would do just as I did. Everyone has been most kind to me here in prison and I have been so thankful for these eight weeks of rest. I was very tired and so pressed with the multitude of petty things that life brings that I have not had time for many years for quiet and uninterrupted meditation. It was a welcome rest for me—before the end. I know now that patriotism is not enough; I must have no hatred and no bitterness toward anyone."[1]

Consternation and horror thus came close, not only to the nurses of the school of the Rue de la Culture, but to all nurses and all people throughout a bewildered world.

Notwithstanding the loss of its matron, the School of the Rue de la Culture continued building on the foundation that she had established. Dr. Depage, however, was to suffer another and greater loss. Madame Depage, returning from a trip to the United States, where she had gone to secure funds for carrying on the widely expanded work of the Belgian Red Cross, was among the victims of the ill-fated ship, "Lusitania."

As a tribute to the two women who met untimely deaths in their efforts to alleviate human suffering, another school of nursing, the Edith Cavell-Marie Depage Foundation, was opened in 1935 in connection with the University Hospital of St. Pierre. With a permanent staff of more than two hundred professional nurses, a number of whom are Augustinian Sisters, a three year course with an extra year for Public Health Nursing, and close association with the University of Brussels, it stands as a fitting memorial to the lifework of the founders of Belgian nursing.

NORTHERN EUROPE

Stories of the development of nursing in the Protestant countries of Northern Europe are similar to those of Protestant Germany. In a region of protracted ice and snow, invigorating climate, and energetic people, where the hours of daylight in midsummer lengthen almost to the exclusion of darkness, is to be found one of the most advanced of European civilizations. *Norway, Sweden, Finland, Den-*

[1] Judson, Helen: "Edith Cavell," 1941, p. 281. By permission of The Macmillan Company, New York, publishers.

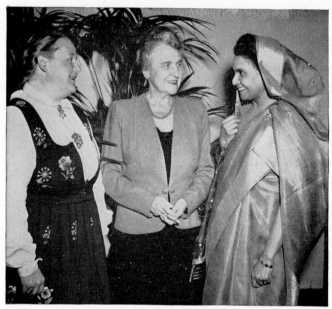

MRS. FRANCES PAYNE BOLTON WITH REPRESENTATIVES OF NORWAY AND INDIA,
CONGRESS OF I.C.N., 1947
(From Trained Nurse and Hospital Review, July, 1947.)

mark, and *Iceland*, benefited by the early founding of religious orders, suffered with the decline of interest in nursing during the Renaissance, and later introduced the modern deaconess movement, modeled after the Motherhouse at Kaiserswerth on the Rhine. As Red Cross hospitals appeared, short courses in nursing were initiated, and eventually an adaptation of the Nightingale System swept aside old traditions.

Association of Northern European Nurses   In order to share their problems and pool their resources, nurses of these five Nordic or Scandinavian countries have developed a regional organization known as the "Association of Northern European Nurses" which meets in convention every four years. By far the greater number of its members are state employed due to the fact that a form of socialism is in force in all of their countries.

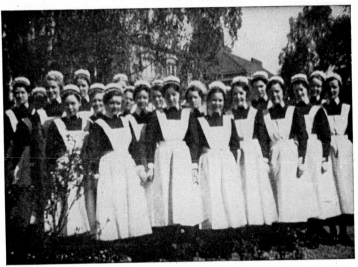

STUDENT NURSES AT SOPHIAHEMMET, STOCKHOLM, SWEDEN
(American Journal of Nursing, December, 1940.)

Measures encouraging breadth of vision and international understanding have been the outcome of integration of interests in the Association of Northern European Nurses. Through its efforts a scholarship for advanced study has been made available annually to one nurse from each country. Arrangements have been made which permit student nurses of one country to take part of their course in another. A system instituted by hospitals makes possible an international exchange of their graduates. Such interchange serves not only as a means of satisfying a desire for travel and new experiences, but at the same time prevents the embarrassments that may be associated with search for new positions.

SWEDEN

Schools of Nursing   A review of the individual history of Sweden reveals a progressive move with establishment of the Sophiahemmet (Sophia Home) in 1884. This nursing school, the first modern one in Sweden, was founded in the city of Stockholm by Queen Sophia. In order to institute Nightingale principles, it was put under the direction of a graduate of the Nightingale School in London. Along with professional courses, the school provides opportunity for a liberal Christian education.

A few years after founding of the Sophiahemmet, a second school of nursing was organized by the Swedish Red Cross and, more recently, a number of other modern schools have come into existence. Uniform policies for all schools of nursing in Sweden are determined by the Royal Board of Health. Entrance requirements are standard, and all schools offer a three and one-half year course, with the block system of arrangement of classes and ward practice. According to this method, no work in the hospital is carried on during periods of classwork and study which total about six months. Tuition is required by the majority of schools and all send their students to large city hospitals for a part of their clinical experience. Upon completion of her course, the new graduate is automatically registered by the state.

Courses in midwifery, developed long ago in Sweden, are offered by some state-conducted schools to young women who have had no previous training as nurses. After completion of a two year course, graduate midwives visit homes of poorer patients to render a specialized service that public health nurses are not prepared to give. In hospitals, the demand is for nurse midwives, and for this service the full time required in preparation is four and one-half years.

State Medicine   While private physicians practice in Sweden, state medicine is far advanced, and state-employed physicians, nurses, and midwives benefit by regulation of work, assured salaries, and a retirement pension scheme. The nurse of fifty-five who has given a minimum of twenty-five years of service is eligible to receive a stipulated income for the remainder of her life. Another pension fund operated by the nurses themselves has been greatly enlarged by endowments.

ITALY

In Catholic Italy, religious orders have remained in control of hospital nursing up to the present time. Few lay nurses, but large numbers of servant-class helpers, are employed and directed by nuns. The Italian Red Cross has been active in the establishment of a number of nursing schools, and it was through its efforts that public health nursing was introduced into Rome soon after the close of the first World War by a group of American nurses working under the leadership of Mary Sewall Gardner.

Long one of Europe's most impoverished countries, Italy has been further handicapped by the devastation which struck the nation in full fury during World War II. Among its many losses, Italy counted the destruction of its famed old monastery, Monte Cassino, for centuries the home of Benedictine monks. The buildings have since been reconstructed according to the most modern type of architecture.

In the struggle toward rehabilitation. Italy was one of the first to test the efficacy of UNRRA. Nurses attached to the Health Division of this organization, along with those representing the League of Red Cross Societies, were active in rendering assistance to a war-weary and poverty-stricken population. As in other devastated countries, these nurses encountered customs and traditions differing from those with which they were familiar, and they, too, must carry on in spite of privations. Those with a sincere desire to cooperate, and the ability to improvise and adjust, were soon in great demand.

THE BALKANS AND THE MIDDLE EAST

The history of nursing in nations around the eastern reaches of the Mediterranean, Greece, Albania, Yugoslavia, Turkey, and Palestine, reveals development along similar lines. Hampered by a low level of education, unaware of the dangers of unsanitary food and water supplies, peoples of these lands have advanced but slowly in the quest for improved medical and nursing practice. Each nation, however, has a few modern hospitals and schools of nursing.

GREECE

In Athens, the School for Hospital and Public Health Nurses of the Hellenic Red Cross, offers a three year course for institutional and public health nurses. The State School of Nursing, also in Athens, provides only classroom instruction, sending its students to the Hippocrateion Hospital for clinical experience. This school is under control of the state and its faculty members are employees of the government. One of its instructors recently was granted a scholarship enabling her to undertake advanced work at the Toronto School of Nursing in Canada.

PALESTINE

In Palestine, near Jerusalem and overlooking the Dead Sea, is the Henrietta Szold School of Nursing affiliated with the great Rothschild-Hadassah University Hospital and Medical School Center. It was opened in 1939 by "Hadassah," the Women's Zionist Organization of America. Modern in all its aspects, this university hospital provides care for Moslem, Jew, and Christian, and affords excellent facilities for teaching student nurses. The basic course of three years may be followed by post-graduate work in midwifery, public health nursing, or surgery. A tuition fee is required. That a cosmopolitan atmosphere prevails is shown by the fact that, on occasion, there have been gathered in one class students of Polish, German, Latvian, Rumanian, and American, as well as of Palestinian, origin.

AFRICA

In Africa, a vast continent combining dense jungle, sun-seared desert, temperate highlands, and seemingly illimitable distances, those engaged in health work must face further difficulty in attempting to educate illiterate, superstitious natives in whose minds evil spirits continue to lurk as finite realities. An explanation to them of the part played by microorganisms in the transfer of prevalent tropical diseases is likely to meet with incredulity and derision.

In certain sections of Africa, however, especially near the Nile delta and at the extreme southern portion of the continent, civilization is more advanced. Nursing schools in South Africa have been developed to such an extent that an exchange of three of their graduates with three from Canada was recently arranged by the national nursing associations of the two countries. Furthermore, interest in nursing education in South Africa, it will be recalled, has been in existence for some time, for Cape Colony was the first country to pass a law, effective in 1891, providing for registration of nurses.

Dr. Albert Schweitzer   The medical and social achievements of Dr. Albert Schweitzer in French Equatorial Africa are world famous. In the year 1913, in the midst of a mahogany grove on the Ogowe River, about three hundred miles from Port Gentil, Dr. Schweitzer and his wife arrived from Alsace-Lorraine to carve out the buildings for a hospital in what has been termed, "the worst climate in the

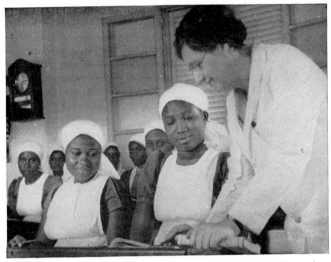

A West Africa Nurse Instructor Checks the Work of Some African
Student Nurses
(Photos courtesy British Information Service.)

world." No other doctor was to be found for miles around. To the
new hospital came at once great numbers of natives suffering from
malaria, dysentery, elephantiasis, sleeping sickness, tuberculosis,
leprosy, and skin diseases of every description. Conditions requiring
surgical procedure were numerous. Patients traveled in canoes or
through jungles, sometimes for weeks, arriving with their families
and friends, all of whom somehow must be housed and fed.

Dr. Schweitzer had abandoned a career in which he had attained
fame as a musician, author, and lecturer, in order to put into practice his theory that every one has *another job* to do in addition to
his art, business, or profession, in serving his fellowmen. His study
of music began at the age of five, and even as a young man he was
well known for his splendid rendition of the composition of Johann
Sebastian Bach. His study of medicine began at the age of thirty in
order that he might "work without talking" in his missionary endeavor. About the same time, a young lady in whom he was interested entered a school of nursing so as to be prepared to work with
him. She became Madame Schweitzer and for many years served as

nurse, anesthetist, and general assistant to her husband. Eventually, the state of her health made it necessary for her to return to their home in Alsace-Lorraine.

Dr. Schweitzer's hospital today comprises approximately forty buildings occupying a cleared area of one hundred ten acres. These are well constructed from the standpoint of ventilation and protection from the intense equatorial heat. Conveniences of electricity, refrigeration, modern plumbing, radios, and daily newspapers are lacking. All supplies must be brought in from a distance. Nurses of Belgian, Dutch, and French origin give devoted service, some of them remaining over a period of many years. Doctors to work with and relieve Dr. Schweitzer, now more than seventy years of age, are difficult to find. Funds to carry on his great humanitarian project are raised through European concert and lecture tours carried on periodically by Dr. Schweitzer, and through the sale of his writings.

Dr. Schweitzer has a deep conviction that, if the lives of fear, disease, and misery of millions of superstitious and backward African peoples could be observed and understood, civilization would acknowledge its great indebtedness to them. The core of his philosophy is to be found in his phrase, "reverence for life," which he believes should be the guiding principle for all social, economic, and political systems. His own reverence for life extends to all living things, and he pays the natives for rescuing and bringing to him, every creature found in distress. He respects the dignity of all men, and recognizes his brotherhood with them. All savages are his brothers and sisters. He lives with them and for them. It is fitting that he has been called, "the kindest man in the world," "the greatest living philosopher," and "a little lower than the angels."

THE ORIENT

The history of Oriental countries bears the universal relationship between Christianity and nursing service, although nursing began here at a later period and has been associated with the missionary movement. By introducing their own medical and nursing practices, Occidental missionaries have been able to gain friendships and, at the same time, to spread teachings of the Christian religion. The major drawback to progress has been a lack of consideration for

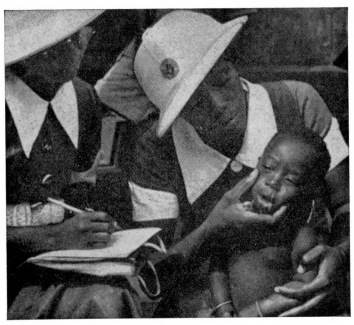

TWO TRAINED NURSES OF THE GOLD COAST, AFRICA, ACTING AS WELFARE
WORKERS

women on the part of Oriental men, and especially for those rendering a personal service.

In China and Japan, women have been traditionally classed as so
socially inferior to men as to be unworthy of the benefits of education, and the nurse has long been regarded, not as the physician's
skilled assistant, but rather as his servant. Consequently, nursing has
been classed among the menial occupations and, as a result, has attracted to its ranks only women from the lowest social strata.

Improvement in nursing method became noticeable with the arrival of increased numbers of professional nurses from Occidental
countries. Soon after the appearance of a group of western nurses,
one missionary doctor, it is reported, nearly wept with joy at sight
of the first anesthetic bed. Along with nursing principles of their
respective countries, these women carried to their native co-workers
a spirit of friendliness and helpfulness which aided in their efforts
to interpret the principles of brotherly love and Christian living.

CHINA

In China, where women have been expected to marry early and live with their husbands' families on terms of strict obedience and respect toward the older generation, foreign ideas have had to generate many changes. It was within this traditional framework that the early missionaries were required to labor.

Impetus to the work of the first missionary nurses was provided by later pioneers. Of special note among the latter was *Nina D. Gage*, a graduate of the Roosevelt Hospital School of Nursing in New York City. As dean of the Hunan-Yale School of Nursing at Changsa, and also as president of the Nurses' Association of China, she was able to bring about reforms in the way of developing a standard curriculum, accrediting schools of nursing, providing for national examinations, and arranging conventions of nurses.

Still other means have been used to introduce modern nursing practices into China. In recent years many young Chinese women, some of them college graduates, have been granted the opportunity to study abroad. On their return to China, they are equipped to institute the modern methods of foreign lands. Among these young Chinese women were *Elsie Mawfung Chung* who graduated at Guy's Hospital, London, in 1909, and *Lillian Wu* who came to America and graduated at the Johns Hopkins School of Nursing, Baltimore. Miss Wu later exerted influence as president of the Nurses' Association of China.

Public health nursing, with all its possibilities for elevation of standards of living, finds an open field in China. Following its inauguration at the Peiping Union Medical College in 1925, public health nursing has advanced into many sections of China. Nevertheless, many setbacks were destined to come. In spite of many years of civil and international war, however, all types of Chinese nursing have progressed to a stage where they will be able to render invaluable service in the years to come.

JAPAN

In Japan, the introduction of western methods by *Linda Richards*, in 1885, has been noted. Under the auspices of the Congregational Board of Missions, she organized at Kyoto the first training school for nurses, and guided it through the first five years of its existence.

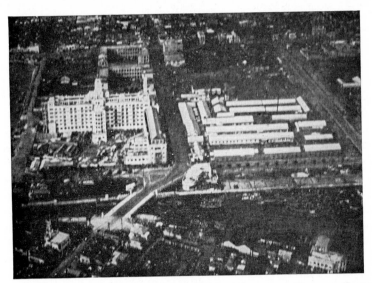

St. Luke's International Medical Center and College of Nursing, Tokyo
(American Journal of Nursing, October, 1933.)

Another major development, founding of the great St. Luke's International Medical Center in Tokyo, was accomplished through the combined efforts of the Protestant Episcopal churches of America and Japan. A school of nursing, established in 1904 in connection with St. Luke's, has become an official college of nursing with a well-planned three year basic course, and a fourth year for those wishing to specialize in teaching, supervision, or public health nursing. This school, planned to meet American standards, has done much to win Japanese tolerance of the education of their women for nursing.

It would seem, strangely enough, that both China's and Japan's nursing services have benefited by the experiences of World War II. Through the presence of many medical and nursing missions and UNRRA workers and material, the best and most modern in medical and nursing practice was offered to these nations. As one of the United Nations, China was given every opportunity to improve its methods for care of the sick and wounded. Likewise, Japan, following surrender, was exposed to up-to-date practices as army, navy and UNRRA doctors and nurses arrived to reestablish services disrupted during the conflict.

KOREA

Korea, a peninsula of eastern Asia, is largely mountainous and in the agricultural stage of development. Little is known of the origin of its people, but because of characteristic features, it is believed that they are a mixture of Mongolian races. Many forms of religion are practiced among them, including animism, ancestor worship, Buddhism, and Confucianism. Christianity was introduced about 1882 with the arrival of European missionaries. Since that time, modern medicine and nursing have been carried on in various isolated centers.

For thirty-five years the Japanese government had control of Korea but lost it at the close of World War II, when it was divided temporarily at the 38th parallel into North and South Korea. For the purpose of gaining control of the entire country, the North Korean army began a drive southward in June, 1950. The Security Council of the United Nations took prompt action, and what is known as the "Korean Police Action of the United Nations" followed until an armistice became effective July 27, 1953.

Almost immediate care for wounded soldiers of all armies was provided by Mobile Army Surgical Hospital (MASH) units. These were so designed as to be capable of moving by jeep and truck closer to the front lines than the field or evacuation hospital. Any available barn, schoolhouse, or church was taken over, or, when necessary, their own tents rapidly set up and equipped. A staff of doctors, nurses, anesthetists, and corpsmen went into action in pre-operative shock wards, post-operative wards, and the operating room. Three or four operating tables were in constant use throughout the day and night until treatment had been given to all the wounded.

Great quantities of whole blood or plasma were used to prevent or overcome shock, and penicillin administered to all with open wounds. Severe chest, abdominal, and extremity injuries were common. To prevent loss of blood and shock, patients were moved as little as possible, litters elevated on blocks often serving as operating tables. By litter, jeep, and helicopter they arrived, to be evacuated as soon as possible in the same manner, or by ambulance or hospital train. The next stop was a field or evacuation hospital, and thence to Japan where they were assigned to army hospitals. Special army hospitals served as neurological centers while others cared for paraplegic,

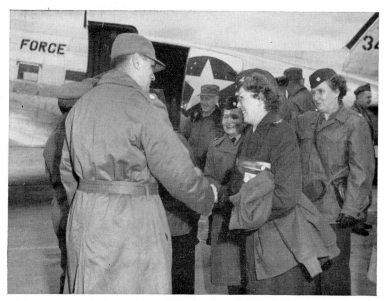

COLONEL MARY G. PHILLIPS, CHIEF OF THE U. S. ARMY NURSE CORPS, ARRIVES AT SEOUL, KOREA AIRFIELD TO BEGIN INSPECTION TOUR OF A MOBILE ARMY SURGICAL HOSPITAL

(From Bulletin of the California State Nurses Association, May, 1951.)

hepatitis, or frost-bite patients. From Japan, those unable to return to their regiments were transported by air ambulance or hospital ship to army hospitals in the United States.

Korean nurses, from both North and South Korea, served with Korean armies. The first foreign nurses arrived one week after the beginning of hostilities, to cope with dust and mud and extremes of temperature as they assisted with a continuous flow of combat casualties. A well-equipped hospital ship with a staff of forty-one nurses, in addition to other personnel, was contributed to the United Nations by the Danish Red Cross. The Swedish Red Cross contributed a hospital unit, equipment, and personnel. A group of Norwegian and Netherland nurses also came to serve in Korea. Nursing Sisters from Queen Alexandra's Royal Army Nursing Corps arrived with equipment for a field hospital. American nurses were stationed with the

United Nations forces in Korea and in army hospitals in Japan, where they worked with and taught hospital corpsmen.

MEXICO

Colorful Mexico, adjoining the southern border of the United States, is possessed of such lavish stores of gold, silver, and petroleum, and such magnificent scenery as to be known as one of the richest and most beautiful of all nations. On the eastern side it is greatly indented by the Gulf of Mexico, has a relatively long, rounded coast line on the western. To the north west, jutting southward from Alta (or Upper) California, is its long, narrow peninsula known as Baja (or Lower) California.

In contrast to its northern neighbor, Mexico has been called the land of "mañana," or tomorrow, where there is ample time for all things, and one never becomes excited or hurried. Situated in the southern Temperate and Torrid Zones, it has tropical vegetation, although, due to high plateaus, atmospheric temperatures in some regions are considerably lower than might be expected. Palm trees and banana plantations are plentiful, while, in the warmer districts, gardenias and orchids may be gathered as wild flowers.

In the vicinity of Mexico City, ancient capital of the Aztec Empire and modern capital of Mexico, are two famous volcanos whose snow-capped outlines may be seen extending high into blue southern skies. Not far away, linking the people of today with preceding generations, are the Pyramid of the Sun and the Pyramid of the Moon. Centuries ago these were ingeniously constructed by Aztec Indians in the location where occurred, according to their legends, the creation of these luminous bodies so universally worshipped by primitive peoples. Immediately surrounding Mexico City is the Federal District, just as the District of Columbia surrounds Washington, capital city of the United States. The nation is a republic composed of twenty-nine states and two territories in addition to the Federal District. A president is elected every six years and is permitted to serve but one term.

In the people of Mexico is to be found chiefly a mixture of Spanish and Indian cultures resulting from conquest of the Indians by Spanish conquistadores. The story of the defeat of Montezuma, last of the Aztec rulers, by Hernando Cortez, invader and conqueror from

Spain, is well known. Mexican tribes had attained so high a degree of civilization before the arrival of their Spanish oppressors as to make them the most cultured of American races. This circumstance inevitably led to the perpetuation of their influence; although their culture was modified, it was not eradicated, by Spanish culture. Then, too, the Indians themselves survived to form about one third of the present-day population of Mexico.

Notwithstanding the early attainment of a high degree of civilization, Aztecs, Toltecs, Mayas, and Incas of Mexico were guilty of a common barbaric practice in offering human sacrifices to their seemingly blood-thirsty gods. Archeologists are discovering and unearthing, one by one, beautiful temples and pyramids of an antiquity that may antedate the better known ones of Egypt, and that were once the scenes of human sacrifice. Sacrificial stones are being brought to light over which many a prisoner-of-war was stretched, as a priest held high a formidable knife before burying it deep into the chest of his victim. Removing the still quivering heart, he would display it to great throngs of worshippers who bowed down to the earth in awe and reverence.

Associated with the names of Cortez and his followers are stories of cruelty and torture designed to extort from natives the location of hidden treasures of gold and silver. Nevertheless, this same Cortez is said to have been appalled by the needless sacrifice of human beings, and to have used his influence to induce the natives to put an end to it forever. As governor of Mexico, he also showed a constructive influence in a number of directions which included the introduction of fruits, vegetables, horses, and mules from Europe. Moreover, as we have already learned, Cortez in 1524, was the founder of the Hospital of Jesus of Nazareth, first on the American continent, and today one of Mexico's most beautiful and modern. Built in a fashion resembling the homes of Mexican and Spanish people of means, it has rooms and porticos encircling two patios or open gardens, one of which contains a fountain. Like many homes, too, it is enclosed by a high wall, the gate of which, from the street, is the only visible evidence of its presence.

In contrast to the luxurious provision for privacy and comfort of a comparatively few affluent citizens, are the abodes of the masses, many of them fashioned of reeds and banana leaves, and containing

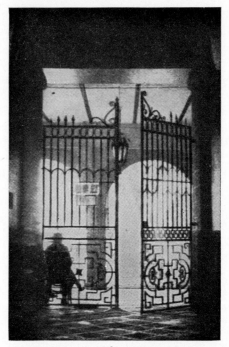

ENTRANCE TO THE HOSPITAL DE JESÚS NAZARENS, BUILT BY CORTEZ IN 1524
(American Journal of Nursing, July, 1940.)

scarcely any household articles. The average Mexican owns little in the way of earthly goods except a sombrero and serape (ser-á-py), the latter indispensable as both overcoat and blanket. He exhibits few desires and has a purchasing power that is almost negligible. Undisturbed by lack of provision for modern principles of sanitation, he is content to have his meat cut from a carcass hanging in the sun and covered with flies, and to drink water contaminated by excreta.

The people of Mexico are predominantly Catholic and for centuries nursing was carried on by Sisterhoods of the church. About the middle of the last century the state wrested from the church greater political control than it had hitherto possessed, and the number of churches and church officials decreased noticeably. This decrease in numbers extended to Sisterhoods and Brotherhoods, and the few nuns who remained in hospitals were required by the state to wear white uniforms and caps instead of habits. As might be expected, the practice of nursing soon became neglected as it had been in Europe during the Renaissance. Lay people of the Sairey Gamp type again flourished.

Reforms in Nursing In 1911 guidance of nursing practice was taken over by the University of Mexico, and nursing education and midwifery were placed under the faculty of Medicine. Classes are now provided for student nurses who affiliate with two nearby general hospitals. Graduate courses in public health nursing, school nursing, and social work are also available.

Not only does the University of Mexico maintain high standards of education for its own students, but it has also assumed jurisdiction over all other nursing schools of the country. According to its dictates, schools must meet stated minimum requirements if they are to achieve official recognition. Graduates of accredited schools, after paying a fee and taking what is known as the "Professional Examination" at the end of their course, are entitled to register with the federal government without further State Board Examination.

Hospitals In addition to two large general hospitals contributing to the education of nursing students of the University of Mexico, Mexico City has a British, a French, and an American hospital, each established for the benefit of citizens of their respective homelands, but now largely patronized by Mexicans. Appropriately situated near the entrance to the British Hospital are beautiful statues of England's two world-famous nurses, Florence Nightingale on the one side, and Edith Cavell on the other.

In Mexico City, also, are a Red Cross Hospital conducting an officially recognized school of nursing, and a beautifully constructed and modern institution maintained by the railroads of Mexico. Public health nursing, and the awareness of possibilities for disease prevention and elevation of social standards associated with it, are relatively new. With roots now firmly implanted in the Federal District, its growth and penetration through the states is anticipated.

SOUTH AMERICAN REPUBLICS

Explorers from Catholic Spain and Portugal traveling in a southerly direction over routes and trails blazed by Columbus and Cortez were the original settlers of the South American Republics. Vast treasures of gold and silver were seized that would flow, along with those from Mexico, back to the mother countries. Lying largely in the Torrid Zone, the interior of South America is an area of great tropical heat and dense jungles, where yellow fever, amebic dysentery, and bubonic plague lurk in readiness to strike at the first opportunity. In the extreme south, as in South Africa and Australia, the summer season falls in the months of November, December, and January.

With coming of the white man, the conception of two classes of society, one slave and the other aristocratic, became entrenched, and even today hired or manual labor has a stigma upon it that is carried over to nursing. On the other hand, a progressive spirit and desire for independence that culminated in the revolutions of the nineteenth century freed almost all the continent of European rule, and started the new republics-in-the-making on a road of development that is bringing them more and more into prominence as members of the family of nations.

As in the settlement of Mexico and the Spanish and French provinces of North America, provision for hospitals and nursing care was a part of the programs of Jesuit and Franciscan padres for conversion and civilization of the Indian. Nursing became a function of nuns or of entirely untrained helpers. Eventually, however, deaconesses from Germany and Sisters of Charity of the Order of St. Vincent de Paul from France arrived to meet the demand for skilled services.

Introduction of Nightingale System of Nursing   Interest in nursing did not become great enough to stimulate introduction of the Nightingale System until after the World War of 1914–1918. Attempts at starting schools were made by several individual doctors, by at least one school teacher, and by various Red Cross societies, the last-named usually proving the most successful. The first important step forward came in Rio de Janeiro in 1923 with establishment of the *Anna Nery School of Nursing*, the first modern school in Brazil and one of the first in all South America. Associated with the Hospital São Francisco de Assis, it exerts considerable influence in the community, and, by way of the new public health nursing and school nursing movements, in many parts of Brazil.

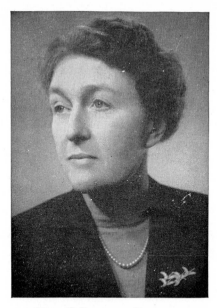

DAISY C. BRIDGES OF ENGLAND
Executive Secretary of the International Council of Nurses

In 1925 the faculty of the Anna Nery School of Nursing furnished leadership for organization of the National Association of Brazilian Graduate Nurses which was formally accepted as an affiliating member of the International Council of Nurses at the Congress of Montreal in 1929. Soon after this, state registration of nurses was put into effect, and the Anna Nery School of Nursing became the official pattern for all accredited schools. Every medical center and university of Brazil is now required to maintain a school of nursing. In 1950, eighteen such schools were in existence.

Another development affecting the advancement of nursing education in South America was the establishment of a nursing school in connection with the *Universidad Nacional del Litoral*, Rosario, Argentina, in 1940. Here entrance requirements are on a level with those for medicine, pharmacy, and dentistry, and the sciences are taught in the university.

In all South American countries, a great handicap in conducting nursing schools has been a dearth of textbooks in the Spanish language. It has been necessary to translate foreign texts and curricula, to use mimeographed material, and to dictate subject matter in the classrooms. Other types of limitation are many. It is reported that in the jungles of Peru nine days of tedious travel by canoe, muleback, automobile, and railroad were necessary in order to transport a patient with acute appendicitis to a not-far-distant hospital.

As modern hospitals and schools of nursing increase in number on this great continent where modern principles of sanitation are not generally accepted, they serve as nuclei from which radiate into concentric areas those social influences which are based on high physical, mental, and spiritual standards.

THE INTERNATIONAL COUNCIL OF NURSES
WITH WHICH IS ASSOCIATED THE FLORENCE NIGHTINGALE INTERNATIONAL FOUNDATION

The International Council of Nurses is a federation of national nursing organizations. These national organizations, not individual nurses, constitute its membership. Nurses from many nations, representing peoples in far-distant corners of the world, meet and exchange greetings at its Congresses, the locations and dates of which have been as follows:

1901—*Buffalo, New York*

> At this meeting, held during the Buffalo Exposition, a constitution was adopted, and election of officers made Mrs. Bedford Fenwick of England, president, Lavinia L. Dock of the United States of America, secretary, and Mary Agnes Snively of Canada, treasurer. Membership was on an individual basis. "Work" was made the first watchword.

1904—*Berlin, Germany*

> Membership was changed from an individual to a national basis, and arrangements made for affiliation with the only three well-organized associations of the time, the National Council of Nurses of Great Britain, the German Nurses' Association, and the American Nurses' Association. A

gracious welcome to Berlin by Sister Agnes Karll was the beginning of a friendship which proved able to withstand the stress and strain of many troubled years. "Courage" was taken as the watchword.

An Interim Conference only was held in Paris, France, in 1907. "The participants in the conference were most notable. The large contingent from Great Britain was led by Mrs. Bedford Fenwick, with Isla Stewart, genial and full of *joie de vivre*. From the United States, Mrs. Hampton Robb, a striking example of beautiful, happy womanhood; Miss M. Adelaide Nutting, earnest and forceful; Miss A. W. Goodrich, witty and charming; dear Miss Dock and many another."[2] Also among the notables present were Mlle Chaptal and Dr. Anna Hamilton of France, Baroness Mannerheim of Finland, and Sister Agnes Karll of Germany.

1909—*London, England*

The national associations of Canada, Denmark, Finland, and Holland were admitted to membership. Among the guests of honor on the platform was Edith Cavell, whose report on "Nursing in Belgium" brought forth a comment on "the quiet, calm, and serene manner in which this small, retiring woman gave her paper."[3] *Sister Agnes Karll* of Germany was elected president. "Life" became the new watchword.

1912—*Cologne, Germany*

The national associations of India and New Zealand were admitted to membership. "The Over-strain of Nurses" was the subject of an address, later published in pamphlet form. A momentous event was a boat trip to Kaiserswerth on the Rhine, where a wreath of flowers was placed on the grave of Friederike Fliedner. At the closing banquet, an educational memorial to Florence Nightingale was pro-

---

[2] The British Journal of Nursing, July, 1937, p. 180.
[3] Judson, Helen: Edith Cavell. New York, The Macmillan Company, 1941, p. 142.

posed by Mrs. Bedford Fenwick and seconded by Mary Adelaide Nutting. The new watchword was to be "Aspiration" and the new president, *Annie W. Goodrich*, of the United States.

Fate had decreed that it was to be thirteen years before another regular session of the International Council of Nurses would convene. War-time conditions made impractical an earlier gathering. In the meantime, however, a meeting of the Board of Directors was held in San Francisco in 1915 at which *Mrs. Tscherning* of Denmark was elected president. In 1922 the Grand Council met in Copenhagen, Denmark, to consider the applications for affiliation of five national associations of nurses, and to elect new officers. The resignation of Lavinia L. Dock as secretary, after twenty-one years of service, was accepted with expressions of deepest regret, and subsequently a beautifully illuminated framed address conveying a deepfelt sense of indebtedness was sent to her. Miss Dock was succeeded by *Christine H. Reimann* of Denmark, and *Mrs. Tscherning* by *Baroness Mannerheim* of Finland.

1925—*Helsingfors, Finland*

The high standards and efficiency of the hospitals and nurses of Finland made deep impression upon all visitors. *Nina D. Gage* of the United States was elected president, and *Ellen M. Musson* of England, became treasurer, an office which she continued to hold for twenty-two years. Desire for unanimity was expressed in the watchword, "Peace."

An Interim Conference was held in Geneva, Switzerland, in July, 1927. Thirty-four countries were represented by more than seven hundred nurses. Business transacted included appointment of a Standing Committee for consideration of the previously proposed educational memorial to Florence Nightingale, and consideration of a proposal for the exchange of nurses between countries affiliated with the International Council of Nurses.

1929—*Montreal, Canada*

In a brilliant ceremony amid many colored flags, the national associations of Sweden, Greece, Jugoslavia, Brazil, and the Philippine Islands were admitted to membership. "Service" was to be the new watchword, and the new president, *Mlle L. Chaptal* of France.

1933—*Paris, France*

High mass at the Cathedral of Notre Dame marked the beginning of the Congress. In her opening address, Mlle Chaptal welcomed the nurses of forty-two countries, and referred to the 200,000 members of affiliating associations as "a pacific army, working unremittingly not only to cure, but to prevent disease." "Concord" was accepted as the new watchword, and *Dame Alicia Lloyd Still*, of England, was elected president.

1937—*London, England*

Among the distinguished visitors to this, the eighth Congress of the International Council of Nurses, were representatives of the League of Nations, the League of Red Cross Societies, the Rockefeller Foundation, the Royal College of Physicians, the Royal College of Surgeons, the Ministry of Health, and the field of education. The presence of Dame Alicia Lloyd Still, retiring president, and Mrs. Bedford Fenwick, the "two great generals of nursing," added distinction to the nursing group which was referred to as the "Nursing League of Nations." *Dean Effie J. Taylor* of the Yale School of Nursing was elected president, and the new watchword was "Loyalty."

Addresses to be delivered at the Congress were printed in English, French, and German, and discussions were carried on in the same languages. A discourse by Sir Kingsley Wood, Minister of Health, contained the following: "The world is at one when it comes to the fight against disease. Nursing is now a definite profession, the members of which are not substitutes for doctors, but fellow workers in medicine."

1947—*Atlantic City, New Jersey*

By train, ship, and plane, nurses arrived from thirty-nine countries to take part in this ninth Congress of the International Council of Nurses. Previous to the regular session, the Grand Council, or voting body, held a three-day session in Washington, D.C. General trends discernible throughout the Congress were as follows:

(a) Assumption of responsibility for world-wide basic and post-graduate education of nurses and subsidiary workers.

(b) Integration of nursing with public health and social service programs.

(c) Interest in regional organization similar to that of the Association of Northern European Nurses.

(d) Provision for meeting the greatly increased demand for nurses resulting from political, economic, and social upheavals.

(e) Provision for securing social and economic security for all nurses.

(f) Cooperation with the World Health Organization (WHO), the United Nations Educational Scientific, and Cultural Organization (UNESCO), the League of Red Cross Societies, and the Florence Nightingale International Foundation.

The new watchword, given at the Farewell Session by Effie J. Taylor, retiring president, was "Faith." Miss Taylor said that it was to be an active faith—in ourselves, in our colleagues, and in God. She then quoted the following lines from Sir Rabindranath Tagore:

> "Faith is the bird that feels the light
> And sings when the dawn is still dark."

Miss Gerda Hojer, president of the Swedish Nurses' Association, was elected to succeed Miss Taylor.

An Interim Conference was held in Stockholm, Sweden, in 1949, when the fiftieth anniversary of founding of the International Council of Nurses was commemorated. The number of active members was increased to thirty by reinstatement of the national nursing associations of Germany, Austria, and Japan, and election of the associations of Haiti, Italy, Korea, Southern Rhodesia, and Turkey. General trends of discussion in which progress was made were as follows:

(a) Development of an international standard of nursing service and nursing education, with a Code of Ethics pertaining to both.

(b) Advancement of knowledge and understanding of the social implications of all illness, mental and physical, with emphasis on the work of prevention.

(c) Promotion of research relating to nursing service and nursing education.

(d) Provision for exchange of nurses between countries for limited periods of study or employment, with the I. C. N. serving as a clearing house for setting up policies and making arrangements.

(e) Consideration of the feasibility of providing means of international contacts for student nurses through their national student organizations.

1953—*Petropolis, Brazil*

This Tenth Quadriennial Congress was attended by about 1300 nurses who represented the 400,000 members of their national associations. The following activities were among those under consideration:

(a) Responsibility for assisting approximately 4000 displaced nurses forced to seek refuge in foreign countries, many of them without identification in regard to professional status

(b) Exchange of nurses by one country with another, the yearly number of which, since 1950, has been about 2000 for salaried employment and 500 for study programs, with the I.C.N. acting as a uniting and supervising center

(c) Responsibility for providing acceptable standards of nursing service in obstetric, tuberculosis, pediatric, and general medical nursing

(d) Measures for relief of the global shortage of nurses

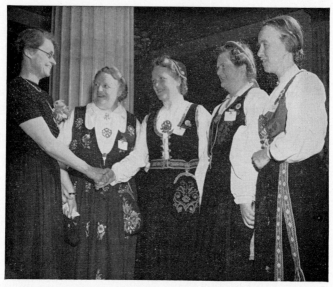

GERDA HOJER, FORMER PRESIDENT OF INTERNATIONAL COUNCIL OF NURSES, GREETING NURSES FROM NORWAY AT THE I.C.N. CONGRESS IN 1947

    (e) Promotion of the economic welfare of all nurses
    (f) Unanimous adoption of an *International Code of Nursing Ethics*[4]
The new president is *Mlle Marie M. Bihet,* director of nursing at the Edith Cavell-Marie Depage Hospital in Brussels. The new watchword, given by Gerda Hojer, retiring president, is "Responsibility." Italy is to be the place of meeting in 1957.

Florence Nightingale International Foundation   The *Florence Nightingale International Foundation*, first conceived during the Congress of Cologne, Germany, in 1912, was put into effect in 1934 as a living memorial to Florence Nightingale. It now operates as the Educational Division of the I.C.N. which has set for itself the twofold purpose of raising educational standards for nurses and strengthening international goodwill.

    In addition to carrying responsibility for a program of advanced nursing education, FNIF activities include development of a center of information on educational facilities as they apply to nursing,

[4] American Journal of Nursing, September, 1953, p. 1070.

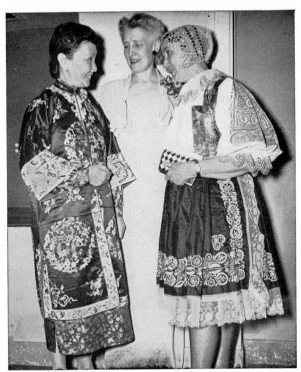

LILLIAN WU OF CHINA AND ANNA RYPACKOVA OF CZECHOSLOVAKIA WITH KATHARINE DENSFORD AT THE I.C.N. CONGRESS IN ATLANTIC CITY, NEW JERSEY (From American Journal of Nursing, June, 1947, by permission of American Journal of Nursing.)

establishment of scholarships and fellowships for selected students, promotion of research in nursing, and development of the section of the I.C.N. library dedicated to Florence Nightingale. When requested, it participates in special studies sponsored by the World Health Organization.

All candidates for admission to courses of study are recommended by special Florence Nightingale International Foundation Committees of their respective countries. Selection is made according to educational background and prospective ability to make future contribution to the nursing profession and to society. A limited number of applicants are accepted from each participating country. Tuition is paid by the students themselves, through scholarships provided by their national associations, or through fellowships provided by the I.C.N.

Upon completion of a course of the Foundation, the graduate is extended the privilege of becoming a member of the group known as the *Old Internationals' Association,* which assures continued contact among them. It is of this group that the living memorial to Florence Nightingale is composed. These women have derived benefit from contact with each other quite as much as from the courses offered. They have come under the influence of a spirit of eagerness to understand peoples of ways and customs differing from their own, and return to their own countries imbued with a desire to share that understanding with their countrymen.

In the performance of their duties, all doctors and nurses exercise a tremendous influence in breaking down barriers of suspicion and ill-will, barriers that have long obstructed world peace. They rank in the vanguard of those forces struggling for universal understanding and goodwill. It is not chance that has placed medicine and nursing in this role, but rather the very core of their philosophies, deeply rooted as it is in the principles of brotherly love, service, and instrumentation of the Golden Rule.

SUMMARY

About sixty nations, working with the World Health Organization, are in agreement with the premise that the promotion of health is fundamental to achievement of a socially adjusted and peaceful world. Through official relationship with the WHO, it has become the privilege of the International Council of Nurses to share in its lofty objectives. Today, nurses fill positions on the WHO Secretariat, are stationed in each of its regional offices, act as nurse consultants, serve on the World Health Expert Committee on Nursing, and act as delegates to World Health Assemblies. Opportunities for preparation to work in special fields are provided by WHO scholarships. The I.C.N. also works in various relationships with other international organizations.

Opportunities for contributing to understanding and teamwork among nations are open to many individual nurses through regional federations of nurses, the exchange of nurses by one country with another, and through foreign assignment with the army, navy, air force, and other federal nursing services.

Nurses from all quarters of the globe meet and exchange views at Congresses of the I.C.N., usually held quadrennially, with places of meeting distributed over the countries whose national nursing organizations make up its membership. The Congress of 1912, held in Cologne, Germany, is notable because it was here that an educational memorial to Florence Nightingale was proposed by Mrs. Bedford Fenwick of England and seconded by Mary Adelaide Nutting of the United States. This proposal reached fruition in 1934 with founding of the *Florence Nightingale International Foundation.*

The FNIF is now the Educational Division of the I.C.N. It provides post-graduate education for a selected group of students, and works closely with the World Health Organization. Headquarters of the FNIF, like those of the I.C.N., are in London, England.

TOPICS FOR DISCUSSION

1. In what department of the United Nations has the greatest degree of international understanding and cooperation been demonstrated?
2. Name several ways in which nurses are enabled to participate in promoting the objectives of the World Health Organization?
3. What opportunities are open to nurses for becoming acquainted with peoples of other nationalities?
4. Compare nursing developments of Catholic France and Protestant Germany.
5. What is the story of the American Nurses' Memorial in France?
6. Make an outline of outstanding events in the development of nursing in the following countries:

France	Italy
Germany	Greece
Belgium	Palestine
Northern Europe (Norway,	Africa
Sweden, Finland, Denmark)	The Orient
Iceland	Mexico
	South American Republics

7. With what country and work is each of the following names associated:

Mlle L. Chaptal	Mary Sewall Gardner
Dr. Anna Hamilton	Dr. Albert Schweitzer
Sister Agnes Karll	Nina D. Gage
Edith Cavell	Linda Richards

8. When and through whose influence was the I.C.N. founded?
9. How does membership of the I.C.N. differ from that of other nursing organizations?
10. When and where are Congresses of the I.C.N. held?
11. (a) When and where was the last I.C.N. Congress held? (b) When and where is to be the next one? (c) Who is now the president?
12. (a) At what Congress of the I.C.N. was an educational memorial to Florence Nightingale first proposed, and when was it finally established? (b) What is its name and what are its objectives?
13. What relationship do you see between world health and universal peace?

REFERENCES

Dock and Nutting: A History of Nursing. New York and London, G. P. Putnam's Sons, Vols. III and IV, 1912.

Dock and Stewart: A Short History of Nursing. 4th edition, New York, G. P. Putnam's Sons, 1938.

Goodnow, Minnie: Outlines of Nursing History. 9th edition, Philadelphia, W. B. Saunders Co., 1953.

Hagedorn, Hermann: Prophet in the Wilderness (Albert Schweitzer). New York, The Macmillan Co., 1947.

Hansen, Helen F.: Professional Relationships of the Nurse. Philadelphia, W. B. Saunders Co., 1942. Chapter 23.

International Aspects of Nursing Education. A series of mimeographed addresses provided through the Annie W. Goodrich Lectureship Fund. New York, Teachers College, Columbia University.

Judson, Helen: Edith Cavell. New York, The Macmillan Co., 1941.

Pavey, Agnes E.: The Story of the Growth of Nursing. London, Faber and Faber, Ltd., 1937.

Schweitzer, Albert: On the Edge of the Primeval Forest. New York, The Macmillan Co., 1931.

Schweitzer, Albert: Out of My Life and Thought (an autobiography). New York, Henry Holt and Co., 1933.

Seymer, Lucy Ridgley: A General History of Nursing. New York, The Macmillan Co., 1949.

Stewart, Isabel M.: The Education of Nurses. New York, The Macmillan Co., 1943.

Journals

American Journal of Nursing
British Journal of Nursing
Canadian Nurse
Nursing World
Nursing Times
International Nursing Review

Index

ABBESSES, famous,
  Radegunde of Poitiers, 125
  St. Clare or Clarissa, 169
  St. Hildegarde, 187
Accreditation of nursing schools,
  national, 501, 509, 511
  state, 426
Accrediting Service, N.L.N., 501, 509
"Activity Analysis of Nursing," 440
Addams, Jane, 379
Affiliations, first, 364, 388, 423
Africa, nursing in, 536
Age,
  Dark, 115–148
  Golden, of ancient Greece, 63
  New Stone, 13, 43, 74, 250
  of Chivalry, 131
  of coma in medicine, 189
  of farmers, 13, 35, 45
  of hunters, 10, 35
  Old Stone, 4, 10, 41
  Pastoral, 35
Aikenhead, Mother Mary, 288
Air Evacuation School, 466
Alcott, Louisa M., 353, 386, 387
Alcuin, 143
Alexander the Great, 19, 62, 68
Alexandria, 19, 62
  museum of, 19
American Association of Industrial
  Nurses, 502, 503, 512
American College of Physicians, 498
American College of Surgeons, 425–
  426, 498
  approval of hospitals by, 425–426
American Hospital Association, 426,
  498
American Journal of Nursing, 398, 427
  early editors of, 398
  founding of, 398, 427

American Medical Association,
  activities of, 425
  committees of, 498
  councils of, 425
  founding of, 225
  publications of, 425
American Nurses' Association, 410–
  411
  membership of, 505, 506
  reconstruction of, 502, 503
  responsible for nursing practice,
    504
  sections of, 505
American Red Cross Nursing Services,
  during World War I, 413
  during World War II, 460
  established, 404–405
  Home Nursing classes of, 416,
    429, 461, 486
  Volunteer Nurses' Aide Corps of,
    461
American Red Cross Society, 157–158.
  See Red Cross.
American Society of Dental Surgeons,
  426
American Society of Superintendents
  of Training Schools for Nurses,
  founding of, 396
  promotes advanced education for
    nurses, 405
  reorganization of, 410, 411
Ancestor worship, 42
  Chinese, 42
  Roman, 72
Animism, 5, 36
Anna Nery School of Nursing, Brazil,
  548–549
Anthony, Susan B., 235
Antoinette, Marie, 212, 230
Apollo, the sun god, 52–53

Apprenticeship System, 132–134
  criticism of, in schools of nursing, 361, 423
  in medicine, 224
  in schools of nursing, 361
Aristotle, 59, 63, 75
Armistice,
  of Korean War, 425
  of World War I, 418
Army School of Nursing, 415, 429
Artemis, sister of Apollo, 53
Aryan tribes, 36
Asceticism, 36, 37, 120, 144
  of St. Catherine of Siena, 183
Asklepiades, 57, 60
Asklepios, 53, 58
Asoka, king of India, 39–40, 47
Association of Collegiate Schools of Nursing, 441, 502
  merges with the N.L.N., 504
Association of Northern European Nurses, 519, 532, 533
Assyria, culture of, 26
Astell, Mary, 233
Atlantic Charter, 472, 487
Augustinian nuns, 242–244
  first purely nursing order, 242
  in Canada, 255–258, 262
  in city hospitals, 242, 246, 255
  in Hôtel Dieu of Paris, 242
  life of, 242–243
Austen, Jane, 235
Avicenna, 14, 189
Aztec Indians, culture of, 74–76, 249

BABYLONIA, 21–26, 46
  Code of Law of, 23
  Hammurabi, king of, 23
  Medicine of, 23–25
  women of, 25
Baggally, Olive, 515, 517
Barclay, Miss, 364
Barton, Clara,
  founder of American Red Cross, 357
  president of American Red Cross, 358
  work during Civil War, 356, 387
Battle of Solferino, 345
Baucq, Philippe, 530

Beard, Richard Olding, 409, 429
Bedouin tribe of Arabia, 137, 139
Beecher, Catherine, 235
Beecher, Dame Ethel Hope, 411
Beggary, 95
Beguines, 173–174, 195
  beguinages of, 173
  visiting nursing of, 173
Behring, Emil von, 384
Belgium, nursing in, 530–531
Bellevue Hospital,
  during the Civil War, 352
  founding of, 271, 280
  reform of, 358, 387
Bellevue Hospital Training School for Nurses, 361, 364
  cap of, 377
  early graduates of, 364–369
  first to adopt Nightingale System, 364
Bertheau, Caroline, 208
Bethlehem Hospital ("Bedlam"), 191
Bickerdyke, Mother, 354, 387
Birth of Reason, 59, 63
Black Death, epidemic of, 181–182, 184
Blackwell, Elizabeth, 352, 387
  and Civil War nursing, 352
Blue Stockings, 232, 234
Boardman, Mabel T., 404
Bolton, Mrs. Frances Payne, 437, 462
Books, sacred,
  of China, 41
  of Egypt, 17, 41
  of India, 36–37
  of Palestine, 29–30
  of Persia, 34
Booth, William, 378
Botticelli, 211
Brahmanism, 36, 39
British Journal of Nursing, 399, 427
Brontë, Charlotte, 235
Brothers Minor, 168–169
Brown, Esther Lucile, 495
Brown Report, 495–497
Browne, Jean, 445
Buddha, 39–41, 46, 79
Bureau of Labor Statistics, 491
Burgess, May Ayres, 495
Burney, Fanny, 235
Byzantine Empire, 136

CABOT, Dr. Richard, 424, 430
Caesar, Julius, 19, 68, 69, 79
    Octavius (Augustus), 19, 68, 69, 75, 102
Cameron, Dr. G. Stewart, 445
Canada, 254–265
    founding of Hôtel Dieu of Montreal, 261
    founding of Hôtel Dieu of Quebec, 255
Canadian Nurse, The, 399, 427
Cannes Conference, 419
Cannon, Ida M., 424, 430
Cape Colony, South Africa, 399, 536
Carnegie Foundation,
    studies medical schools, 386
    studies nursing schools, 494–495, 511
Carrel, Alexis, 385
Castles of feudalism, 129
    life in, 130
    nursing by lady of, 130
Catholic Social Reform, 283, 331
Cavell, Edith, 413, 530
    at I.C.N. in London, 551
Celsus, 100
Cervantes, 209
Chadwick, Sir Edwin, 228, 314, 330
Chaptal, Mlle, 521–523
Charity Hospital of New Orleans, 266, 279
Charlemagne, 142–143, 147
China, ancient, 41–45
    ancestor worship of, 42
    Buddhism and Taoism of, 44
    Confucianism of, 41, 44, 47
    medicine of, 44
    status of women in, 41
China, nursing in, 540
Chivalry, 131, 177
Christian Church, early, 90
    care of the sick by, 94
    deacons and deaconesses of, 86
    democratic ideals of, 95
    orders of women of, 88–90
    organization of, 86
    teachings of, 81–82
Chung, Elsie Mawfung, 540
Churchill, Winston, 487
Cicero, prose writer of Rome, 69

Civilization, beginnings of, 11
Clara Weeks Shaw, 369
Clubs, women's, growth of, 393, 427
Code, International, of Nursing Ethics, 556
Code of Law,
    of Hammurabi, 23, 46
    of Moses, 28
Colleges founded in America, 269. See also names of specific colleges.
Columbus, Christopher, 71, 177, 277, 547
Committees, medical,
    for study of nursing education, 434, 495
    on costs of medical care, 449, 453, 454
    to study the nursing problem, 496, 512
Committees, nursing,
    for improvement of nursing services, 500–501, 511
    on distribution of nursing service, 444, 453
    on function of nursing, 491, 498, 511
    on grading of nursing schools, 437, 451, 495
    on institutional nursing, 410
Confucius, 41–43, 46, 63, 66, 79
Constantine the Great, 91, 107
Constantinople, 135, 175
    capital of Roman Empire, 104
    fall of, 189
Cortez, Hernando, 249, 277–278, 544–545, 547
    establishes first hospital in America, 252–253
Council of Trent, 215
Cowley Brothers, 310
Creelman, Lyle, 515
Crusades, 155–201
    Children's, 175
    gains and losses of, 174, 201
    hospitals of, 199
    social changes associated with, 175
Culture, European, transferred to America, 215
Curie, Pierre and Marie, 384
Curriculum for schools of nursing, 410, 440, 444

DANCING mania, 181
Dark Ages, 115–148
Darrach, William, 438–439
Dartmouth College founded, 269, 279
Daughters of American Revolution, 401, 428
David, ruler of Hebrews, 28
Deaconess Order, early, 86–88
    modern, founded, 299–309
Deborah, 31
de Bullion, Madame, 261, 278
de la Peltrie, 256, 260, 278
Delano, Jane A.,
    organizes Red Cross Nursing Service, 404–405, 428
    with Red Cross in Florida, 368
Depage, Dr. Antoine and Marie, 530–531
Diakonia and xenodochia, 95
Dickens, Charles, 132, 297
Dioscorides, 99
Dispensaries of Rome, 71
Dispensary, Philadelphia, 274, 280
Distribution, uneven,
    of medical and nursing services, 449
    of nurses, 440, 444, 449
Divination, 25
Divorce, common in Rome, 69
Dix, Dorothea Lynde,
    in care of mentally ill, 236, 295–297, 332
    organization of army nursing, 355–357, 387
Dock, Lavinia L., 367
Domesday Book, 155
Dominican Order, 188, 222, 250, 277
Drake, Sir Francis, 207
Duchess d' Aiguillon, 255, 278
Dunant, Henri, 346–349, 357
    member of Y.M.C.A., 379

EBERS' Papyrus, 17
Ecole Florence Nightingale, 520, 523
Economic Security Program, 491
"Economic Status of Registered Professional Nurses," 491
Edith Cavell-Marie Depage, Foundation, 531
    Hospital, 556

Education for nurse specialists, 405–406
Egypt, ancient, 12–21
    calendar of, 13, 45
    Hebrews in captivity in, 27, 46
    medicine of, 17
    mummies of, 18
    museum of, 19
    nursing in, 20
    papyri of, 17, 41
    priest-physicians of, 15–17, 20
    pyramids of, 19
    temple-women of, 20, 21
Ehrlich, Paul, 384
Eliot, George, 235
Endowment of nursing schools, 436–437
Epidauros, temple of Asklepios, 57
    hospital of, 58–59
    priest-physicians of, 58
    sacred serpents of, 59
Epidemics,
    in Canada, 255
    in New World, 252, 254
    of leprosy, 164
    of malaria, 98, 102
    of measles, 252
    of smallpox, 252, 278
    of yellow fever, 368
Erasmus, 209
Eustochium, 93
Exchange of nurses, 516, 555

FABIOLA, 92–93, 97, 107
Factories,
    large numbers of, 290–291
    working conditions in, 291
Far East or Orient, 35, 46
Far West or Occident, 73
    first settlers of, 73–74
    Indian medicine of, 74
    Indian women of, 74
Farrand Training School for Nurses, 423
Feminism, rise of, 233
Fenwick, Mrs. Bedford,
    at St. Bartholomew's Hospital, 372, 388
    at World's Fair in Chicago, 395
    founder of I.C.N., 397

Fenwick, Mrs. Bedford, (*Continued*)
  founder of Royal British Nurses'
    Association, 394, 427
Fertile Crescent, 21, 34, 45
Feudalism, 116, 127, 212
  agriculture of, 131
  effect of break-up of, 218
  progress toward social recovery
    of, 131
  three social groups of, 128
Fisher, Alice, 364
Fist hatchet, 4
Flexner, Abraham, 386
Fliedner, Friederike, 299–308
Fliedner, Pastor Theodor, 299–308, 332
Florence Nightingale, 311–331
Florence Nightingale International
  Foundation, 556, 559
Four Freedoms, 471
France,
  founding of nursing schools in,
    520
  nursing in, 519
Franciscan Order, founding of, 168,
  199
  in Canada, 254, 255
  in New Spain, 250
  in New World, 222, 277
Friars, black, 168
  gray, 168, 188
Fry, Elizabeth Gurney, 309, 310, 331
  founder of Protestant Nursing
    Sisters, 309, 310
  reformer of prisons, 235, 292–295,
    300, 331
Fuller, Samuel, 268
  wife of, as midwife, 269, 279
Fund, Nightingale, 327, 333, 336

GAGE, Nina D., 540
Gainsborough, Sir Thomas, 211
Galen, 101, 188, 220
  his teachings lost sight of, 144, 219
Gardner, Mary Sewall, 535
General Federation of Women's Clubs,
  393, 427, 486
Germany,
  motherhouse system of, 526
  nursing in, 525–529
  Red Cross hospitals of, 426

Ginzberg, Eli, 498
Ginzberg Report, 498, 511
Gold, discovered in California, 226
Golden Age of Greece, 63
Goldmark, Josephine, 434, 495
"Good Samaritan," parable of, 82
Goodrich, Annie W.
  at National Health Conference,
    451
  at Teachers College, 406–407
  at Western Reserve University,
    437, 453
  Dean, Army School of Nursing,
    415, 429
Grading of medical schools, 386, 389
Grading of nursing schools, 437–443
Gray, Carolyn E., 437
Greece, ancient, 52–66
  iatrion of, 54
  mythology of, 52
  philosophers of, 52
  temples of, 54
  women of, 63
  xenodochion of, 54
Greece, nursing in, 535
Grellet, Stephen, 292
Grenfell, Dr. Wilfred T., 380–381, 389
Guilds, 117, 132–134
  classes of workmen in, 132
  nursing for members of, 146
  of barber-surgeons, 189, 220

Gunn, Jean I., 445

HADASSAH, 536
Hamilton, Dr. Anna, 520, 524
Hammurabi, king of Babylonia, 23, 46
Harvard College, founding of, 269, 279
Harvard Medical School, founding of,
  225
Harvey, William, 200
Health Education, 423, 430, 433
Hebrew people, 26–34
  charity of, 33–34
  Old Testament of, 29
  prophylaxis of, 31
  religious teachings of, 28–30, 33
  tithing of, 33
Helen, Sister, 360, 387
Henrietta Szold School of Nursing, 536
Henry VIII, 238
Henry Street Settlement, 370

Herbert, Sir Sidney, 317–318
    aids Florence Nightingale, 333
    as military hygienist, 330
    as sanitarian, 228
    meets Florence Nightingale, 314
    writes to Florence Nightingale, 317–318
"Hiawatha," animism of, 5
Hieroglyphics, 13, 45
Hippocrates, 59–61
    as "Father of Medicine," 61
    assisted by women, 60, 76
    ethical principles of, 61
    scientific principles of, 61
    teachings of, forgotten, 144, 245
Hojer, Gerda, 554, 556
Holmes, Oliver Wendell, 226
Homer, 52
Horace, poet of Rome, 69
Horus, 14, 45
Hospital of Immaculate Conception, 252
Hospital of Jesus of Nazareth, 252–253, 277–278, 545
Hospital of St. John at Valletta, 191–194
Hospital São Francisco de Assis, 548
Hospital(s). See also under names of specific hospitals.
    army, of Rome, 71
    city, 195, 196, 240
    European model of, in New World, 289
    first Christian, of Rome, 271
    first in America, 252
    first in Canada, 278
    first in United States, 271
    for mentally ill, 296
    growth of, in Late Middle Ages, 190–193
    growth of, in New England, 271, 279–280
    Moslem, 140–141
    of Crimean War, 318, 322, 324
    of Knights Hospitallers, 190–194
    of Renaissance, 240
    of Revolutionary War, 273
    of Rome, 191
    of secular orders, 190
    of Seven Years' War, 279
    of Sisters of St. Lazarus, 194

Hospital(s). See also under names of specific hospitals. (Continued)
    of St. Mary Magdalene, 159, 194
    of St. Mary of the Teuton, 159
Hôtel Dieu,
    of Lyons, 146
    of Montreal, 261–262, 278
    of Paris, 146, 242–244
    of Quebec, 255–260, 262, 278
Howard, John, 291, 331
Howe, Julia Ward, 238, 314
Hull House, 379
Hunan-Yale School of Nursing, 540
Hunayn, 140
Hunt, Leigh, 298
Hygeia, 53
Hygiene, Personal, 99, 180

Iatrion of Greece, 54
Illinois Training School, 423
Imhotep of Egypt, 17, 57
Inca Indians, culture of, 74, 76, 249
India,
    asceticism of, 36, 37
    Brahmanism of, 36
    Buddhism of, 37–39
    caste system of, 36, 39
    early medicine of, 40
    King Asoka of, 39–40
    Vedas of, 36, 37
    women of, 40
Individualism, doctrine of, 176
Industrial nursing, 466–468
Infanticide, 165
Interstate licensure, 508
Institutes for medical research,
    Pasteur, 385, 389
    Rockefeller, 385, 389
Instruction of nurses, first on American continent, 278
Insurance, group, 449–450
Interim classification of nursing schools, 500, 511
International Council of Nurses, 550–557
    founding of, 396–397
    relationship with other organizations, 515, 516
    studies nursing shortage, 491
International Red Cross, 420

Isis, mother earth, 14, 45
Islam,
    elements of, 137
    holy city of, 135
    Koran of, 138
    medicine and science of, 140
    mosques of, 137, 138
    prophet of, 135
    rival of Christianity, 134
    Seljuk Turks of, 156
    status of women under, 141
Italian Red Cross, 534
Italy, nursing in, 534–535

JAMESTOWN colony, 267
Janus, temple of, 66, 68
Japan, nursing in, 371, 540
Jenkins, Helen Hartley, 407
Jenner, Edward, 221
Jesuit Order, founding of, 214, 215
    in Canada, 254, 255
    in Colonial America, 222
    in New Spain, 251, 277
    "Relations" of, 251
John, King of England, 176
Johns, Ethel, 440
Johns Hopkins Hospital Training School, 365, 422–423
Johns Hopkins Medical School, 385, 389
Joint Commission for Care of Patient, 499
Jones, Agnes, 344
Journals, nursing,
    founding of, 398–399
    of U. S. today, 507, 512
Juno, 66
Jupiter, 66

KAISERSWERTH Deaconess Institution, 299–308
    daily routine of, 305
    ethical teaching of, 305
    facilities for instruction, 303–304
    instruction at, 302
    system regulating school of, 304–305
    uniform dress of, 305
Karll, Sister Agnes, 526–527

King's College Hospital, 209
King's Touch, 222
Kircher, Athanasius, 220
Knighthood, education for, 153
Knights Hospitallers, 158–162
    military influence of, 159, 162
    of St. John of Jerusalem, 159, 191–194
    of St. Lazarus, 159, 164
    Teutonic, 159
    uniforms of, 161–162
Koch, Robert, 383, 389
Koran, bible of Moslems, 138–139, 141
Korea, 542–544
    MASH units of, 542

LABOR unions and professional organizations, 398
Lazarettos,
    for women, 197
    increased, 145
    of Knights of St. Lazarus, 164
    of Late Middle Ages, 159, 190
League of Nations, 420–421, 429
League of Red Cross Societies, 419–420, 421, 429, 486
Leonardo da Vinci, 210
Leone, Lucile Petry, 515
Leprosy, 168, 194–195
    a major medieval problem, 164
    at xenodochium of St. Basil, 96
Licensing of nurses, 446–448, 508, 513
    agency for, 509
    New York law in regard to, 447
    permissive or mandatory, 508, 513
Lister, Lord Joseph, 384, 389
Livingstone, Nora, 369
Long, Dr. Crawford, 226
Louis XIV, 212
Louis XVI, 212
Loveridge, Emily L., 368
Loyola, Ignatius, 214
Lucia della Robbia, 209
Luther, Martin,
    dissolves monasteries, 238
    led revolt, 209, 214
    mendicant monk, 214
    translated Bible, 209
Lying-in Hospital of New York, 275

MACDONALD, Margaret, 413
Machiavelli, 209
Magic, black and white, 9
Magna Charta, 176, 212
Malaria, 98, 102
Mance, Jeanne, 260–262, 278
Manuals of nursing procedures, early, 300, 302
Manuscripts, 122–123
    medical, of Moslems, 188
Marcella, 92, 107, 117
Marco Polo, 177
Mars, god of war, 66
"Martin Chuzzlewit," 297–298, 332
Massachusetts General Hospital, 424, 430
Massachusetts General Hospital Training School
    cap of, 377
    founding of, 361
    preliminary course of, 373
Mather, Cotton, 269
Matilda, wife of William the Conqueror, 155
Matron's Council of Great Britain and Ireland, 394
Maxwell, Anna Caroline, 371
    at camp hospital in Georgia, 401, 428
Maya Indians, culture of, 74, 76, 249
McCarthy, Dame Maude, 412
McGee, Anita Newcomb, 401
McIsaac, Isabel, 416
McManus, R. Louise, 498
Mecca, holy city of Moslems, 135, 137
Medical missionaries, 380
Medical practice, survey of, 448
Medical Social Service, 424, 430
Medicine,
    age of coma in, 189
    Babylonian, 23
    Byzantine, 187
    early Christian, 98
    Egyptian, 17
    enters the university, 239
    Hebrew, 30
    in colonial America, 222, 223, 267, 268
    in the ascendant, 196
    of ancient China, 44
    of ancient India, 40

Medicine, (Continued)
    of ancient Rome, 70–71
    of early Middle Ages, 143
    of Islam, 140
    of Late Middle Ages, 185
    of Moslems of Spain, 188
    of New Spain, 250
    of Renaissance, 219, 226
    primitive, 6
    revolution in, 382
    withdraws from monasteries, 239
Medicine man,
    of ancient Egypt, 17
    of Indians of Americas, 76
    of New Spain, 250
    of primitive peoples, 9, 10
Memorial,
    to American nurses of World War I, 523–525
    to Florence Nightingale, 555–557; proposed, 551
Men nurses,
    Brotherhood of Mexico City, 278
    Brothers of St. John of God, 284
    Cowley Brothers, 310
    of knights hospitallers, 159
    recruitment of, recommended, 497
Mendicant Orders, 165–170
Mental hospitals,
    Bethlehem, 191
    development of, 275
    Dorothea Lynde Dix and, 296, 332
    Linda Richards and, 371
    Sara Parsons and, 371
Mental illness,
    care for patients with, 241
    in New England, 272
    reform in care of patients with, 295
Merryweather, Miss, 342
Mexico, nursing in, 544–547
Michelangelo, 210
Middle Ages, 115
    middle class of, 201
Military rank, first granted, 428
Milton, John, 209
Minna, at Kaiserswerth, 301
Missions, of New World, 251, 277
Modern nursing established, 340
Mohammed, 135, 136, 137, 141, 147

Monasteries, Benedictine, 118–127
  activities of, 121
  attracted scholarly men, 197
  classes of monastics in, 120
  daily routine of, 121
  dissatisfaction within, 123, 163
  dwindling population of, 154
  manuscripts of, 122–123
  preservation of knowledge in, 122, 186
  Rule of St. Benedict in, 119
  suppression of, 238, 246
Monasteries, Buddhist, 40
Monastery at Cluny, France, 123
Monasticism, Christian, 117–118
Money, Miss, 364
Montezuma, 249
Montreal, founding of, 260–262
Montreal General Hospital Training School, 363–364, 369
More, Hanna, 234
More, Sir Thomas, 209
Mores or customs,
  Greek, 64
  tribal, 3
Moses,
  developed Mosaic Law, 28
  laws of, governing camp life, 30, 164
  led Hebrews to Palestine, 27, 46
  pharmacists in time of, 17
Moslems, 137, 138, 139, 140
Motherhouse System, of Germany, 526
  of Kaiserswerth, 307, 308
Muhlenberg, Reverend, 276
Murdock, Dr. Thomas P., 498
Murdock Report, 498–499, 512

NATIONAL accreditation of nursing schools, 501
National Association of Colored Graduate Nurses,
  disbanding of, 503
  organization of, 397
National Council of Nurses of Great Britain and Northern Ireland, 397
National Federation of Business and Professional Women's Clubs, 486
National Federation of Licensed Practical Nurses, 512

National Health Conference, 451
National Health Program, 451
National Inventory of Nurses,
  by A.N.A., 492, 511
  by U.S.P.H.S., 462, 485
National League for Nursing, 503, 504, 505–506, 512
  divisions and departments of, 505–506
  membership of, 505, 506, 512
  responsible for nursing services and nursing education, 305
National League of Nursing Education, 410, 411, 429
National Mental Health Act, 483, 487
National Nursing Council,
  for war service, 460, 485
  projects of, 491, 495, 511
National Student Nurse Association, 506
Nationalism, 212
Near East, 12, 41, 73
New England, 266–273
New England Hospital for Women and Children, 359, 387
New France, 216, 217, 254–266
New Spain, 216, 217, 249–254
New Testament of Bible, 30
New York Hospital, founding of, 272, 280
New York Hospital Training School, 369–371
New York State Charities Aid Association, 358
Newgate Prison reform, 291, 300
Nightingale, Florence, 311–331
  as world consultant, 331, 333
  at Kaiserswerth, 315, 316
  at Scutari, 318–322
  birthplace of, 209
  books by, 328, 329
  Crimean war service, 317–326
  death of, 409, 429
  early interest in nursing, 236
  early life, 311
  first position of, 316
  living memorial to, 409, 555–557
  papers of, on sanitation, 330
  post-war activities of, 326
  presented with Badge of Honor, 327

Nightingale, Florence, presented with Nightingale Fund, 327
  promotes district nursing, 341–343
  promotes expansion of army nursing, 322
  promotes non-sectarian reform of nursing, 336–341
  promotes reform of workhouse infirmaries, 343–345
  promotes sanitation in India, 330–331
  romance of, 314
  social work of, 322
Nightingale Fund, 327, 333, 336
Nightingale School of Nursing, 336–341, 386
  basic principles of, 337
  probationers of, 338, 340
  social groups of, 338
  time-schedule of, 339
Nightingale System,
  principles of, 337, 361
  spread of, 358–364, 548
Nirvana, 39, 47
Noguchi, Hideyo, 385
Northern Europe, nursing in, 531–534
Noyes, Clara D., 407, 418
Nurse Draft Bill, 468, 487
Nurse Society of Philadelphia, 275, 280
Nurses' Associated Alumnae of U. S. and Canada, 396, 401
"Nurses, Patients, and Pocket-Books," 439
Nursing,
  as a separate occupation, 195
  declining interest in, 238–246, 422, 479–480
  early Christian, 95, 101
  in city hospitals, 196, 272
  in guardianship of secular orders, 239
  lacking in New England, 267
  medieval, 195–197, 201
  methods exposed, 297–299
  not a separate occupation, 47, 145
  of Civil War, 349–357
  of Crimean War, 324
  of early American period, 381–382

Nursing, (Continued)
  of feudal castles, 130
  of Korean War, 542–544
  of military orders, 158
  of Revolutionary War, 273
  of South African War, 402
  reform of, after Civil War, 358–378
  reform of, by Florence Nightingale, 336–341
  socio-economic study of, 491, 511
  surveys of, in Canada and Great Britain, 445–446
  surveys of, in U. S., 433–445, 494, 497, 500
  trend in, 1893 to 1920, 422–423
  women lose control of, 240
"Nursing and Nursing Education in the United States," 434
"Nursing for the Future," 511
Nursing Functions, study of, 492
Nursing organizations, membership of, 512
Nursing practice acts, revision of, 508, 513
"Nursing Schools at the Mid-Century," 501
Nursing technicians, 499
Nutting, Mary Adelaide, at Johns Hopkins Hospital, 366, 373
  at Teachers College, 406–409

"OLD Internationals," 557
Old Testament of Bible, 29, 30, 46
Order(s),
  Beguines of Liège, 173
  Deaconess, early, 86–89
  Deaconess, modern, 299–308, 332
  Dominican, 166, 169
  early Christian, of women, 86–91
  Franciscan, 168–170
  military nursing, 158–162
  of St. John of Jerusalem, 191
  of St. Ursula, 215, 256–262, 278
  of Virgins, 88–90
  of Widows, 88–90
  Poor Clares, 169
  Protestant Nursing Sisters, 309
  secular, 170–195

Order(s), (*Continued*)
  Sisterhoods of English Church, 309
    Sisterhood of All Saints, 309
    Sisterhood of St. John's House, 309
    Sisterhood of St. Margaret, 309
    Sisters of Mercy, 309
  Sisters of Charity, 284–289
  Tertiaries of St. Francis, 171
Organizations, medical,
  American College of Physicians, 498
  American College of Surgeons, 425–426, 498
  American Medical Association, 225, 425, 498
  American Society of Dental Surgeons, 426
Organizations, nursing,
  alumnae associations, 394–395
  American Association of Industrial Nurses, 502–503, 512
  American Nurses' Association, 410, 411, 504–506
  American Society of Superintendents of Training Schools, 396
  Association of Collegiate Schools of Nursing, 441
  Association of Northern European Nurses, 532–533
  Canadian Nurses' Association, 410, 411, 429
  German Nurses' Association, 526
  growth of, in New World, 394–398
  International Council of Nurses, 550–557
  Matron's Council of Great Britain and Ireland, 427
  National Association for Practical Nurse Education, 508
  National Association of Brazilian Graduate Nurses, 549
  National Association of Colored Graduate Nurses, 397, 603
  National Association of Graduate Nurses of France, 523
  National Council of Nurses of Great Britain, 397

Organizations, nursing, (*Continued*)
  National Federation of Licensed Practical Nurses, 512
  National League for Nursing, 503, 505, 512
  National League of Nursing Education, 410, 411, 429
  National Organization for Public Health Nursing, 410, 411, 504
  National Student Nurse Association, 506
  Nurses' Associated Alumnae of U. S. and Canada, 396, 411, 427
  Regional associations, 518–519
  Royal British Nurses' Association, 401, 427
  Six formerly in existence, 502
  Three now in existence, 504, 512
Orient, nursing in, 538
Osiris, 14, 45

Palestine, 26–34, 46
  child's nurse in, 47
  medicine of, 30
  nursing in, 536
  people of, 27
  women of, 31
  xenodochia of, 34
Palmer, Sophia, 398
Panacea, 53
Paracelsus, 219
Paré, Ambroise, 220
Parsons, Sara, 371
Passavant, Rev. William, 276
Pasteur, Louis, 330, 383, 385, 389
Paula, 92, 93–94, 97, 107, 117
Pavlova, Grand Duchess, 323
Peiping Union Medical College, 540
Pelton, Garnet, 424, 430
Peltrie, Mme de la, 256–257, 260
Pennsylvania Hospital, 272, 280
Permanent Army Medical Corps Nursing Service of Canada, 402, 413
Permanent Court of International Justice, 411
Persecution of Christians, 90
Persia (Iran), 34, 45, 46
  morality of, 35
  Zendavesta of, 34
  Zoroaster of, 34

Pfefferkorn, Blanche, 440
Philadelphia General Hospital, 271, 280
Philip of Macedonia, 62
Phoebe, 86, 87, 106
Pilgrimages,
    to Mecca, 135
    to Palestine, 152
Pinel, Philippe, 245
Plagues,
    of Middle Ages, 179
    of third century, 97
Plato, 59, 63, 75
Pope, Georgina F., 402, 428
Pope Innocent III, 190
Pope Urban II, 156, 157
Poverty in England, 213, 214
Practical nurses, 446, 480, 508, 512
Preliminary course,
    at Simmons College, 373
    first in America, 373
    first in Scotland, 373
Preservers of medicine during the Middle Ages, 186–188
Priest-Physicians,
    of American Indians, 76
    of ancient Egypt, 15, 16, 20, 45
    of ancient Greece, 58, 60
    of Palestine, 30
    of primitive man, 9, 10
Princess Mary's Royal Air Force Nursing Service, 412
Printing, invention of, 208
Prison(s),
    condition of, 241
    German, Association, 301
    Newgate, 291, 300
    reform of, 291, 331, 332
Prisoners' refuge at Kaiserswerth, 301
Probationers,
    at Kaiserswerth, 301–302
    at Nightingale School, 338, 340
Procurement and Assignment Service, 460, 485
Professional Counseling and Placement Service, 506
Protestant Hospital at Bordeaux, 520
Protestant Nursing Sisters, 309
Protestant Social Reform, 289
Psychiatry, rise of, 482
Psychosomatic medicine, 483, 487

Public Health Movement, 227–228, 341–345, 450–452

QUEBEC, founding of, 255–260
Queen Alexandra's Royal Army Nursing Corps, 403, 411
Queen Alexandra's Royal Naval Nursing Service, 412
Queen Elizabeth, subjects of, as pirates, 266
Queen of Sheba, 28
Queen Victoria, 236

RADEGUNDE of Poitiers, 125, 197
Rank for nurses, 402, 403
Raphael, 211
Rathbone, William,
    befriends Dorothy Lynde Dix, 295
    inaugurates modern district nursing, 341–343, 386
    inaugurates reform of workhouse infirmaries, 343–345, 386
Reconstruction, following World War I, 419
Red Cross, French, 525
Red Cross Home Nursing, 461
Red Cross Hospital of Mexico, 547
Red Cross Societies,
    American, 357, 387
    birth of, 345
    flag of, 348
    League of, 419–420, 421, 429, 486
    spread of, 348, 387
    Treaty of Geneva, 348
Reform in nursing,
    Catholic, 284–289, 331
    Nightingale, 336–345, 360–361
    of workhouse infirmaries, 343
    pre-Nightingale, 359
    Protestant, at Kaiserswerth, 299
Reform, social, 283
Reformation, The, 214, 239
Regional associations of nurses, 518–519
Registration of nurses,
    and licensing, 446–448, 453
    early agitation in regard to, 399
    first laws enacted, 399
    spread of, 423

Rehabilitation,
  following World War I, 419
  following World War II, 468
"Relations" of the Jesuits, 251, 260
Rembrandt, 211
Renaissance,
  art revival of, 209
  classic revival of, 208, 242
  decline in nursing of, 238–241
  included medicine, 219
  industrial revolution of, 213
  political revolution of, 211
  women of, 228
Research and Statistics Unit of
  A.N.A., 491
Research, nursing, 490–494, 510
Reserve Nurses of Canada, granted
  relative rank, 428
Revolutions, political, 211–213
  American, 213, 234, 273
  French, 213, 234
  Industrial, 213
  Latin-American, 213
  Napoleonic, 213, 234
Reynolds, Sir Joshua, 211
Rhazes, 140
Richards, Linda,
  as nurse missioner, 371, 387
  first trained nurse in America, 359,
    387
  in Japan, 540
Robb, Isabel Hampton,
  at Illinois Training School, 364
  at Johns Hopkins Hospital, 365,
    394
  books of, 366
  inaugurates affiliations, 364, 388,
    423
Roberts, Mary M., 398, 438
Rockefeller Foundation, 434, 495
Rockefeller Institute, 385, 389
Rockefeller Survey, 434, 444, 452–453
Rogers, Lina L., 371
Roman Empire, 68, 79
  fall of, 102–104, 109
Roman matrons, 92–94
Rome, ancient, 66–73
  army hospitals of, 71
  dispensaries of, 71
  medicine of, 70
  sanitation of, 70

Rome, ancient, women of, 71, 92
Roosevelt Hospital School of Nursing,
  540
Roosevelt, President Franklin D., 487
Royal British Nurses' Association, 401,
  427
Royal College of Nursing, 419
Rubens, 211
Rue Vercingetorix Private School, 521–
  522
Rule,
  of St. Augustine, 159
  of St. Benedict, 119
Russell, Kathleen, 445

SALADIN, Moslem leader, 175
Salon, French, 234
Salvation Army, 378, 389
Sanitary Commission of Civil War,
  349–351
Sanitation,
  era of, 227
  of English army, 328
  of Hebrews, 46
  of India, 330
  of Romans, 70
"Santa Filomena," 323
Santo Spirito Hospital, 146, 191
Saul, ruler of Hebrews, 27
School Data Survey, 500, 511
School of the Rue Amyot, 521
School of the Rue de la Culture, 530,
  531
School(s), medical,
  attempts at reform of, 385
  development of, in America, 225
  established in Mexico City, 217
  grading of, 386, 389
  Johns Hopkins founded, 385
  Salerno, established, 146, 147, 188
School(s), nursing,
  Carnegie study of, 494–497
  curriculum for, 410, 440, 444
  early American, 361
  first modern, 336
  grading of, 437–444
  national accreditation of, 501
  organization of, early, 362
  prevailing methods in, 375
  Rockefeller survey of, 435
  school data survey of, 500

School nursing, beginnings of, 370
    Lillian D. Wald and, 370–371
    Lina L. Rogers and, 371
Schweitzer, Dr. Albert, 536–538
Scriptorium, 122
Seaman, Dr. Valentine, 273, 280
Seljuk Turks, 156
Semitic tribes, 26
Semmelweis, Ignaz, 226
Serpents, of wisdom, 53
    sacred, 59
Serra, Father Junipero, 254, 277
Seton, Mother Elizabeth, 276, 288
Settlement Houses, 379, 388
Sewall, Samuel, 269
Shakespeare, William, 209
Shattuck, Lemuel, 228
Shaw, Clara Weeks, 369
Shortage of nurses,
    during World War I, 416
    following World War II, 479,
        487
    in rural areas, 440
Sieveking, Amalie, 300, 308
Sisterhood of All Saints, 309
Sisterhood of St. John's House, 309
Sisterhood of St. Margaret, 309, 310
Sisterhoods of English Church, 309
    introduced to America, 276
Sisters of Charity,
    founding of, 284–289, 331
    instruction by St. Louise de
        Marillac, 285
    organization of school, 289
    uniform dress of, 286
Sisters of Mercy,
    Catholic Order of, 276, 317, 324
    Protestant Order of, 309
Sisters of St. Lazarus, 194
Slaves,
    first from Africa, 267
    Greek physicians as, 68, 98
    Greek scholars as, 68, 75
Smith, Captain John, 267
Snively, Mary Agnes, 366, 367
Social groups of Europe,
    aristocrats, 229
    industrial, 239
    lower class, 236, 237
    middle class or bourgeois, 229
Social problems of England, 290

Social problems of Middle Ages, 163
    abandoned children, 165, 194
    infanticide, 165
Social Security Act, 450–452, 454
Social Service,
    founded, 283
    medical, 424, 430
Socialized medicine, 452, 534
Society of Roman women, 72
Society of St. Joseph de la Flêche,
    261
Socio-Economic Study of Nursing,
    491, 511
Socrates, 59, 75
Solferino, battle of, 345
Solomon, ruler of Hebrews, 28
Sophiahemmet, The, 533, 534
Soranus of Ephesus, 99
South African War, 402
South American Republics, nursing
    in, 547–550
Spanish-American War, 401, 428
St. Bartholomew's Hospital, 191
St. Basil of Caesarea, 96–97, 109, 145
St. Benedict, democracy of, 119, 163
    rule of, 119
St. Catherine of Siena, 182–185, 197
St. Clare or Clarissa, 169
St. Elizabeth of Hungary, 171
St. Francis of Assisi, 166–173, 199
    Franciscan Order of, 168, 199
    mission in honor of, 254
    Second Order of, 169, 199
    Third Order of, 170, 199
St. Hildegarde, 187
St. Jerome, 92, 104, 107, 117
St. Louise de Marillac, 286–296, 331
St. Luke's International Medical Cen-
    ter, 541
St. Paul, 83–106
    a prolific writer, 84
    attitude toward women, 85
St. Peter, first Bishop of Rome, 86,
    106
St. Radegande, 125, 197
St. Thomas' Hospital,
    founding of, 191
    Nightingale School founded, 336
St. Vincent de Paul, 283–289, 331
Stanton, Elizabeth Cady, 235
State Board Test Pool, 509

State Boards,
of Medical Examiners, 385
of Nurse Examiners, 426
Stewart, Isabel M., 428
Stewart, Isla, 372, 388
Stimson, Julia C., 418
Stowe, Harriet Beecher, 235
Strong, Rebecca, 373, 388, 405, 423
Structure changes in organized nursing, 502–507
Stuart, Mary of Scotland, 230
Student Nurse Association, National, 506
Student Nurses' Association of Royal College of Nursing, 419
Studies of nursing shortage, 491, 511
Study of Nursing Functions, 492, 512
Study of organized nursing, 502
Suffrage, woman, 235, 513
Surgery, status of, during Late Middle Ages, 189
Survey of medical practice, 448–450
Surveys of nursing,
by American Medical Association, 498
by Carnegie Foundation, 494–497
by Grading Committee, 437–444
by Rockefeller Foundation, 434–437
in Canada and Great Britain, 445–446
Sweating sickness, 181
Sweden, nursing in, 533–534
state medicine in, 534
Sydenham, Thomas, 221, 382

Teachers College,
advanced courses at, 405–409, 423, 428
proposes nursing technicians, 499
Temple(s), 20–21
of Asklepios, 57
of Egypt, 20
of Epidauros, 54, 55, 57
of Greece, 54
of Karnak, 20
of Rome, 66, 68
Territorial Nursing Service, 412
Textbooks for nurses,
dearth of, 550
first to be used, 329, 374, 388

Toltec Indians, culture of, 74–76, 249
Toynbee Hall, 379
Training Schools for Nurses, first modern, in America, 388
Tribes, primitive, 3
Aryan, 36
barbarian, 103
Bedouin, 137, 139
Semitic, 26
Truce of God, 153
Tuke, William, 221, 245

Uniform dress,
adoption of, 376–378
army, of Crimean War, 325
lack of, in early convents, 125–126
lineage of the cap, 377
of Beguines of Belgium, 174
of Dominican Order, 168
of Franciscan Order, 166
of Kaiserswerth deaconesses, 305
of Knights Hospitallers, 161–162
of monasteries of Late Middle Ages, 197–198
of nuns of early Canada, 264
of Protestant Nursing Sisters, 309
of secular orders, 198
of Sisters of Charity, 286
United Daughters of the Confederacy, 486
United Nations, 472–479, 487
Economic and Social Council, 474–477
F.A.O., 477
U.N.E.S.C.O., 477
W.H.O., 475–477
General Assembly, 473
International Court of Justice, 474
Secretariat, 478
Security Council, 473
Trusteeship Council, 477
Universal Declaration of Human Rights, 510
Universities, rise of, 188
University,
of Bologna, Italy, 188
of Cambridge, England, 188
of Mexico City, 217, 547
of Minnesota, 409, 429
of Montpellier, France, 188

University, (*Continued*)
of Oxford, England, 188
of Paris, France, 188
of Pennsylvania, 422
University of Pennsylvania Hospital Training School, 422
U.N.R.R.A., 486, 535
Ursuline nuns, 256–262, 265, 278
first instructors on American continent, 259
founding of Order, 215
in New Orleans, 266
in Quebec, 256–260, 262, 265
U. S. Army Nurse Corps,
established, 403, 428
first gathered by Dorothea Lynde Dix, 355–356
U. S. Cadet Nurse Corps, 462, 486
U. S. Department of Labor, 511
U. S. Navy Nurse Corps, established, 403, 428
U.S.P.H.S., 462, 485

VAN DYCK, 211
Van Leeuwenhoek, Anton, 220
Van Rensselaer, Euphemia, 376
Van Schurman, Anna, 233
Vassar Training Camp, 416, 429
Vedas, sacred, of India, 36–37
Veils, wearing of, 126, 510
Velasquez, 211
Versailles, 212
Vesalius, Andreas, 219, 220
Virgil, historian of Rome, 69
Virgins, Order of, 89, 106
Visiting nursing,
founded in Liverpool, 341–342, 386
founded in London, 342–343
of Beguines of Belgium, 173
of deaconesses of Kaiserswerth, 308
of Friends of Poor of France, 300
of Phoebe, 87, 106
of St. Catherine of Siena, 182
of St. Elizabeth of Hungary, 172
of United States, founded, 370–371
Volunteer Aid Detachment, 413
"Vulgate" translation of Bible, 92, 104

WALD, Lillian D.,
founder of visiting nursing, 370–371
instructor at Teachers College, 407
Waldron, Martha M., 360, 387
War(s),
American Civil, 349–357
nursing in, 349–357, 387
Sanitary Commission of, 349–351
French and Indian, 212, 262, 279
Napoleonic, 213, 234
Revolutionary, 273, 280
South African, 400–401
Spanish-American, 400–401
Thirty Years, 215
World I, 411–418
World, II, 457–471, 485
Wardroper, Mrs., 336
Warrington, Dr. Joseph, 275, 280
Weir, Professor George, 446
Western Reserve University School of Nursing, 437, 451
Widows,. Order of, 88, 106
Willard, Frances E., 235
William the Conqueror, 154, 155
Wilson, President Woodrow, 420
Winslow, C. E. A., 434
Winslow-Goldmark Report, 434–436, 452
Woman's Hospital of Philadelphia, 359–360, 387
Women,
a new status for, 509, 510
attitude of St. Paul toward, 85
barbarian, 151
employment of, in industry, 236–237, 509
interest in charitable work, 172
interest in feminism, 233–236
lose control of nursing, 240
of American Indians, 74, 250
of ancient Babylonia, 25
of ancient China, 41
of ancient Greece, 63–64
of ancient India, 40
of ancient Palestine, 31
of ancient Rome, 71–73, 76
of China and Japan, 539
of early Christian Church, 86, 90, 106

Women, (*Continued*)
  of industrial class, 239
  of Industrial Revolution, 236
  of knights hospitallers, 169
  of Middle Ages, 178
  of monasteries, 124–127
  of Renaissance, 228, 231, 232, 245
  of Revolutionary War, 273
  of the temples, 20, 45
  organization among, 393
  pioneer life of, in America, 262
  position of, in Early Middle Ages, 147
  primitive duties of, 8
  upper and lower classes of, 245
  veils of, 126–127, 510
Workhouse infirmaries, 343–345, 387
World Federation for Mental Health, 482, 487
World Health Expert Committee on Nursing, 515
World Health Organization, 475–477
  cooperation in, 515
  regional offices of, 515
  studies nursing shortage, 491

World's Fair of Chicago, 395–397, 429
Wu, Lillian, 540

XENODOCHIA,
  of ancient Palestine, 34, 46
  of St. Basil of Caesarea, 96–97, 109, 149
  predecessors of modern hospitals, 34, 95, 97
Xenodochion of ancient Greece, 54
Xenodochium of St. Basil, 96–97, 109
  segregation of lepers at, 145

YALE University School of Nursing, 437, 451
Y.M.C.A. and Y.W.C.A., 379–380, 388–389
  Henri Dunant, member of, 379

ZENDAVESTA of Persia, 34, 46
Zoroaster of Persia, 34, 46, 79